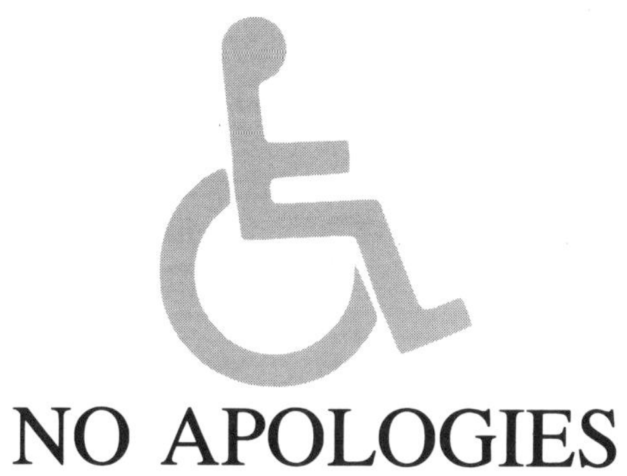

NO APOLOGIES

NO APOLOGIES

Florence Weiner

St. Martin's Press
New York

Book design by Lennox Robinson

If You're Thinking About Having a Disability by William Roth, Ph.D., used by permission of The Exceptional Parent, 605 Commonwealth Avenue, Boston, MA 02215
My Daughter is Leaving Home, What Do I Do Now? by Betty Pendler used by permission of The Exceptional Parent.
Deprived, Exhibited by Albert Davidson reprinted by permission of The New York Times
Into the Land of the Myths by S.L. Rosen reprinted by permission of The Disability Rag.
The Job by Frances Lynn reprinted by permission of The Disability Rag.
A Way for Frances by June Price reprinted by permission of The Disability Rag.
The interview of Phyllis Rubenfeld was reprinted by permission of The Exceptional Parent.

Every effort has been made to secure permission from people who were interviewed.

Library of Congress Cataloging in Publication Data

Weiner, Florence.
No Apologies.

1. Handicapped—United States. 2. Handicapped—Services for—United States. I. Title.
HV1553.W45 1986 646.7'00240816 86-3688
ISBN 0-312-57523-8 (pbk.)

First Edition
10 9 8 7 6 5 4 3 2 1

Cover/Charles Sabatier and his bride Peggy Griffin return from altar.
He is the Executive Director of the Commission on Handicapped Affairs, and she is a manager of the Main Street Project of Norwood, Massachusetts Chamber of Commerce.
Charles Sabatier was wounded in Vietnam, and Peggy Griffin is partially sighted.

Back Cover/Harriet Bell, a contributing editor, enjoys the birthday party of her granddaughter, Heather.

Cover photos
Front-Sylvia Stagg-Giuliano
Back Cover-Agnes Zellin

For Richard, the brightest light of all

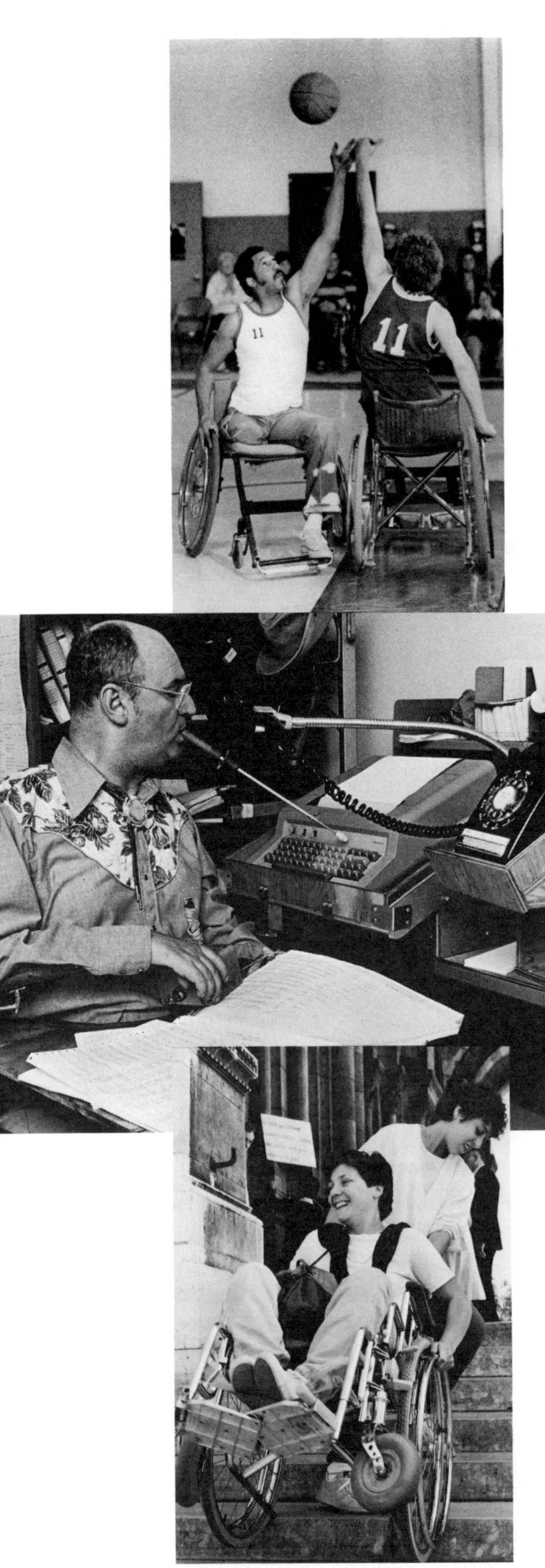

Contents

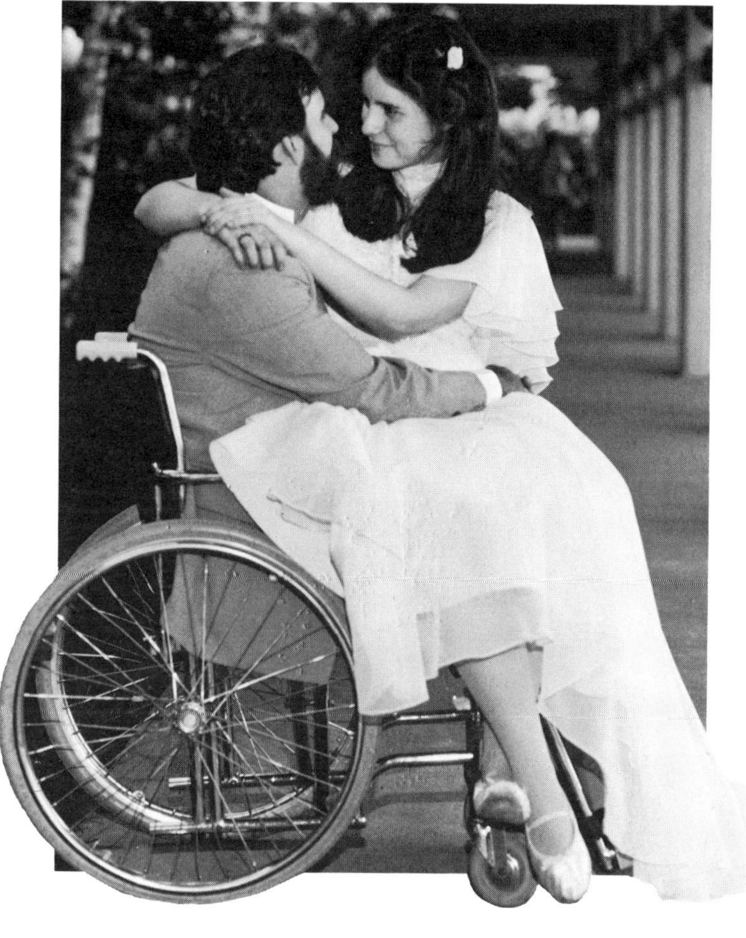

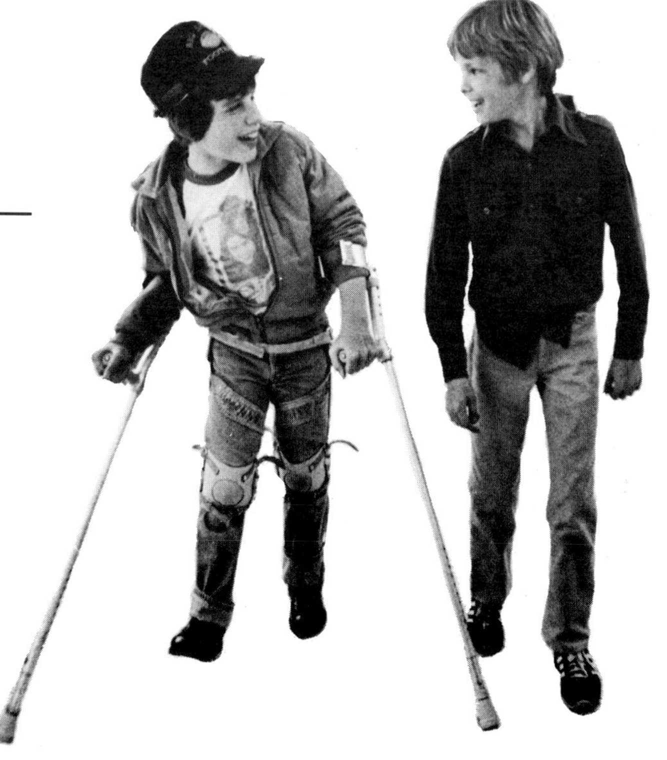

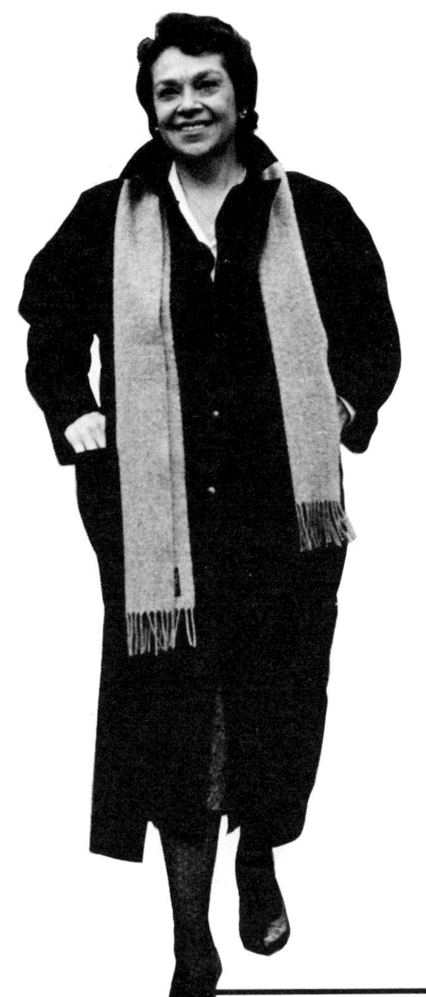

Florence Weiner is a disability rights activist, a member of the American Coalition of Citizens with Disabilities and co-founder with Harriet Bell, Ph.D., of the Polio Information Center, Roosevelt Island, New York. Her books include *How to Survive in New York with Children, Peace Is You and Me,* and *Help for the Handicapped Child.*

The interviews and research in *No Apologies* were conducted over the last four years throughout the United States and in England, France, and Germany.

No Apologies grew out of the belief that people with disabilities have valuable insights and information for everyone.

HARRIET BELL, PH.D., contributor, is a health advocate, public member of the New York State Board for Nursing, and co-founder and director of the Polio Information Center. Dr. Bell, who lived at Goldwater Memorial Hospital, Roosevelt Island, for 25 years after contracting polio, served as president of the hospital community board for four terms and contributed to the writing of the Patient's Bill of Rights. It was for her work on behalf of patients' rights that she was a recipient of the Wonder Woman Foundation Award in 1982.

WILLIAM ROTH, PH.D., who has written the introduction and is a contributor, is chairperson of the Department of Public Affairs and Policy, Nelson A. Rockefeller College of Public Affairs and Policy, State University of New York, Albany. He is the coauthor of *The Unexpected Minority: Handicapped Children in America* and author of *The Handicapped Speak*.

Acknowledgments

Many people made this book possible. After we talked, people suggested I see a friend, a colleague, a parent of a disabled child, or an advocate who would know more people. This went on for four years.

Harriet Bell has worked with me from the beginning with unmatched generosity of spirit. Together, we established the Polio Information Center.

I met people I might never have met, people who touched my life, and I touched theirs. One thing is certain, I will never be the same.

Contributors	**Harriet Bell, Ph.D.** **William Roth, Ph.D.**
Manager	**Barni Smith**
Research Staff	**Fay Daniels** **George Lieberman**

If, during your reading of *No Apologies*, you recall an incident that results in a laugh or a tear or a sudden insight, let us hear from you, even though we may not be able to answer all letters. If you have discovered a way of coping with a disability, write to us.

***No Apologies* is a combination of practical advice, personal observations, and authoritative references. Everyone involved—from the author to the guest speakers to the technical editors—either has a disability or has a close family member with a disability.**

Florence Weiner
St. Martin's Press
175 Fifth Avenue
New York, New York 10010

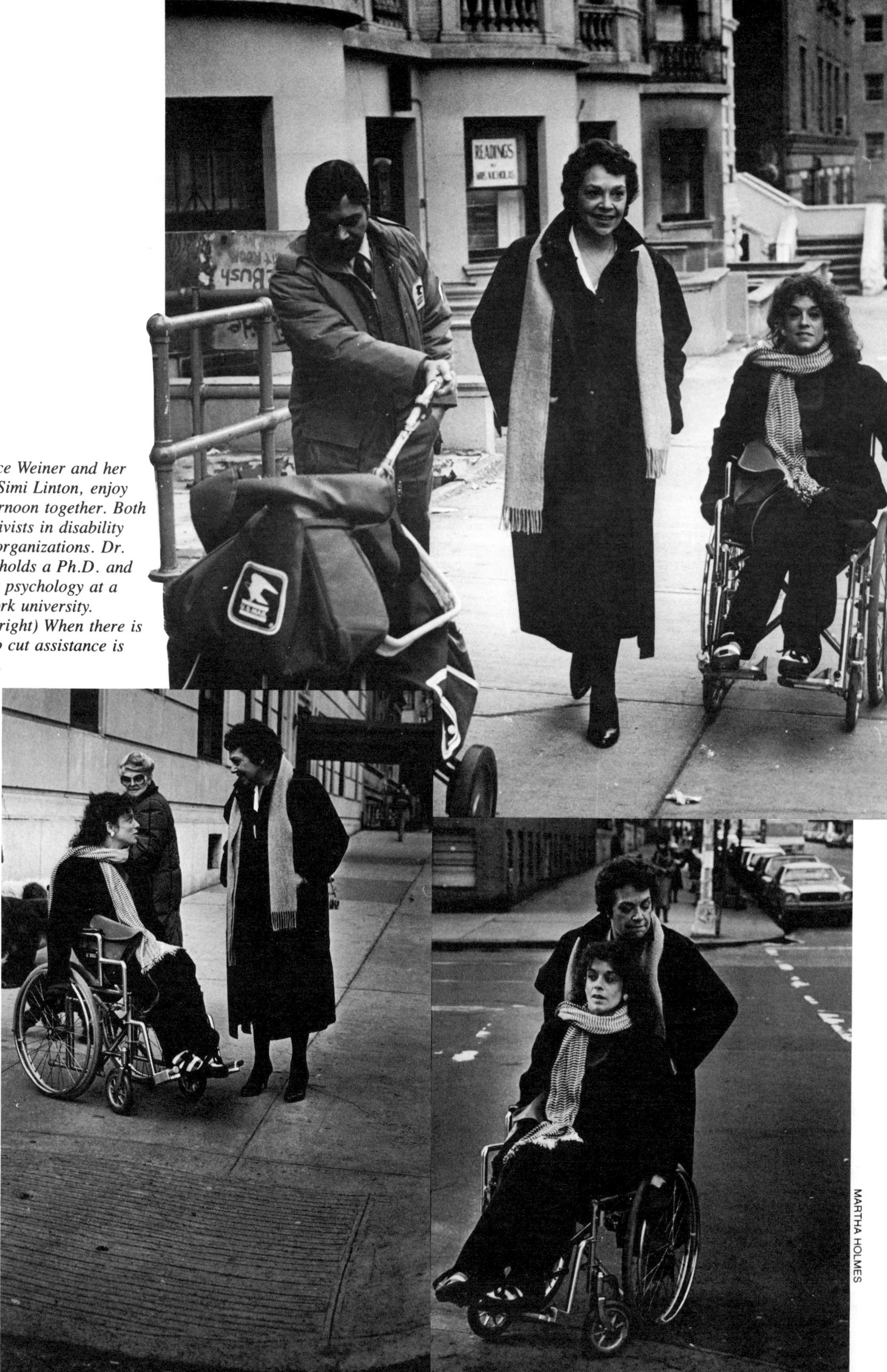

Florence Weiner and her sister, Simi Linton, enjoy an afternoon together. Both are activists in disability rights organizations. Dr. Linton holds a Ph.D. and teaches psychology at a New York university. (lower right) When there is no curb cut assistance is needed.

MARTHA HOLMES

Author's Words

People with a disability are not "those people," set aside from everyone else. We and our families make up the statistics. Someone came up with a figure of 36 million disabled people in this country, but that is only a statistic.

What about the estimate of more than 43 million people with heart conditions, or the 36 million with arthritis, or millions of us who are alcoholic, have emotional disabilities, drug addiction, high blood pressure, asthma, diabetes, kidney disease, cancer, strokes, pain, hearing and visual impairments that never get reported to statisticians?

"We are living longer because of medical progress and modern technology, and we outlive chronic disabilities that once killed us or kept us hidden away."

We are living longer because of medical progress and modern technology, and we outlive chronic disabilities that once killed us or kept us hidden away. Yet each year there are 10,000 new spinal cord injuries, mostly young men, resulting from sports or car accidents.

Television takes us right to the scene and aftermath of shootings of public figures and private citizens, to fires, and to accidents of all kinds; and we realize we live with disabilities.

Disability cuts across every economic class, age, ethnic, religious, and racial boundary, and it is a group that one can join in a moment. People with a disability, then, are not "those people," they are ourselves and those dear to us.

The statistics became very real to me when one Sunday morning my phone rang too early.

Before the message was given, I received it. My sister had been badly hurt in an automobile accident and she was in an intensive care unit. Exploratory surgery revealed a severe spinal injury. She would never walk again.

At 24, my sister became one of 10,000 people who sustain disabling spinal injuries in this country each year. The statistics are not simply interesting but become terribly real when they hit home; it doesn't only happen to other families.

I had just completed a book called *Help for the Handicapped Child,* intended for families faced with the problems surrounding a child with a disability. I began to live what I had written as I spent time with my sister.

The early stages were marked by a period in the hospital and then, later, almost seven months in a rehabilitation institute.

At a rehab center, families cluster in the corridors when they visit. A common bond encourages friendship: genuine caring, sharing victories (return of sensation in an arm or leg), sharing defeats (lost bladder or bowel function). There is a willingness to do for others, qualities usually experienced only in a disaster.

Helplessness, anger, guilt, embarrassment, a feeling of loss are also there. The family does not basically change. How they react to one another is the same; that there is a victim is the difference. In the hospital or rehab center, the family members become actors on a new stage playing unfamiliar roles with people they have never before met. Doctors, nurses, attendants often seem not to be allies but rather people to whom one must show inordinate deference in exchange for kindness to the person you love who is their patient.

"Disability cuts across every economic class, age, ethnic, religious, and racial boundary, and it is a group that one can join in a moment."

The easy camaraderie on the floor suggested passengers on a trans-Atlantic crossing. Everyone was in it together, at least while there. I believe there are things so deeply personal that they can be revealed only to strangers. People on my sister's floor shared enough of how they ended up there for everyone to know. The most personal aspects of everyone's life were available to the staff on charts.

A nurse shared: "A lot is going on inside, observations, and conclusions. Family and friends are important—necessary—but when visiting hours end, they leave and, in fact, walk out of here."

Psychologists have labeled the emotional stages an individual goes through after extreme shock or crisis. They are denial, anger, bargaining, depression, and acceptance. The staging of human emotion does not take place in any specific order. The feelings can occur all at once, in any order, or may be delayed for years.

I could only guess what stages my sister was experiencing. I did not ask her directly. We spoke about our feelings but unrelated to her injury. Similarly, I doubt that she knew the upheaval inside me. My concern was to not burden her, to keep a certain expression on my face that said all was well. It was not. Was it "denial" I was experiencing when I did not believe for a minute that my sister would not walk? Was it "bargaining" when I stood over a continuously flushing toilet praying? Was that "anger" I felt when her physical therapist told me with finality that my sister could not and would never walk? Perhaps the spirit of willingness to accept what *is* falls somewhere in those staged categories. But then what is the loss and mourning that remains with me long after my sister has put the pieces of her new life together?

One Saturday, I arrived at the institute. The sun was high in a cloudless sky. For the first time, my sister could go out in the neighborhood. How excited we were! The automatic doors swung open and she glided her wheelchair to the curb, which had a perfect curb cut.

Down two more streets, no more curb cuts and a step too high to negotiate safely to get into a coffee shop for lunch.

As I walked alongside my sister, what suddenly became clear was that everyone was staring. And there was no way of knowing what they were thinking as they stared at my sister, her wheelchair, her legs, and then at me. I became frightened at my own rage, uncertain I could contain it.

What also became clear to me on that excursion was that my sister had joined a group that society censures. And, in some way, I, too, was inexorably bound in the struggle. . . .

In the thirteen years since that day, laws have been passed stating that equal rights and equal access are inalienable rights: token accessing of some curb cuts, Braille numbers in elevators, a parking space set aside for drivers who are disabled, a lowered telephone here and there, an enlarged restroom to accommodate a wheelchair user, a ramp for access to some buildings. But it is not good enough.

Disabled citizens pay taxes and are entitled to get into the post office, the library, to churches and synagogues, the courthouse, department stores and shopping malls, the YMCA, train stations, through the checkout aisles of supermarkets, and on the bus.

Disabled citizens will bring about the changes needed to make the society work for everyone. We have learned lessons from the struggles of other minorities, and we will never again be shut out or hidden away.

No Apologies is a guide written by the *real* authorities—people with disabilities and their close family members. Therefore, this book differs from books written by and for professionals who look at people with a disability as patients who someone other than themselves must do something to, for, or with.

The feeling of being entitled was a thread that ran throughout every exchange, no matter whom I spoke to, even though it was often not perceived at the moment.

Most of us are optimists at heart. We give birth with full hope that our children will be healthy, free of a disability. And our expectation is that we and they will remain so.

How we cope determines the quality of our life. How we answer and go beyond the question and create a meaningful, fulfilled life is the focus of this work.

What I have learned about making it with a disability is that in order to go beyond "Why me?" one needs to ask, "Why not me?" Why not me to believe I am entitled to what everybody else in this society has? Why not me to believe I am capable, worthy, and intelligent—with the ability to fight for my rights without giving the responsibility to anyone else, to know the rights of one represent the rights of all, both disabled and nondisabled? Why not me to educate others by letting them know who I am, why I am, and what I believe is just?

Ultimately, I have learned that it is a matter of faith—faith in oneself, faith in others, and faith in the righteousness of all good human beings.

Florence Weiner

Introduction

Florence Weiner has put together a book that tells who disabled people are and where we are going. Most important of all, it does so with no apologies, affirming that we who are disabled need not apologize for our existence, our rights, our needs, our contributions, our love, our independence, our citizenship, our humanity.

Like women, blacks and Hispanics, people with disabilities are an oppressed minority. Recognition of this fact has come late. Disabled activists like Helen Keller and Franklin D. Roosevelt fought largely for others, as if unaware that people with disabilities had a fight of their own.

Their struggle for social justice may have been influenced profoundly by the biological caprice and social injustice of their own disabilities. It is fitting now that disabled people be seen as a group upon whom fundamental injustices have been perpetrated.

If we do not vote consistently or organize effectively, it may be less from apathy than from barriers in architecture and transportation, barriers that make exercising our rights to vote and assemble difficult, if not impossible. If we do not earn as much as others, it may be less from a lack of productivity than prejudice. If we do not consume as wisely, that may be because we have less access to a market that is rigged for people with able bodies. If we are not married as often, it may not be because we cannot love but because the social lesson is that we can't. If we are not seen at movies, discos, baseball games, or concerts, it may be less that we are uninterested than that these events are physically, socially, and economically inaccessible to us.

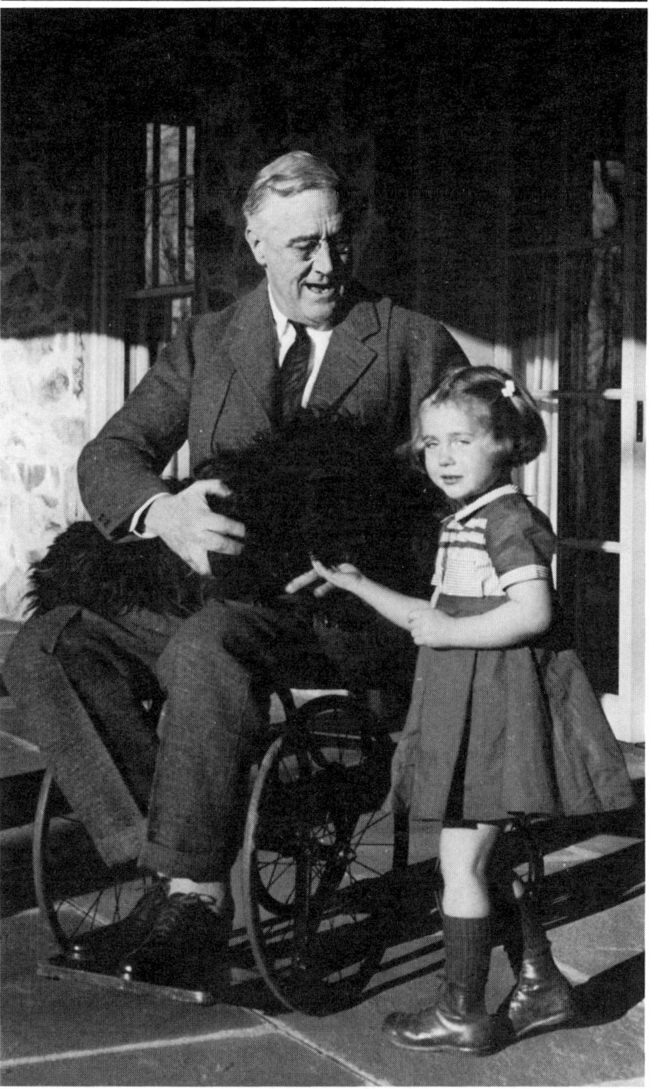

MARGARET SUCKLEY/FRANKLIN D. ROOSEVELT LIBRARY

A rare photograph of President Franklin D. Roosevelt in his wheelchair at Hilltop College, Hyde Park, with Ruthie Bie and Fala, February, 1941. (Courtesy of Margaret L. Suckley and Franklin D. Roosevelt Library)

This book amplifies our voices into speech that commands a hearing.

We speak of many things.

We speak of our public lives and of our private lives. We speak of what is in our hearts and of the social oppression that makes our hearts heavy. We speak of what we do and what we think. We speak of how our lives have been and of how we are directing them.

No Apologies describes the resources that we need for getting what we want from work to play, from childhood to parenthood, from birth to death, from sexuality to political participation, from travel to telephones, from housing to taxes.

This book empowers us, conveying to us the words of our brothers and sisters, telling us where the resources are that we can use to come out of the closet, escape from the clinic, vault and vanquish the numerous vestigial barriers that society dares us with. Thus, this book will further the disability rights movement.

Born in the discovery that people with disabilities share a struggle, the disability rights movement still has obstacles to overcome. We seek access to people's *minds and hearts*.

It is hard to date the beginning of the disability rights movement, but, undeniably, we began to enter ourselves via our own struggle. Not always, but sometimes—many times—we began to win a court case here, curb cuts there, mainstreamed schooling elsewhere. We began to recognize that we have rights. And obligations. And legitimate claims. And talents. And organization. And, yes, even power.

Where is the disability rights movement today?

The truth is that we have accomplished much, but we are in trouble.

We have begun to access systems of education from prekindergarten through graduate school. There are more of us with jobs, fewer of us in institutions. We have engraved our claims into the tablets of the law, changing that law forever. We are getting it together, learning about liking ourselves and each other in the process. And, sometimes contentiously, we have come to regard as rights what we once regarded as favors. For us, there is no turning back.

The summation of our disability rights movement is expressible in a simple word: human. Regarded for years as subhuman, antihuman, ahuman, and unhuman, we have finally won recognition of our humanity. As with blacks, women, and other oppressed people, achievement of social recognition of our humanity was a sea change. Before it, almost anything was justified; little was wrong, and, when wrong, wrong for the wrong reasons.

Human beings sure of the justice of our claims will struggle to preserve legislation and regulations that have brought forth those claims. Recognized as human beings, we in turn recognized the humanity that we share with others.

We must attend to social justice for all human beings. We must all make our journey together.

But the economic and social situations jeopardize all of us. A wedge has been driven between the rich and the poor, and it is not a matter of pure chance that most disabled people are poor.

Many of us have learned in our personal lives that it is possible to live, prevail, and win beyond the confines of hope. Hope and leaders make things easier, yet many have individually struggled in their absence, and, indeed, their absence has characterized much of our struggle. Matters may change, but we should not be too surprised should we find that by the time they do change, we have already won.

Won what? What do we want? What sort of world are we struggling for?

We want a world where employment is not denied us. We recognize that discrimination seldom issues from bigotry but from ignorance. Work is no less important to us than to anyone else.

We want a world where we have a right to an education. Too long have we been denied an education. Too long has that education been inappropriate. Too long have we been kept from our brothers and sisters. At last, the situation is improving, though that improvement is not yet complete.

We want a world where we are not locked in nor out of buildings nor barred from transportation. Like other human beings, we have places to go and things to do.

William Roth, Ph.D.

No other qualified disabled individual in the United States . . . shall, solely by reason of his disability, be excluded from the participation in, be denied the benefits of, or be subjected to discrimination under any program or activity receiving federal financial assistance.

Section 504
Rehabilitation Act of 1973

The law is an endless becoming.

Benjamin Cardozo

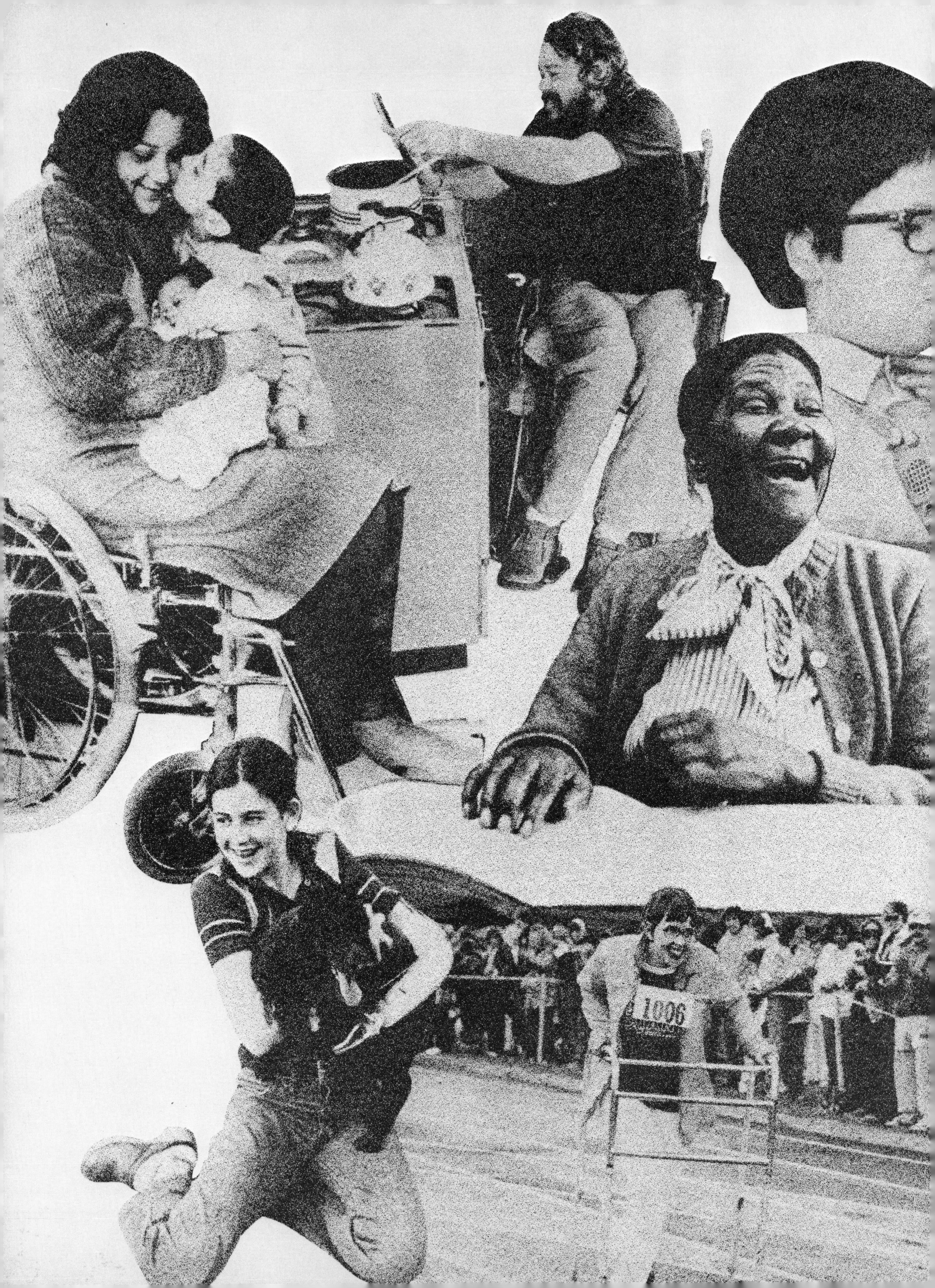
1006

Chapter 1
Who We Are

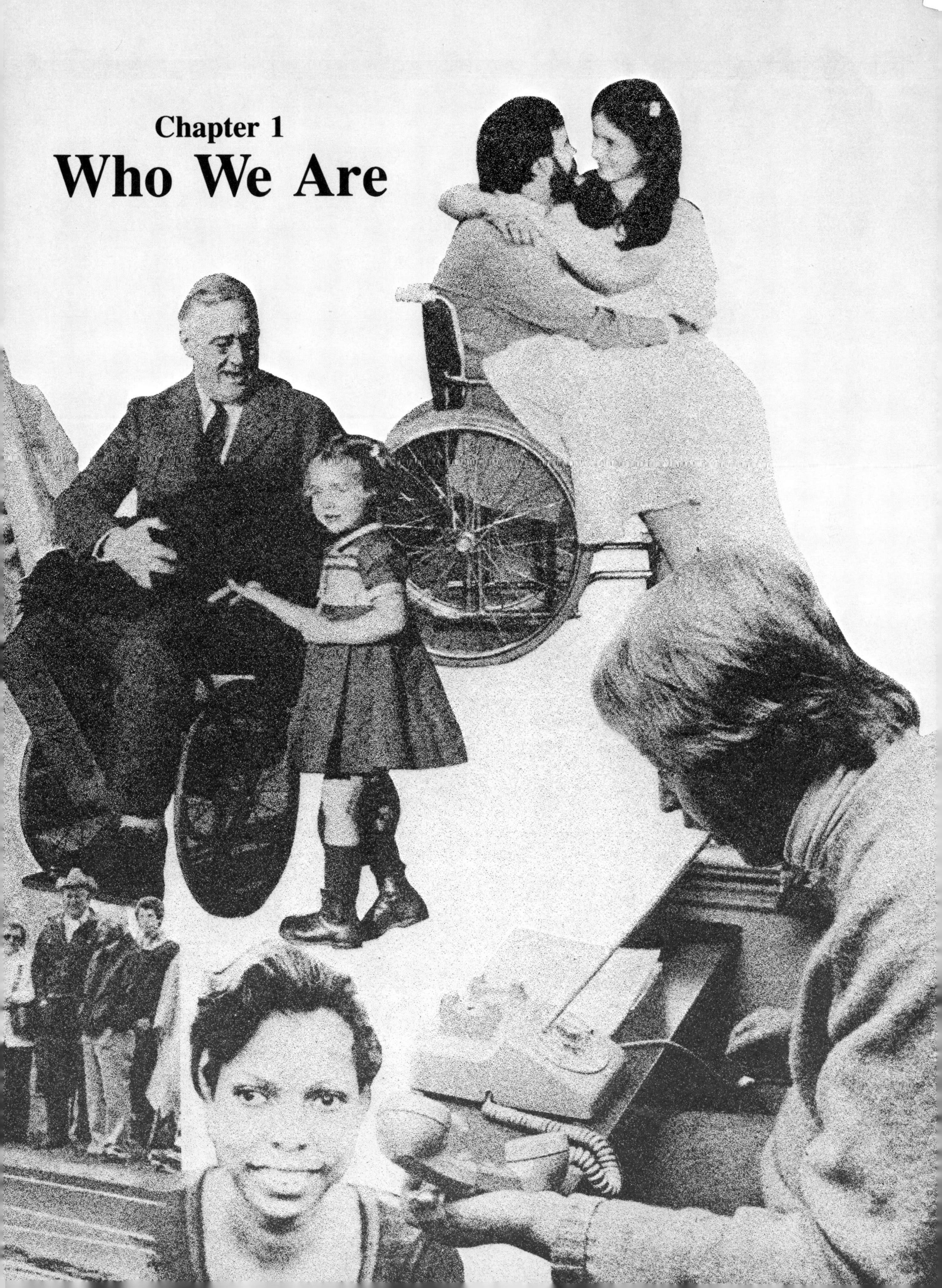

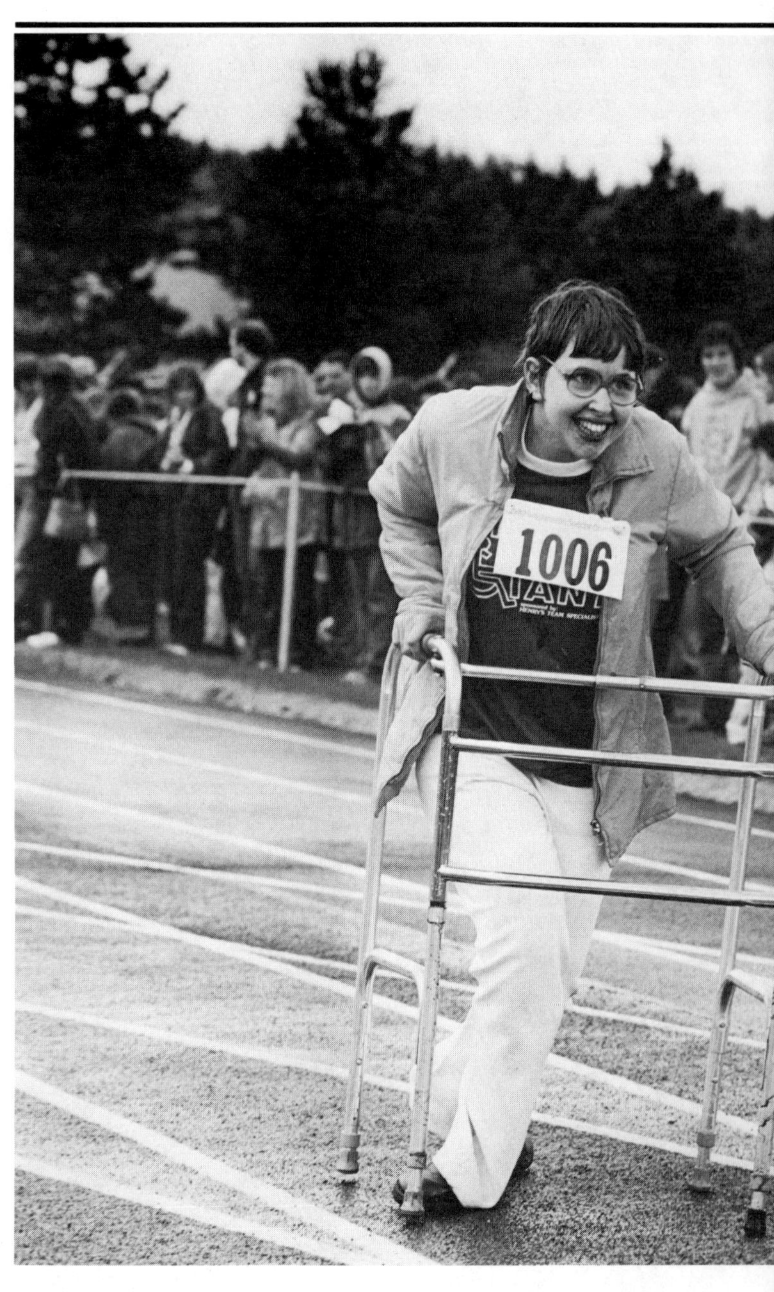
1006

Who We Are
Harriet Bell, Ph.D.

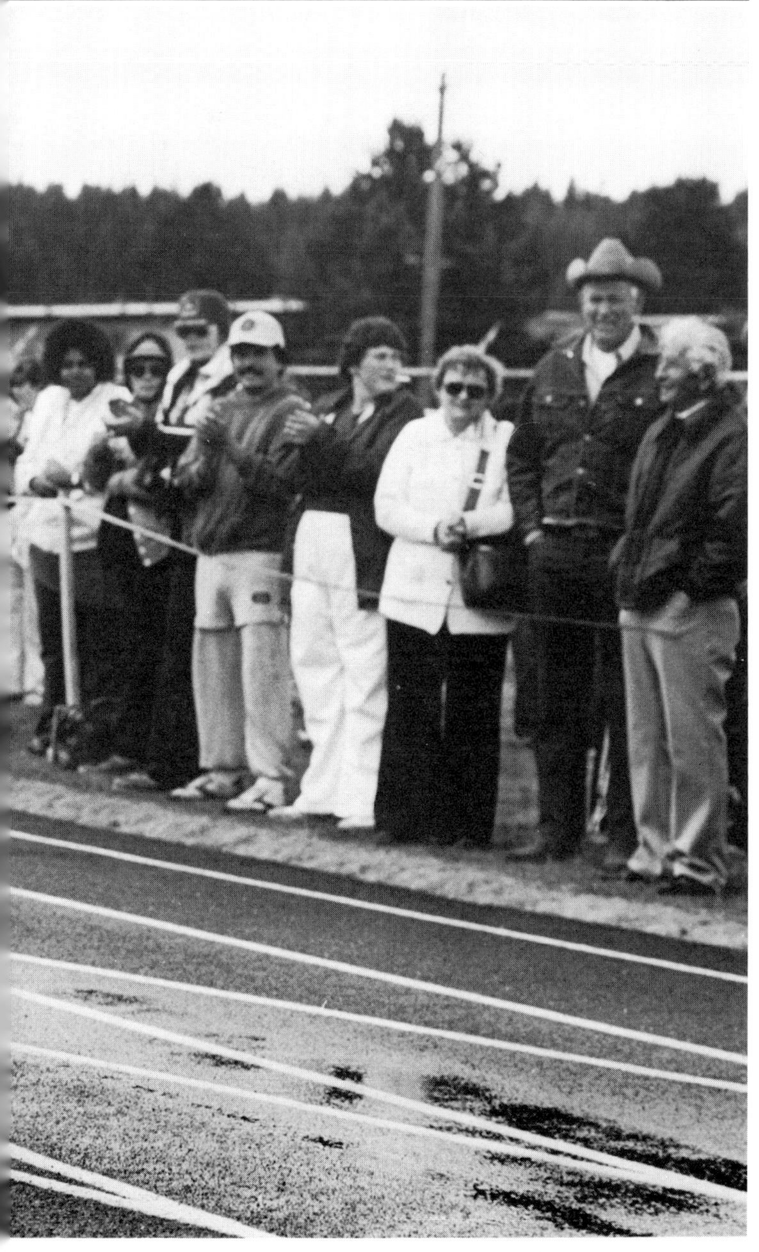

When we were growing up, we never got to know anyone with a disability unless they were in our family, and sometimes not even then. We certainly didn't have a chance to go to school with anyone who had a disability, such as muscular dystrophy, heart condition, hearing impairment, kidney disease, cerebral palsy, or someone who survived a polio epidemic.

I remember a girl in my class who didn't return after the summer. It made a big impression on me when I learned she had had polio and could not return to school again. Her name was Helen, and she wore braces on her legs. Although she lived in my neighborhood, we didn't play together after that.

Regular classes were off limits to children who could not participate in activities without any assistance. Some schools had special classes set aside for disabled children, but those children never ate in our cafeteria or went to assembly with us.

The message was clear. Disabled children were different, not part of our lives. We did not sit next to them in class, invite them to our parties, or ask them to join our scout troop.

The civil rights movement in this country began with a fight for equal opportunity in education, and it is not surprising that the disability rights movement also began with a fight for equal opportunity in education.

It is now a decade since laws mandating equal rights and equal access for all children have been passed, and yet the delivery of necessary services for disabled children is uneven and varies from community to community.

School boards report that they do not have enough money to educate children with a disability, but somehow these same schools find money to build football stadiums, hire a coach at a good salary, and outfit the cheerleaders.

Forty years ago, we were disabled veterans returning from World War II, then Korea, and, later, Vietnam. We cut across all racial, religious, ethnic, age, and socio-economic groups. We began to be mainstreamed, leaving home for the first time to attend college, coming together with others who were disabled. Political activism thrived in this environment.

Most people have treated disabled people paternalistically, and many of us have accepted the role of perennial children. But as disabled citizens learn about rights and realize what a powerful group we are, we will vote for elected officials who understand our needs and who are willing to work in our behalf.

Disabled citizens of the 1980s have families to raise and work to be done. Now that people are living longer, most of us have some chronic disability. Disabled people, then, are no longer "those people." They are us.

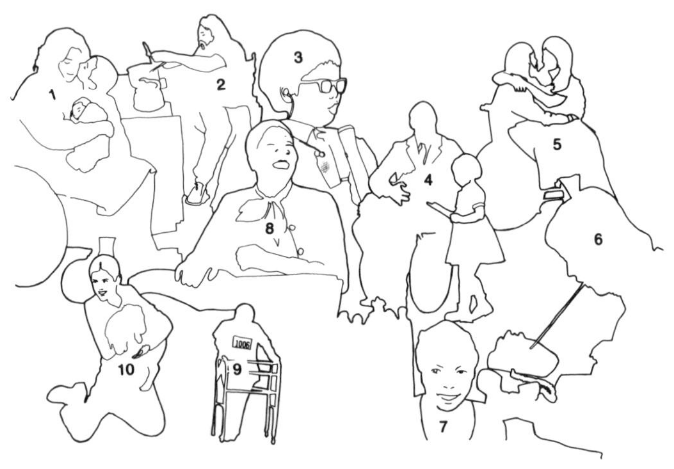

1 NANCY DURRELL MCKENNA/PHOTO RESEARCHERS

2 BRIAN PAYNE/BLACK STAR

3 PHILIP MANHEIM/PHOTO RESEARCHERS

4 MARGARET SUCKLEY/FRANKLIN D. ROOSEVELT LIBRARY

5 SYLVIA STAGG-GIULIANO

6 RUSS KINNE/PHOTO RESEARCHERS

7 FLORENCE WEINER

8 GUY GILLETTE/PHOTO RESEARCHERS

9 H. ARMSTRONG ROBERTS

10 FREDA LEINWAND/MONKMEYER

M.J. Schmidt

M.J. Schmidt is on her way to Rochester to see her daughter, who has just given birth. Before going to the airport, she meets me in the cocktail bar of the office building where she works as a computer programmer.

It is five-thirty; the place is filled with people from the offices above. Beeping sounds from video games and rock music compete. We sit in a booth; her Seeing Eye dog squeezes in under the table, waiting for the popcorn M.J. slips her as we talk.

M.J. is very exciting to be with; her full voice is undoubtedly that of a singer, her easy laughter catching. She is a "ham" and is the first to admit it.

By her suitcase are packages filled with gifts for the new baby. The conversation shifts back to the birth of her first grandchild. Suddenly, she remembers the time she told her mother that she was pregnant.

I had never been very tolerant of people with disabilities who couldn't accept and deal with life. Give people a little while to grieve—six months, a year—and then they ought to shape up. It is just like losing anything else; you have got to grieve about it. That is the way it is. My attitude was, "Get off your ass and do your thing. Find something new. Build a new life." I never realized that sometimes people couldn't cope.

My mother overprotected me and I had to fight for all of my independence. When I got pregnant, she really thought I should not have; she felt she had gone through a lot to raise her child, me, and now she was going to have to raise another one! That, of course, infuriated me; it gave me a very negative attitude toward her having anything to do with my child, something she could not understand. I knew that, by God, I was going to do it myself. I wasn't going to let my mother get her hands on my kid until she had enough respect for me to know that she should just take a normal grandmotherly role and not try to take anything away from me.

I had these marvelous opinions on what it was like to be blind that, of course, no one else had thought about. My marvelous opinion was, "Deal with it." It is there and it is not going to go away no matter how many aspirin you take, no matter how many people pat you on the top of your head.

I did not know much about kids—I had read Dr. Spock—so I was apprehensive about a child. I wanted one but I didn't have any sisters or brothers; therefore, I didn't have any nieces or nephews, and the only kids I'd ever baby-sat for were seven and nine years old. I really didn't know anything about little babies.

So I had my own fears and doubts about this unborn baby—I really didn't want to drown it in the bathinette—and I didn't really feel very secure, but the people who I should have been able to count on were the people I didn't dare count on because I was afraid they were going to take over my life. My husband was positive I would be fine, no problem, which was a great help; he really believed in me.

"I had these marvelous opinions on what it was like to be blind that, of course, no one else had thought about. My marvelous opinion was, 'Deal with it,' It is there and it is not going to go away no matter how many aspirin you take, no matter how many people pat you on the top of your head.

I had a reasonably easy labor, but when they handed me that child, the most terrible, the most awful feeling of hopelessness overcame me. Here I was, almost twenty-five years old, and I was holding this child and doing the usual things—counting her fingers and her toes and everything—and realizing that I couldn't see her and that I wanted to see her. Suddenly I realized the kind of anguish that people go through when they have to make an adjustment. Because I had been blind all my life, I never had to make that adjustment. I can't tell you the enormity of my anguish; I just wanted so much to see and I was so angry and so hurt.

I looked at her and I thought, "I will never be able to see you at bedtime, or see you make your first communion, or see you graduate or get married, and I am going to have to deal with this."

Well, I am a pretty well-adjusted blind person, and this feeling didn't last long. It was like a wave just passed over me. It was grow-up time for me because suddenly I realized, this is what people go through: they had sight all their lives and had it snatched away from them; or they could walk one day and were suddenly faced with the reality of a wheelchair the next. It was as if I had suddenly grown up in so many ways.

I said to my husband the next day, "I will never again be hard on the disabled person who has a difficult time adjusting. Maybe I won't mollycoddle them, but I will have an understanding of the terrible feeling they must have. I think I am lucky to have lived almost twenty-five years and never needed, never wanted, to see that badly before."

But there are days you dread: the day some kid says, "Your mom is blind." That is not a price my child should have to pay because she didn't ask to be born to a blind parent. But, like anything else, the things you dread, the things you worry about, never really turn out the way you worry about them.

Ann was three going on four; it was October 1959. I remember because I am a Dodger fan and the Dodgers were in a playoff with the Milwaukee Braves and I had the TV on because I like TV coverage better than radio. I was ironing. It was a rainy day. Ann and her girlfriend Marsha were sitting out on our front steps playing a game and I was ironing near the door so that I could keep one eye, one ear, on the girls and the other ear on the game. At some point, Ann said, "My mama's reading me a story about a little lame prince." Marsha said, "Ann, you lie." Ann, being shy and retiring like her mother, said "I do *not* lie." "Oh, yes, you *do*. Your mom can't read. She's blind."

Well, here's the day I had dreaded. I put the iron down and I wanted to run out and gather up my kid in my arms and say, "I'm sorry; it's not your problem." But I couldn't, I knew I couldn't. Then, before I could have even gotten to the door, my kid turned around and said, "Well, Marsha, you cuckoo clock, my mom reads Braille and I bet your mom can't do that!" And I walked into the dining room because I was blinking the tears back, and I thought, "I have worried for three and a half years, and if you teach that being blind is an okay thing, your child will accept it; but why didn't *I* know enough to know that? Why didn't *I* know enough to have confidence?"

"I have worried for three and a half years, and if you teach that being blind is an okay thing, your child will accept it; but why didn't I *know enough to know that? Why didn't* I *know enough to have confidence?"*

To this day, if someone stares at me, Ann will stare them down. If anybody asks a question, she will sit and talk about blindness for hours.

Dan was a different kind of kid. He was very sensitive, and when he was three, he ran up to me one day and jumped up onto my lap—you know how kids will kneel up on your lap and scream into your face—and he said, "Mommy, how come you be blind when other mommies can see?" I wanted to say, "Beats the hell out of me, kid," but I looked at him and I said, "Well, Dan, that is not a very easy question. God just decided, I guess, that a certain amount of people are going to have to be blind. I am one of them, and I am blind with my eyes. I want you to understand right now that I am never going to change. Grandma and Grandpa spent thousands and thousands of dollars on my eyes to try to make them work, but there is no way that I am ever, ever going to see. So that is not going to go away or change. But there are other ways to see. You see with your ears and with your mind."

And he said, "Yeah, and besides, Mom, you can do anything anybody else's mom can."

If You're Thinking About Having a Disability

William Roth, Ph.D.

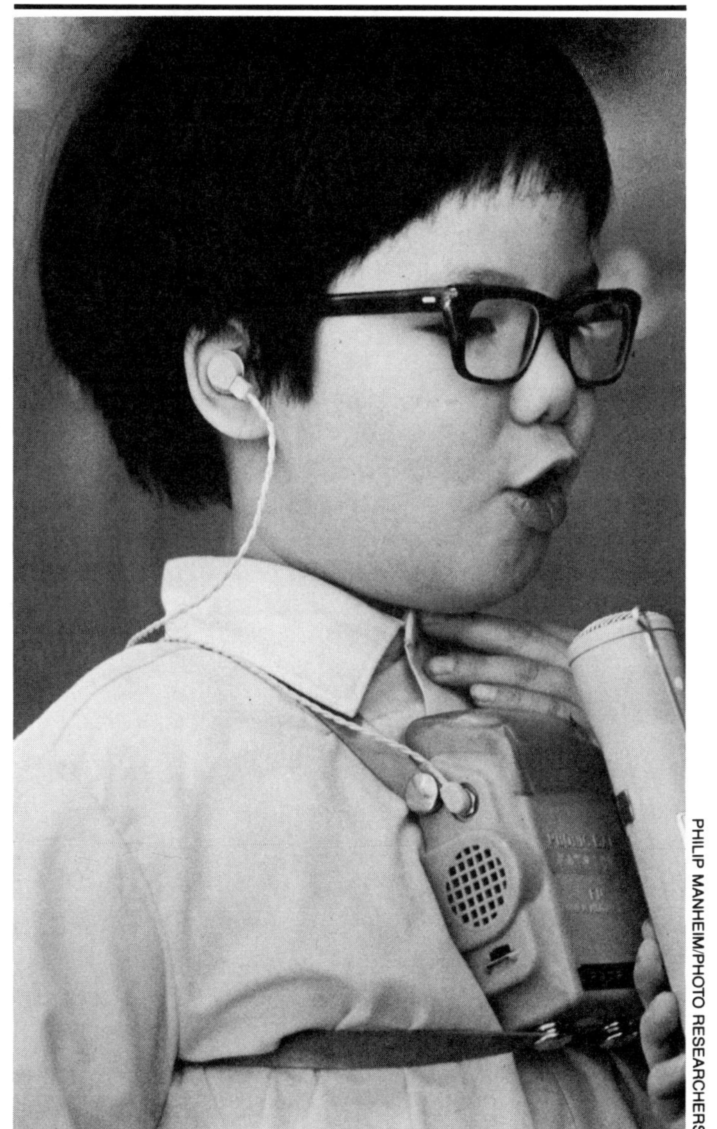
PHILIP MANHEIM/PHOTO RESEARCHERS

First grade student with a hearing impairment uses a microphone, and hearing aids for amplification. He is learning sound formation by touching his vocal chords.

First things first. Just between the two of us, all things considered, it is best that you choose not to be disabled. Although it is possible to make a virtue of your disability, it isn't easy and nobody really knows how to do it. Therefore, play it safe and aim for health, wealth, and wisdom. It's never too early to think about these matters, so, at the moment of conception:

Choose your genetic message with care. Be sure that it does not signal even a susceptibility to a disability. Since only a few disabilities are straightforwardly hereditary, your choice of genetic message is no guarantee, but it is prudent to employ patience, hard work, and foresight, nonetheless. Time is short, so act fast.

Choose your womb with care. Housing is important. Be sure the utilities are adequate. Be sure the mother whose womb you live in has adequate nutrition, that she is not under distracting emotional or physical stress, and that she checked in early with a doctor or a midwife. Prepare her to take motherhood seriously and, at the same time, assure her that she shouldn't worry.

Try to attain a reasonable weight and height. Under no circumstances should you wander from your womb before your nine months' lease is over. Of course, you are curious about what is happening outside. But trust your mother; many are the babies who have come out to take a peek only to find that there is no way back. Prematurity, as we on the outside like to call it, can be dangerous. Prematurity and low weight or height for term bring increased odds of your being born with a disability. Since we don't know which causes which, you may as well play it safe.

Welcome to the world. Once you have decided to

come out, don't be nostalgic and linger. You can't go home again, and you will be needing air. Be nice to your mother; help her in her labor. She is prepared and ready to love you, and you should do nothing to jeopardize that. An easy, well-timed birth under normal circumstances should be your goal.

Be a good baby. As a junior human being, you should know that the young of our species are dependent on others for longer than are other animals. So make things easy for your parents; they will reciprocate, and this will stimulate attention, decrease the chance of your being left in dangerous situations, and help insure that you do not become a battered child.

Do unto others as you would have them do unto you. Remember that you are now a part of a team and pay heed lest you incur rancor from older siblings, fatigue from your mother and father, vices from any of them. Developmental psychology says that now you are egocentric. You will find this rule to be valuable as gold.

The above suggestions, presented in the belief that it is better not to be disabled, are biologically oriented. Should you have been perverse enough not to follow them, you should follow these next suggestions, which are increasingly oriented to the overwhelmingly social world of disabilities. It is not too late; as a baby and child with a disability, you can lead a good life. Indeed, precisely because of your disability, it is important that you do so. Never forget that life is a precious gift, to be lived passionately, lovingly, and wisely. Having a disability, you may become more aware than most children of how lucky you are to be alive.

Life is likely to go much easier for you if your parents are rich. It is time that you recognized some realities. Rich families can command good medical care, good therapy, good education, good services. Although the best things in life may be free, money is a good second best. Further, the wealth your parents command may one day be yours, and life may be easier if you can afford extravagant (if necessary) adjustments from your environment.

While you are designing your family, make sure they have the prestige to demand respect by professionals and the knowledge of when professionals are wrong. You should request the same omniscience and omnipotence from parents that you expect from your God.

Never forget, first and foremost, you are a child; you will develop as a whole child. Physical maturation is only one aspect of your development. Therefore, choose a family that recognizes this and is not overly protective; on the other hand, they should not let you wander into danger. You will have to be fiendishly clever to insure that your parents know where to draw the lines.

Eat well, benefit from medicine, avoid lead paints, and fasten your seat belt while traveling in cars. But, all the while, you must remember your psychological, emotional, and intellectual development; don't sacrifice them to your physical development. Don't despair; difficult decisions like this are a part of life.

Make sure that your family learns how to respond appropriately to your disability. This includes not only your mother, but your father, brothers and sisters, and most importantly, you. It is hard to describe what an appropriate response is, but you will probably develop intuitions about it.

As you grow up, you will encounter situations where the social demands on your unique body are different. You will have to learn how to bob and weave and make sense of conflicting demands. Sometimes you may feel that people react to you as someone other than yourself; learn how to inject your true self into situations. This isn't easy, and you will probably become an expert social scientist while still a child. You will face many situations where social savvy is necessary. Take heart, there are rewards. You will discover much that is concealed to your able-bodied friends. As for your own actions, be careful that you don't use your disability as an excuse for not doing what you can, for getting attention, and, in general, for not living. There are too many difficulties in growing up disabled for you to invent new ones.

Institutions are usually bad; try to stay away from them. Since you have already provided yourself with an intact rich family, this should be easy. But situations may develop in which your family concludes that it must send you to an institution. Try your best to impress on them that you want to stay with them. But if you are sent to an institution, be sure that it is a good one and that the decision to institutionalize is reversible. You are too young to make decisions that may jeopardize your future. Under no circumstances should you allow yourself to go to an institution that will warp your mind, injure your body, or break your soul. Remember that you are a human being with inalienable rights; never let yourself be put in the situation where your humanity is betrayed.

"Remember that you are a human being with inalienable rights; never let yourself be put in the situation where your humanity is betrayed."

Be sure your parents don't make endless rounds looking for cures that don't exist; make just as sure that

they find all the cures that do exist. Chances are that you will have more contact than your able-bodied friends with people outside your family trying to help you. Make sure they are competent, inform them of all they should know about you, insure that your parents and they respect each other and you. See your doctor from time to time and stay tuned for advances in medicine.

Depending on your temperament, you may be hopeful or hopeless about changes in your body. Should you opt for hope, do not fantasize a disability-free future, which almost surely will never come. Invest your jelly beans shrewdly and don't put them in one basket, especially if the basket is an illusion.

You have to educate society as well as yourself. You are probably starting to realize that your situation of disability not only describes characteristics of you but characteristics of your society. Education starts at home, moves to the school, and finally to the broader world. As you come to realize that your situation is in large part a fabrication of other people and not of your own making, it may seem easy to give up any responsibility for yourself. Don't. If you do, you are giving up your humanity.

You are in school. Congratulations! If you have handled your situation properly, you will have secured whatever you needed in the way of preschool education. You have informed your parents that the later social effects of many disabilities can be ameliorated by proper and uniquely designed preschool programs. Should these opportunities not exist, you have asked your parents to move or get together with other parents of disabled children to create such opportunities. Now you must decide whether to go to a school for disabled children or a school for able-bodied children. Life may seem easier in a school with disabled children. However, in the long run, you may wish that you had gone to an integrated school. Your decision should be reversible: change your mind, change your school. Should you opt for an integrated school, you may meet resistance from teachers, administrators, or pupils. Usually, this resistance comes from ignorance, and you will have to teach those by whom you would be taught. The world of school is different from the world of your family. Don't expect the same love, attention, and understanding from your teachers and classmates as you would from your parents and siblings. But remember the law is on your side. Unless you are lucky, there will be situations in which you will be teased by other children and discriminated against by teachers. Don't let it break you. Learn how to fight and learn that this does not mean being obnoxious. Don't forget, in spite of your disability, you are a child like other children. You share far more with these children than you don't.

Check that the principal and teachers and others know the unique characteristic of your disability and that your peers learn how to react to you. They will have an opportunity to grow as you do, learning from you as they teach you. This is important not only for you but for other disabled children and people whom your classmates will meet in the course of their lives. It is a hard burden to take on the role of teacher while so young, to exercise the responsibility of citizenship while disenfranchised, to work with those who sometimes may try to exclude you. It is your life to live, and decisions like this can only be made by you.

Learn how other people perceive you and how you perceive others. This is an important part of your development. These perceptions are taken for granted amongst the able-bodied. They cannot in general be taken for granted in interactions involving you. It is important to pay this some heed, since you are a social being.

Learn to distinguish between disappointments derived from the situation of disability and disappointments shared by all children. You will have many disappointments throughout childhood. Every child does. You may be tempted to attribute these disappointments to your disability. Search out whatever virtues are unique to your disability. Given the deficits of disability, exercising these virtues is crucial. This is not to suggest "compensation," a word you will no doubt hear till you vomit. Instead, search out your strengths and use them, not as compensation but for their own sake.

"After all is said and done, your situation is a riddle. Your birth was a riddle. Your childhood is a riddle. Your adolescence and adulthood will be riddles. You will know riddles as few able-bodied people know them. Learn how to laugh at yourself even as you cry. At the same time, do not become a mere passive spectator of your own life. It is you who are living it."

Develop a sense of humor. After all is said and done, your situation is a riddle. Your birth was a riddle. Your childhood is a riddle. Your adolescence and adulthood will be riddles. You will know riddles as few able-bodied people know them. Learn how to laugh at yourself even as you cry. At the same time, do not become a mere passive spectator of your own life. It is you who are living it.

An important riddle of your life is that you are a disabled person in an able-bodied society. There will be a tension between developing your own unique personality, predicated to an appropriate (but not inappropriate) degree on your disability, and complying with the demands of those around you that you follow the rules of able-bodied society, make that society feel at ease with you, and be as much like other people as possible. Some "normalization" is necessary to make you accepted by your society. However imperfect it is, it is the only society you have, and it is composed of human beings as fallible as you are. An ideal society would not require "normalization," but your society frequently will not tolerate difference and will demand "normalization." Just how you sail the course between being one of the gang and being yourself is your decision. But avoid the extremes of selling your soul to be like everyone else and of being a misanthrope.

When you have grown up, deciding about whether to help change society is your decision. Your disability will give you unique perspective on family, school, and society. This perspective, although painful, is invaluable, and it is to be cultivated. But you should not remove yourself from society: Your perspective is a unique way to involve yourself in it. Just avoid the vices of perspective: cynicism, rancor, and distance. Your childhood is not only a childhood. You are growing up every day and one day will become an adult. You should enjoy the unique opportunities of childhood at the same time that you prepare yourself for the opportunities of adulthood. Your society may try to hide your future from you for reasons of its own, but that does not mean that the future is any less real nor any less to be prepared for.

As an adult, you will be a free man or woman. You must see to it that your path to adulthood makes you aware of your freedom. Do not allow yourself to become a perpetual child. There comes a time in life when it is no longer appropriate to follow parents, teachers, and friends unquestioningly.

There comes a time when life becomes your responsibility. Of course, because of your disability, you may have special cause to be dependent frequently on others. This does not change your ultimate responsibility for your own situation. Your life will always be a paradox, not the easiest of lives. It is stupid to fool yourself and to think your life in some fundamental sense different, to delude yourself into thinking it impossible, to propagandize yourself into believing it worthless. You are a human being living in the society of human beings. This entails responsibility, provides opportunity, defines dignity, and denotes promise. Don't let yourself be duped into thinking otherwise.

There will be few adults in whom you can see your future. Don't let the absence of "role models" deter you from growing up. It may take effort on your part to construct a future that will welcome you. It will take imagination, vision, and work. But a little work never hurt anyone. Occasions will rise when your parents, siblings, schoolmates, teachers, and others will not have answers to your questions. This is because, in all probability, they will not have grown up with your disability, and parts of your development will confuse them. This is but one fact that makes you a member of a unique minority.

You should make of your life a fuller one than it would have been without your disability. How this is done is a mystery. This is not to say that suffering is good. But many people with a disability add to their lives, making something richer and more complete than would have been possible without having surmounted an obstacle.

William Roth, Ph.D., is chairperson of the Department of Public Affairs and Policy, Nelson A. Rockefeller College of Public Affairs and Policy of the State University of New York at Albany. He is coauthor of *The Unexpected Minority: Handicapped Children in America*, and author of *The Handicapped Speak*.

Permission was given by the *Exceptional Parent* where this first appeared.

Harilyn Rousso

Harilyn Rousso is a therapist in private practice in New York City. An activist in disability rights, she founded Disabilities Unlimited, a counseling and consultative service for people with disabilities and their families in the New York area. Rousso is chairperson of the Association of Mental Health Practioners with Disabilities and a member of the board of the Coalition of Sexuality and Disabilities.

I think some disabilities are more tolerable than others. Cerebral palsy, for example, is a special kind of disability that is not very pleasant to look at at times. It's unfortunate, but it is a reality. Cerebral palsy creates gestures and movements that people are not accustomed to handling.

So, in my mind, having cerebral palsy meant that I should be a researcher, a librarian, do the type of thing where I would be away from people . . . hidden. That is how I perceived it.

"Most people have tremendous potential to do many creative things, but because of 'the critic' inside us, many of us seem to feel lousy about ourselves and never quite get it together. However, if we allow ourselves the pleasure of feeling successful, our self-confidence will be reinforced. Helping to put 'the critic' to rest is important."

There are some assumptions about what disabled people's lives are like: We are all unhappy; the world is cruel; there is no real potential to move beyond the experience of being disabled. Common for disabled and nondisabled alike is the fact that a lot of people just don't feel good about themselves. Most people have tremendous potential to do many creative things, but because of "the critic" inside us, many of us feel lousy about ourselves and never quite get it together. However, if we allow ourselves the pleasure of feeling successful, our self-confidence will be reinforced. Helping to put "the critic" to rest is important.

Sometimes, too, success is scary. "Making it" can have a lot of implications. Maybe that means you have to be a "superperson" or very independent; you can't be a kid anymore or be needy, dependent. I think a mistaken idea of what it is to be successful is that you have to feel "together" all the time. That's a very scary prospect.

With a disability, you don't even have a fighting chance if you don't believe—100 percent—that you can fight. You are still going to have a fight even if you feel good about yourself. Sometimes kids tease me when I walk down the street. The teasing has had varying impacts, depending on where I've been in my life. At times, it has been extremely painful and has set me back because it reinforced some of my own feelings of disgust at being "the freak."

People with disabilities, like myself, were trained to accept that they have to be "nice kids" and know all the rules. Many people do not like it if you speak up. They feel it is enough that people tolerate you; you shouldn't put any extra pressure on them. This can keep you in a very passive position, a hard mold to break out of. Assertion is a natural outgrowth of feeling good, feeling worthwhile, thinking, "Why shouldn't what I want be valid?" But learning self-esteem is often slow and difficult.

In this learning process, one of the fears that comes up is that passivity is the only way you have gained any acceptance at all. That makes you feel very angry so another fear is that you will open your mouth, talk a blue streak, scream, yell. In fact, that is what you feel like doing. Sometimes you have to learn some tricks, techniques, for helping yourself deal with these emotions.

The real trick is finding a technique that suits you, makes you comfortable, and that doesn't put you into a second-class position.

Katherine Corbett

Katherine Corbett is a blend of the best qualities of New England and California: dependability and easy informality. Corbett is cherished by many friends and respected for her commitment, particularly to the needs of disabled women.

She is the creator and coordinator of the Disabled Women's Project of the Disability Rights Education and Defense Fund, Berkeley, California. Their primary objective is to determine the educational needs and the type of employment best suited for disabled women. From the results of thousands of questionnaires and interviews, there is evidence that disabled women in this country experience a "double disability."

No one ever said to me, "You are handicapped." We never talked about it, even in my family. No one ever said, "It is hard for me to be with you because then I will be reflected badly in other people's eyes." No one ever talked about it; no one ever sat down and asked me, "Is it hard?" There were never any feelings expressed about my disability. Things were never said to me that I needed to hear. I was never told that I was, in fact, "handicapped." I am different—I will always be different—and this is my norm and I am going to work from this norm. There is better within this.

I think of myself as putting down my head and plowing through things. This has been a mixed blessing. It has given

"No one ever talked about it; no one ever sat down and asked me, 'Is it hard?'"

me a drive—an intense, pushing, burning energy that results in my accomplishing a whole lot in a lot of different ways. I am very, very strong because of that, in terms of really being able to persist and do hard work, both personal work and work work. I attribute this to the work that was done with my body when I got polio, the physical therapy; it was participatory. I had to do it; I had to take responsibility. I think that is what gave me that perpetual push to be better, to get better, to do better. You can look at anything and it can be better. As a child, I was faced with what would be an impossible task—moving muscles that really didn't move. I would watch my body substantially change and get, in fact, better. So I had the sense that if you worked at it long enough and hard enough, you would get what you wanted.

Not talking about my disability made me very upset sometimes. People would say I was just like everybody else, and I would think, "How come they don't go to the hospital for checkups? How come they don't go in for surgery? How come, if I am just like everybody else, people stare at me in the street?" I was forced by my family and by my culture to be nice to people. A stranger would be standing at a bus stop and would watch me walk down the street and would turn to me and say, "What's wrong?" It happened all the time because I was just about the most disabled person they would see on the street where I lived. My mother would make me stand there and be nice to them. I wasn't allowed to feel angry or embarrassed.

What always felt bad to me, especially as a child being stopped on the streets, is that I always felt I was being ripped off—somebody was taking something away from me and giving me nothing in return. They might tell me stories about their sister or their brother who had such and such disease, but they never gave me anything; they just took. There was no reciprocity. I always had to do the work. I had to take care of them. I had to take care of their feelings. The conversation always went, "What's the matter with you?" If I told them, they would say, "Oh, that is awful," and I would reply, "No, it is not so awful. It is really okay. I am fine." They would ask if it hurt, if it could be fixed, because it was not okay for me to be the way I was—I had to be "normal." So I would answer, "No, I am really quite fine. I have come a long way. I really like myself now."

The Lively Arts

Victoria Ann-Lewis

I was three years old in the summer of 1949 when a polio epidemic swept through the Midwest. No swimming pool was safe, drinking water was suspect, and physical contact was discouraged. Despite precautions, I contracted polio.

One of my first distinct memories was of Halloween that same year. I am dressed in pink Doctor Denton pajamas with a little pig mask and my father carries me from house to house while I whisper, "Trick or treat." Another memory: Though shy, I organize the whole kindergarten class into a train ride and, playing conductor, take them on a trip to Kansas City, my previous home. Another: In grade school, I make braces, tiny wooden crutches, and a small wheelchair for my dolls, and with these images of myself, I act out little plays.

"I won best thespian all four years in high school. But, though praised, I always understood that a professional acting career was out of the question due to my postpolio limp and withered leg."

Looking back on these incidents, I recognize the beginning of my desire to perform, to create other realities, and to act out my own reality. I am struck by the lack of shame I felt about my disability at that time. This was not the case later in my life.

I performed throughout grade school and high school, took classes in acting and singing, and wrote plays and poetry. I won best school thespian all four years in high school. But, though praised, I always understood that a professional acting career was out of the question due to my postpolio limp and withered leg.

When I entered college, I majored in English literature. My college didn't even offer theater arts. But every fall and spring there were school festivals for which I wrote and directed satirical one-act plays. The one-acts were fun, but the obligatory yearly productions of drama classics were pretty dull affairs, with male actors and directors jobbed in. I had roles in a few of these plays, but most of the time I hid my nose in a book.

After receiving a masters degree, I taught high school English for two years. I enjoyed it but still felt unsatisfied and guilty about not trying to do the one thing that meant the most to me—acting. I decided to change careers before it was too late.

I wanted professional theatrical training, so I applied to the Neighborhood Playhouse in New York City. When they discovered I was disabled, they refused to accept me until my limp was corrected. I went into physical therapy and was able to correct the limp somewhat, but when I called the school I couldn't get past the secretary. At the time I thought, "I can't blame them. I can't really be a professional actress."

It wasn't until I moved to Portland, Oregon, that I got my first acting job. I did community theater through local universities and eventually was hired full-time by Family Circus Theater, a touring theater group.

Family Circus was one of the most exciting performing groups in Portland. They had a distinctive style—fast, funny, and choreographed—a style demanding many hours of tedious rehearsal. Equally important, however, was the message encased in the polished comic form—for example, concern about global pollution in *Garbage: An S.O.S. from Outer Space* or antinuclear politics in *Superman Meets the Plutonium Tycoons*.

The group extended their critical attitude to traditional theater practices. Performances were offered in nontraditional settings—parks, prisons, schools, rest homes. Competition within the group was frowned upon. In fact, they didn't even audition me. I was interviewed. What I said about my skills and experience was assumed to be true until proven otherwise.

Years later, one of the company members confided to me that he had wanted to oppose my joining the company because of my disability. He didn't think I could "keep up." But this was the early '70s, idealistic and iconoclastic, and small-minded objections were not well-received.

Luckily for me Family Circus was my first big break. The three solid years of performing and touring not only made up for some of the professional training I had missed but also gave me real credentials as an actress. Never mind that people who met me offstage assumed I was an administrator or costumer when I said I worked for a theater group. People who saw me perform had no doubt I was an actress. Family Circus took a gamble with me, but they never regretted it.

"My first reaction was, 'Wait a minute. I'm not crippled. I'm an actress. Don't put me in that world of ugliness and freaks and abnormality.' Nervous and embarrassed, I stammered out a polite thanks: I didn't want to offend a disabled person. It would take some years before I would understand what had happened that night, before I would feel positive about having experiences in common with another disabled person."

It was at this time that I began to train physically. I was hellbent on developing every part of my body not "involved" in the polio, as they say medically. I studied mime and dance—modern, jazz, and ballet.

My sister was a terrific dancer. She and my mother had "the legs for it," as my father used to say, meaning very nice to look at. Maybe Daddy thought I felt left out when he said things like that or maybe he actually believed it, but when I was little, he used to tell me that he wanted me to be one of the Rockettes, the precision chorus line dancers at Radio City Music Hall in New York, when I grew up.

I didn't think *that* was possible, but out of all the people in my family, I, the one who had gotten polio, decided to become a professional performer.

So there I was, on the road with Family Circus. I never called myself disabled at that time. I was trying to prove myself as an actress despite my disability. It was a shock to me after a performance when a woman approached me and said, "You were really an inspiration to me. I've been trying to cover up my disability [she had also had polio] in order to act, but you didn't hide anything and totally involved the audience." My first reaction was, "Wait a minute. I'm not crippled. I'm an actress. Don't put me in that world of ugliness and freaks and abnormality." Nervous and embarrassed, I stammered out a polite thanks: I didn't want to offend a disabled person. It would take some years before I would understand what had happened that night, before I would feel positive about having experiences in common with another disabled person.

Of course, I never actually *forgot* that I was disabled. That would have been impossible with people staring at me and my feet every day. Every step of my theatrical career was colored by that fact. But there didn't seem to be much sense in calling more attention to it.

I left Family Circus Theater and Portland, Oregon, and moved to San Francisco, hoping to broaden my professional horizons. I was afraid I wouldn't find work, aware as I was that the majority of roles in western theater are for white, able-bodied males. One's career possibilities significantly decrease if one is a woman or black or disabled. The necessity for commercial success makes it too risky for most professional theaters to cast somebody who doesn't fit the norm. I knew that my legs and my limp severely limited my chances of theater employment.

It's no coincidence that I found work with Lilith, a woman's theater company. The company was named after Lilith, Adam's first wife in the earliest versions of the Bible. Lilith refused to lie beneath Adam and had to leave paradise. At the beginning, she was simply a woman who didn't fit into the cultural norms of her time.

So here in San Francisco was a theater company that embraced "misfits." I was a natural.

When the company began to revise *Moonlighting*—a

play about women and work—for a European tour, I was encouraged to work up a piece on disability and work. It was frightening, but with my director, the work was done. When *Moonlighting* opened in Germany, my experiences as a disabled actress were part of the script.

Hamburg, April 1979. A cold wind is blowing off the lake, beating against the huge, heated circus tent. I walk into the spotlight and begin:

> Polio is an acute viral infection of the nervous system. The primary area of attack is the spinal column, *die Wiebersalle*. Polio causes nerve degeneration resulting in muscular paralysis and weakness.
>
> I got polio when I was three years old. I have two different sized legs and a limp. I am disabled. *Ich bin behindert.*

I raise my pant legs and show the heavy-calved, pink-tighted left leg and the yellow-tighted, bony stalk of a right leg. There are gasps. I feel the audience suffering a collective psychic contraction: This is taboo; this is forbidden.

I continue. I make them laugh by showing them how I try to cover up my limp. They understand this—everyone has tried to cover up an imperfection, a pimple, a balding head. I turn somersaults.

I try to explain, doubling my efforts by using sign language, that I've had trouble because I don't fit the cultural norm. But why? After all, "Theater is supposed to reflect life," I say, "and life is more than conventional beauty." And before I can get the next sentence out, the audience—700 people—burst into applause. Not for me but for themselves, for the infinite potential for beauty and freedom that every human being carries, which is at war with the competitive, death-embracing standards of our society.

During the European tour, I gave this speech in German, I gave it in Italian, I gave it in French. Sometimes I couldn't wait to get out in the spotlight; other times, I'd stand backstage in dread, my old need to be "normal" taking over. All I had ever wanted out of life was to be a good actress.

Unfortunately, due to the demands of costume changing, the monologue had to appear early in the show. The audience had barely seen me act. I feared the speech was too loaded and bullied them into liking me *because* I was disabled, the last thing I wanted.

What would get me out on the stage was thinking about the disabled people I knew at home, or those who might be in the audience and how hard they were struggling for visibility, and out I'd go to raise my pant legs.

The piece is easier for me to perform now, particularly to disabled audiences, who laugh more. I know how it makes them feel to see a real disabled person on stage, not some stereotyped, pitiful character.

The American stage is in a transition period for the integration of minority actors into traditional theater.

"When I get discouraged, when I'm tired of being a pioneer, when I'm disgusted by my fear of auditioning, when I'm frustrated in a dance class, I remember that Sarah Bernhardt performed for the last decade of her life with only one leg."

Recently, San Francisco's American Conservatory Theater (ACT) cast a black man as Scrooge in a production of *A Christmas Carol*. Not so long ago, roles for blacks in legitimate theater were restricted to waiters and maids or parts in all-black productions (interestingly, this has been less true of opera, where the voice is everything). Disabled persons are still at square one in terms of access to American theater.

Still, I'm glad I'm trying this today. A half-century ago, my only performing opportunities would have been carnival sideshows. But now I have a chance to make it as an actress.

When I get discouraged, when I'm tired of being a pioneer, when I'm disgusted by my fear of auditioning, when I'm frustrated in a dance class, I remember that Sarah Bernhardt performed for the last decade of her life with only one leg.

Victoria Ann-Lewis is a fine actress with an abiding respect for her craft. From San Francisco, which has been her home base for a number of years—with frequent stops at Berkeley, where she served as editor of the *Independent*, the magazine of the Center of Independent Living—Ann-Lewis went down to Los Angeles, where she is an artist-in-residence at the Mark Taper Forum and appears frequently on television.

David

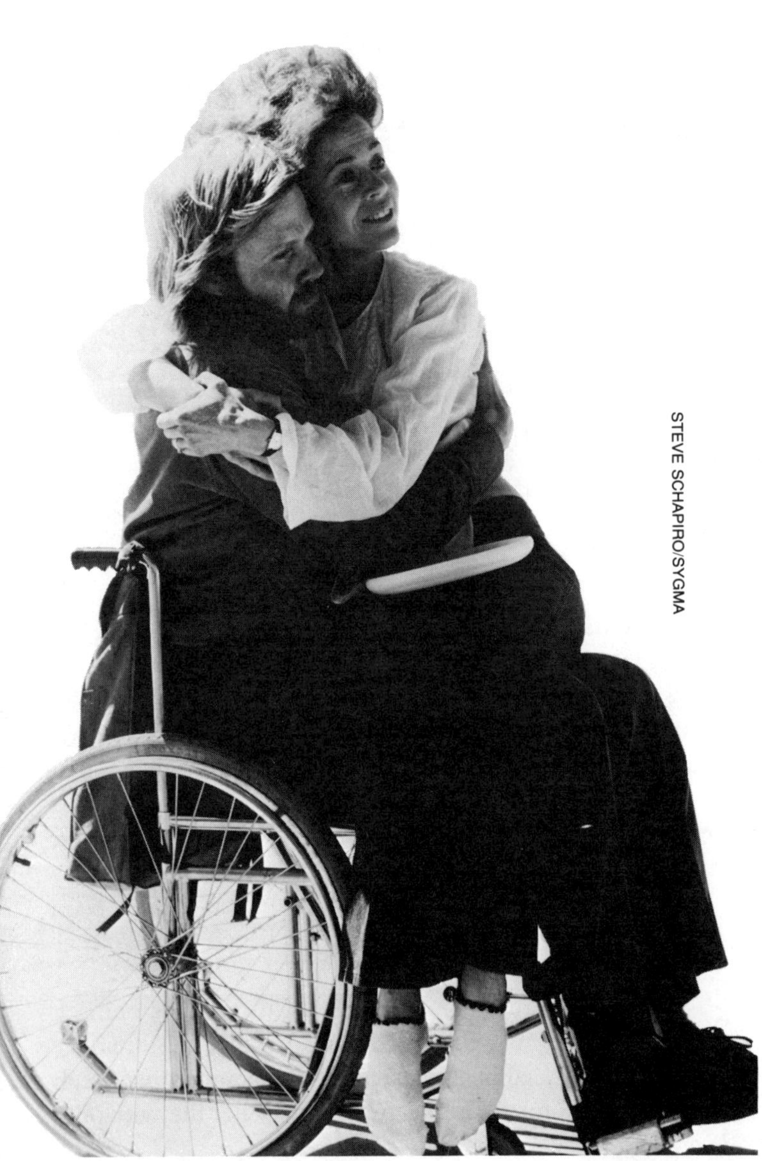

STEVE SCHAPIRO/SYGMA

Jon Voight as a paraplegic with Jane Fonda in the movie, Coming Home.

The movie *Coming Home* exploits the feelings and emotions of people in wheelchairs, and yet the movie was not about a guy in a wheelchair, Luke, as much as it was about the character portrayed by Jane Fonda. Luke was an angry young man who adjusts to his wheelchair, but the film was not about that adjustment. I found the sex parts half-exhilarating and half-disturbing. I was an atypical audience for a lot of reasons. I was overly critical of its accuracy. When he came out wearing only a towel and went into the bathroom, I thought, "Thank God, they are educating the general public." But he came through as Jon Voight and not as a guy in a wheelchair. And too often he was too full of jargon, textbook and clinical answers. I know Voight did a good job before the film trying to research his role, but the result was still too "Hollywood."

In the scene where he wheels himself with his two canes and she bumps into him and his leg bag breaks, the audience laughed, but it was nervous laughter. We are so toilet trained in our culture and so aware of toileting that the bag breaking became a dishonor. His urine spills all over the place and the audience needs that comic relief. They can't really handle it.

I also saw it in another way because I so strongly identify with Luke. He was, for all intents and purposes, a disabled man, a man in a chair, who was really turning Jane Fonda on. This man was disabled and it was not possible to say if he was neuter. He may not have been having sex the same standard way—whatever that is—but there was electricity and love, so much as to be almost tangible.

The most erotic place for me, where he was most a man in the traditional sense, was the scene where he had the courage to face her husband. He told him he loved that man's wife and was sorry and yet not sorry.

To me, it was where everything came together, including the sex.

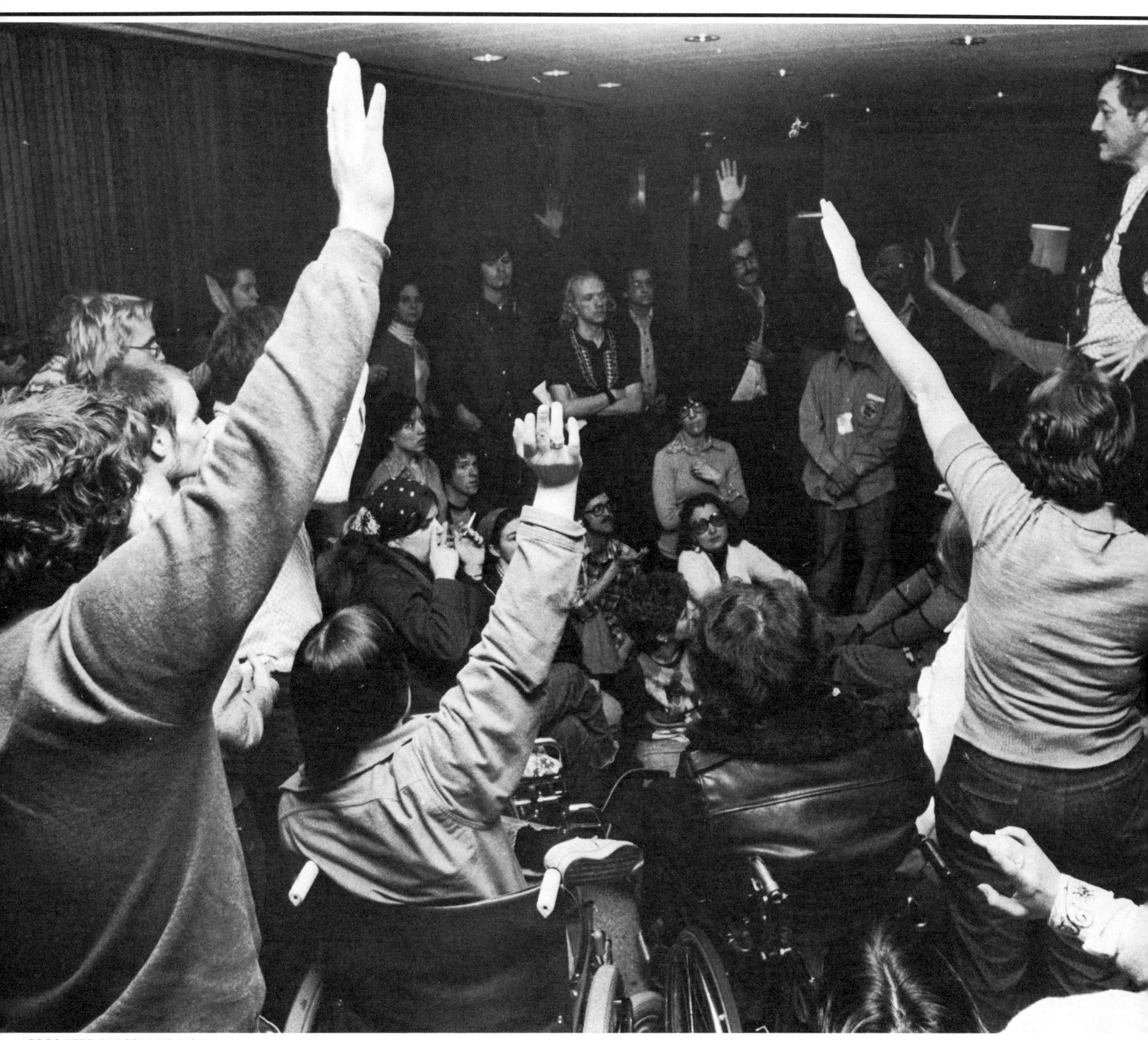

ASSOCIATED PRESS/WIDE WORLD

Washington, April 6, 1977 Taking a vote outside the office of Secretary of Health, Education, and Welfare, Joseph A. Califano Jr. whether to remain. The group stayed for 28 hours to protest the delays in the implementation of the Civil Rights Act, known as Section 504.

On May 7, 1977, Secretary Califano signed the first implementation regulations.

Chapter 2

Living/Making It With a Disability

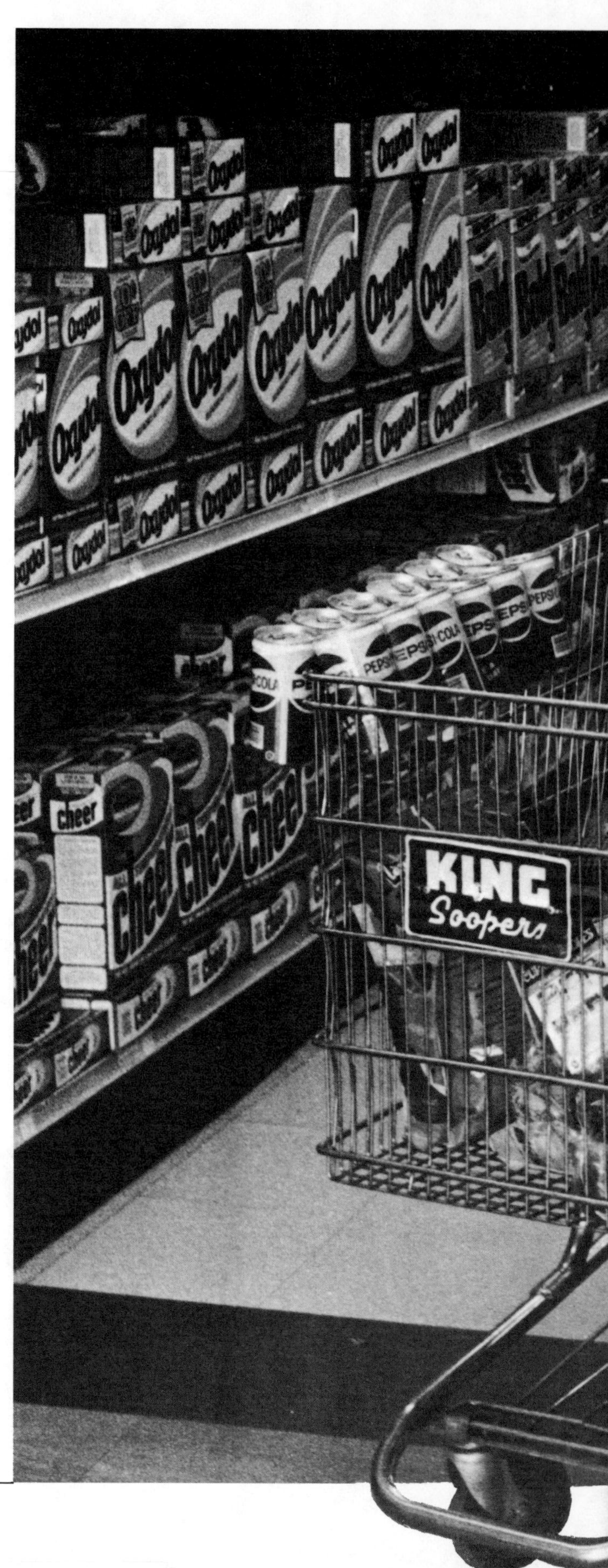

Beyond the problems of finding a place to live that is large enough to move around in and money to pay the rent, there is the need to feel wanted on a street, in churches and synagogues, in McDonald's®, and anyplace where everyone else goes

A soap opera is the highlight of the day if someone with a disability can't get out of the house, get on a bus, get into a movie theater or department store, or take the children out to play.

Disabled taxpayers have the right to use what their money supports—municipal buses and trains, libraries, post offices, police stations, parks and playgrounds, swimming pools, museums, and community centers.

How can a society whose public parks, playgrounds, beaches, and recreation areas cannot be enjoyed by disabled citizens be a society that upholds its Constitution?

How can a society that has inaccessible museums, historic landmarks, theaters, concert halls, stadiums, and attitude barriers against disabled artists, be a society that redeems the promise of its Constitution?

It cannot.

In Denver, a woman fills her shopping cart and pushes it from her motorized chair.

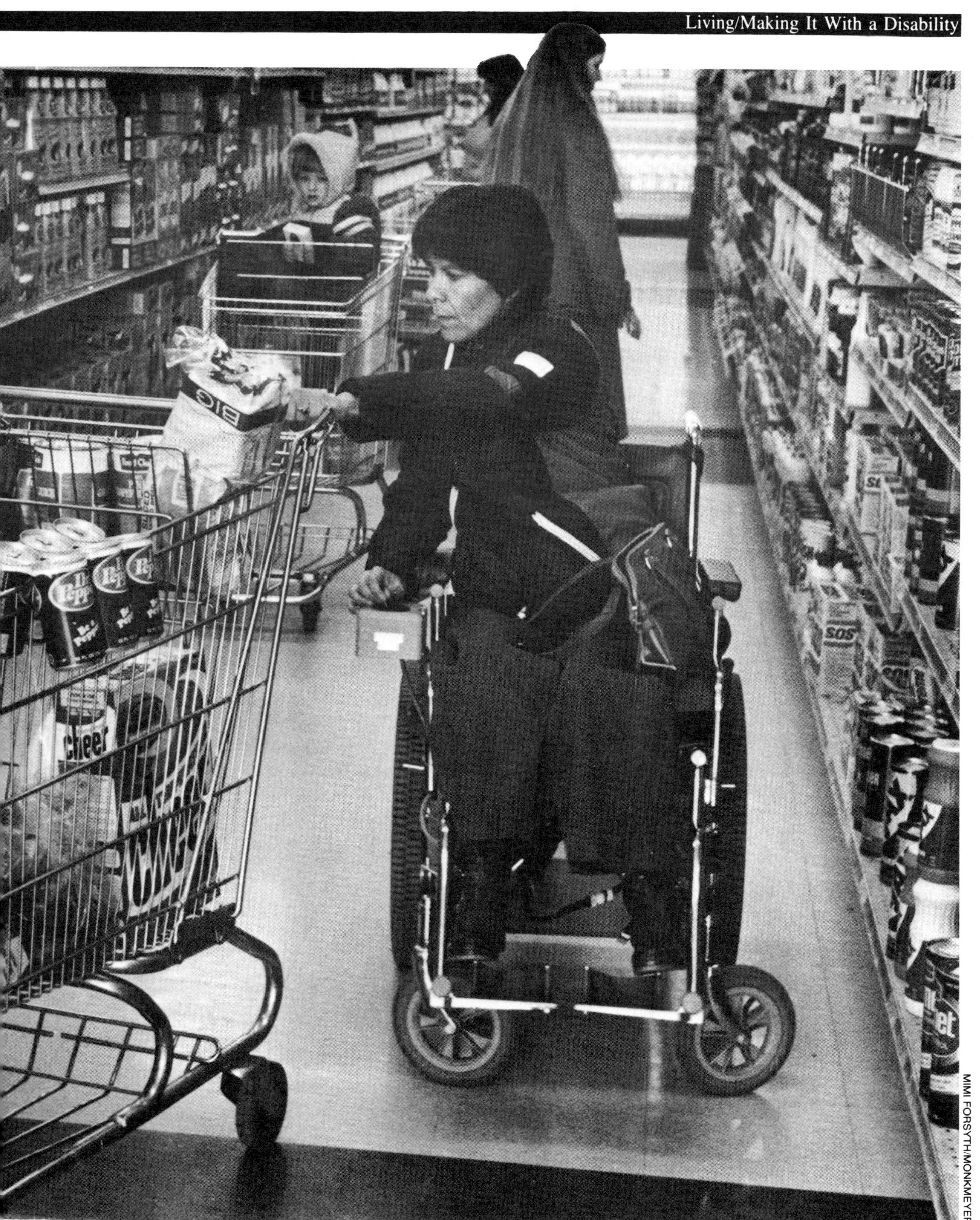

MIMI FORSYTH/MONKMEYER

Centers of Independent Living

The Movement to Living Independently

A movement to independent living for disabled citizens was bound to happen when it did—in the early seventies. Perhaps it was a combination of forces that brought it about: the end of the Vietnam War, sending home thousands of disabled veterans; the effective organizing of disabled citizens; and the deinstitutionalization of a large number of people who would, with support services, live for the first time outside a hospital.

It is difficult to point to an exact time when, or a place where, the movement for independent living began. Certainly, the foundation for this movement reaches back to the returning disabled veterans of the Second World War and to two bills passed in 1943: the World War II Disabled Veterans' Rehabilitation Act (Public Law 78-16), which provided vocational rehabilitation for disabled veterans; and

The climate in the country was one of appreciation, particularly to individuals who had become disabled fighting in the war. This was expressed by efforts to train and employ disabled veterans.

the Servicemen's Readjustment Act, known as the "GI Bill" (Public Law 78-346), which provided for the education and training of men and women whose education or career had been interrupted by military service.

The climate in the country was one of appreciation, particularly to individuals who had become disabled fighting

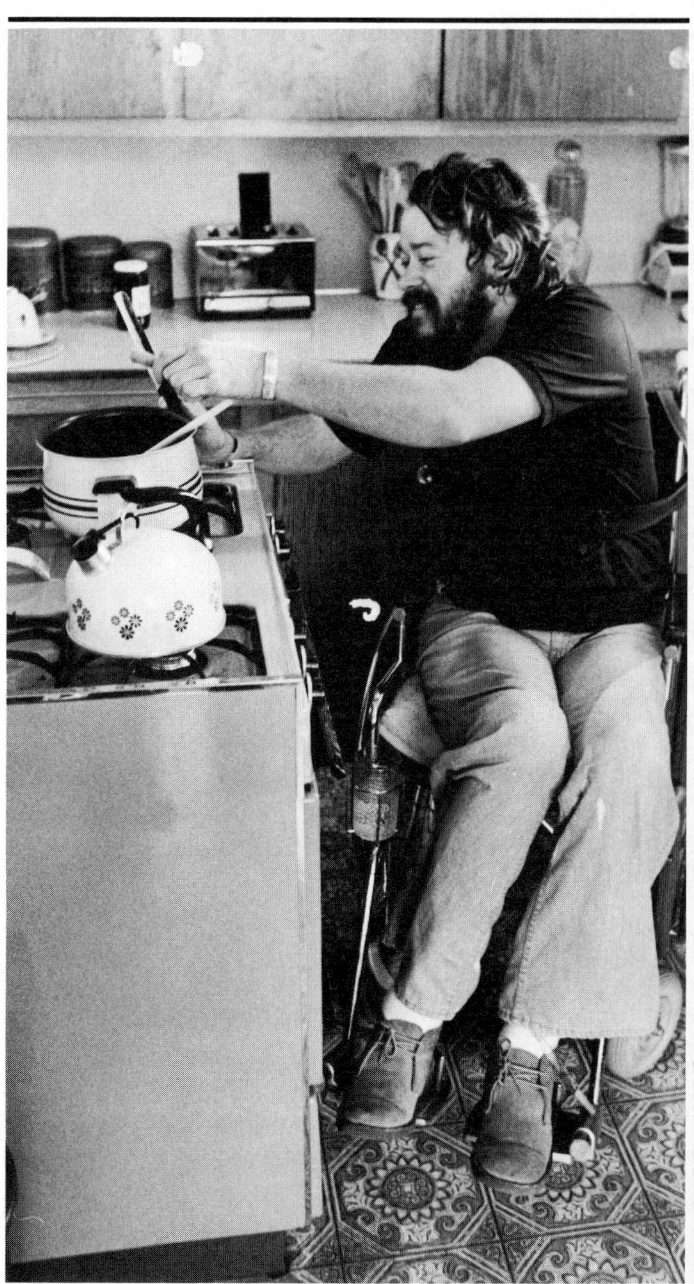

Preparing dinner in an accessible kitchen with pots, pans, cooking utensils and food supplies within reach.

in the war. This was expressed by efforts to train and employ disabled veterans.

Major polio epidemics swept the country from 1946 to 1955. Franklin D. Roosevelt, a polio survivor, had begun the National Foundation for Infantile Paralysis and proved a person with a disability could handle the job of being President.

The National Foundation–March of Dimes provided financial support and equipment so that people who had contracted polio could leave hospitals and rehabilitation centers and return to their homes.

Tim Nugent started the first program to accommodate severely disabled students in higher education in 1947 at the Champaign-Urbana campus of the University of Illinois. By 1962, several students were transferred from a nursing home to modified housing near campus.

The civil rights movement in the 1960s raised questions of the rights of all members of society. Many leaders now in the disability rights movement were committed to the work of the civil rights movement . . .

The civil rights movement in the 1960s raised questions of the rights of all members of society. Many leaders now in the disability rights movement were committed to the work of the civil rights movement, and many large academic communities where strong political activism took place are presently the sites where many centers of independent living are now based.

The movement for independent living and the emergence of independent living centers flourished at the same time that several other complementary social movements also developed: self-help, demedicalization/self-care, deinstitutionalization/normalization, and mainstreaming.

Definitions of independent living centers abound. They have been referred to as service stations with the purpose of enhancing the will and the way to self-determination. One definition of an independent living center is: a community-based program that has substantial disabled citizen involvement and leadership and provides directly, or coordinates indirectly through referral, those services necessary to assist disabled individuals to increase self-determination and to minimize unnecessary dependence.

There are more than 200 independent living centers

BILL OF RIGHTS

We believe that all people should enjoy certain specific rights. Because people with disabilities have consistently been denied the right to participate fully in society as free and equal members, it is important to state and affirm these rights. All people should be able to enjoy these rights, regardless of race, creed, color, sex, religion, or disabilities.

1. *The right to live independent, active, and full lives.*
2. *The right to the equipment, assistance, and support services necessary for full productivity, provided in a way that promotes dignity and independence.*
3. *The right to an adequate income or wage, substantial enough to provide food, clothing, shelter, and other necessities of life.*
4. *The right to accessible, integrated, convenient, and affordable housing.*
5. *The right to quality physical and mental health care.*
6. *The right to training and employment without prejudice or stereotyping.*
7. *The right to accessible transportation and freedom of movement.*
8. *The right to have children and a family.*
9. *The right to a free and appropriate public education.*
10. *The right to participate in and benefit from entertainment and recreation.*
11. *The right to communicate freely with all fellow citizens and those who provide services.*
12. *The right to a barrier-free environment.*
13. *The right to legal representation and full protection of all legal rights.*
14. *The right to determine one's own future and make one's own life choices.*
15. *The right to full access to all voting processes.*

This Disabled Citizen Bill of Rights was written by members of the Center of Independent Living in Berkeley, California, for Disabled People's Civil Rights Day, October 20, 1979.

strung across the country, reaching from Anchorage, Alaska, to Yonkers, New York, and back to Hilo, Hawaii. The centers—with names such as Our Way, Inc. in Little Rock, Arkansas; The Whole Person, Inc. in Kansas City, Missouri; HIP, the acronym for Handicapped Independence Program; DIAL, Disabled Information Awareness and Living, in Clifton, New Jersey—have become, for disabled citizens, the primary self-help units. The centers attempt to serve both as adjuncts to the present human service system and as alternative service providers. As an adjunct to the system, the centers may provide peer counseling and advocacy not supplied by mainline human service organizations.

Definitions of independent living centers abound. They have been referred to as service stations with the purpose of enhancing the will and the way to self-determination.

Picture a Chevrolet showroom in the '50s, floor to ceiling windows, but with the space now partitioned off into offices marked with handmade signs: "attendant care," "transportation." Double doors burst open admitting first a young man in a motorized wheelchair and then a mother singing to a small child; there is lots of laughter, conversation, hard work, with physically disabled people in the majority. This is the Center of Independent Living (CIL) in Berkeley, California.

By contrast, the independent living center in lower Manhattan is housed in an office building; the center in Santa Barbara, California, is in a frame house; and Cathedral CIL in Jacksonville, Florida, is in the Memorial Regional Rehabilitation Center.

No matter the architecture, the objective is the same—to have a center run by and for individuals with disabilities.

Enormous interest from countries in Central America, Sweden, Germany, France, India, Japan, and Australia will undoubtedly lead to an international consortium of disabled citizen-run independent living centers.

The Easter Seal Society, United Cerebral Palsy, or other community voluntary organizations can give you the names of independent living centers and disabled citizen organizations in your area.

Independent Living Research Utilization (ILRU), a national center for information, training, and technical assistance in independent living, has compiled a registry of independent living programs. You can purchase a copy of the directory by writing ILRU Project, P.O. Box 20095, Houston, TX 77225.

Independent living centers are being added and may not be included in this list. Some centers have merged or disbanded. Every effort has been made to list the most current addresses available.

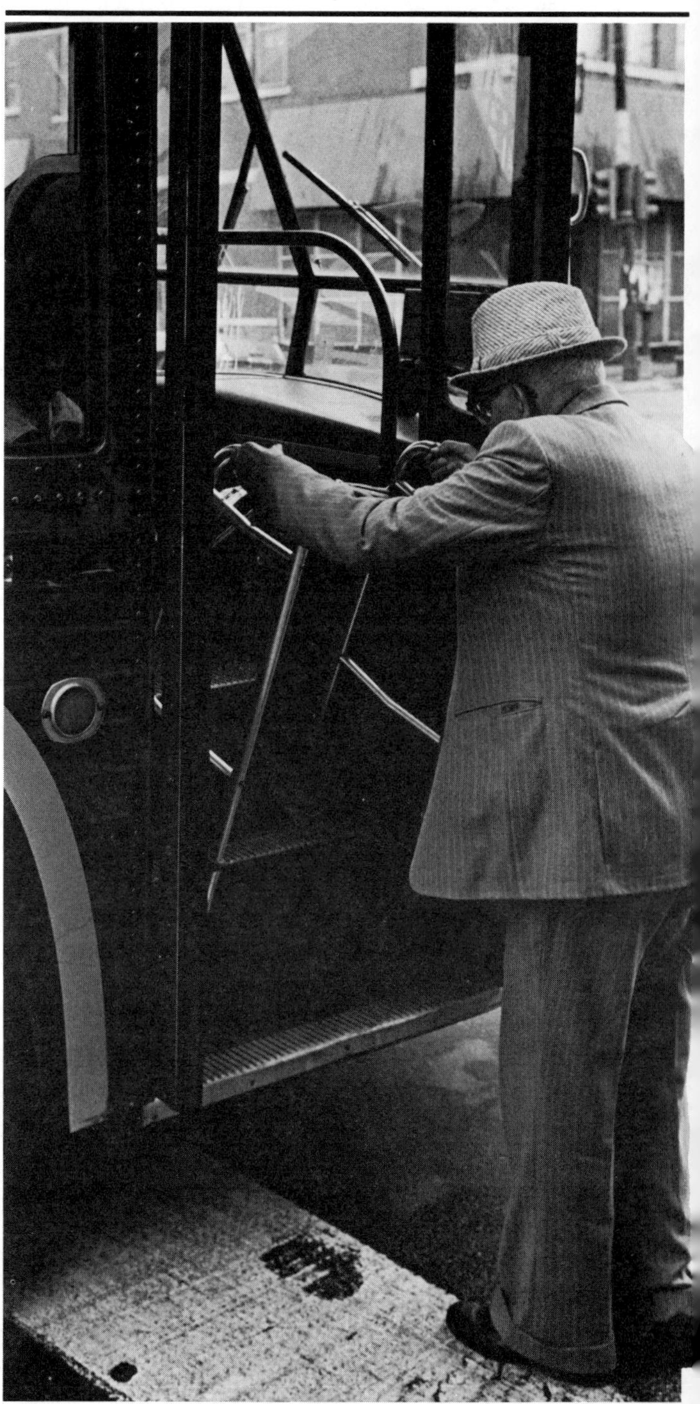

Man tries to board a non-accessible public bus in Chicago.

Centers of Independent Living

(Addresses are in order by state abbreviation.)

Hope Cottages, Inc.
2805 Bering Street
Anchorage, AK 99503

Access Alaska, Inc.
3710 Woodland Drive, Suite 900
Anchorage, AK 99517

Access Alaska—Outreach Office
500 First Avenue
Fairbanks, AK 99701

Independent Living Center
3421 Fifth Avenue South
Birmingham, AL 35222

Our Way, Inc.
10434 W. 36th Street, Room 314
Little Rock, AR 72204

Independent Living Services Center
5800 Asher Avenue
Little Rock, AR 72204

Arizona Bridge to Independent Living
3130 E. Roosevelt
Phoenix, AZ 85008

Community Outreach Program for the Deaf
268 W. Adams Street
Tucson, AZ 85705

Metro Independent Living Center
161 N. Sixth Avenue
Tucson, AZ 85701

Darrell McDaniel Independent Living Center, Deaf Services
18 South Chester
Bakersfield, CA 93304

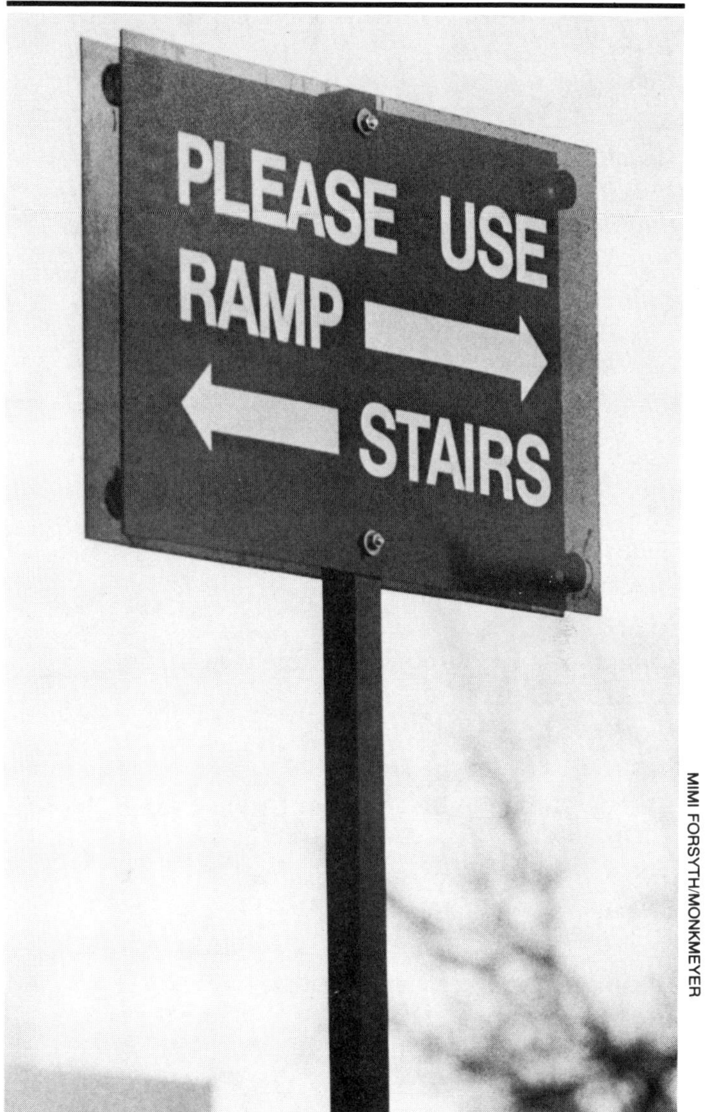

MIMI FORSYTH/MONKMEYER

Center for Independence of Disabled
875 O'Neill Avenue
Belmont, CA 94002

Center for Independent Living
2539 Telegraph Avenue
Berkeley, CA 96704

Northern California Independent Living Project
555 Rio Lindo Avenue
Suite B
Chico, CA 95926

Center for Independent Living—San Gabriel Valley
114 East Italia Street
Covina, CA 91723

Southeast Center for Independent Living
12458 Rives Avenue
Downey, CA 90242

Humboldt Access Project, Inc.
712 Fourth Street
Eureka, CA 95501

California Association of Physically Handicapped Service Center
605 W. Home Street
Fresno, CA 93728

Dale McIntosh Center for the Disabled
8100 Garden Grove Boulevard
Suite 1
Garden Grove, CA 92644

Community Resources for Independent Living
26633 Jane Street
Hayward, CA 94544

Darrell McDaniel Independent Living Center, Branch Office
44815 Fig Avenue, Suite B
Lancaster, CA 93534

Disabled Resources Center, Inc.
1045 Pine Avenue
Long Beach, CA 90813

Community Rehab Services—Independent Living Center
4716 Brooklyn Avenue, Building B, Room 15
Los Angeles, CA 90022

Good Sheperd Center for Independent Living
4323 Leimert Boulevard
Los Angeles, CA 90008

Westside Center for Independent Living
12901 Venice Boulevard
Los Angeles, CA 90066

Spanish Speaking Task Force for the Handicapped
4716 Brooklyn Avenue, Building B, Room 75
Los Angeles, CA 90022

Independent Living Project/Mt. Diablo Rehabilitation Center
490 Golf Club Road
Pleasant Hill, CA 94523

Resources for Independent Living
1230 H Street
Sacramento, CA 95814

Rolling Start, Inc.
443 W. Fourth Street
San Bernardino, CA 92401

Community Service Center for the Disabled
1295 University Avenue
San Diego, CA 92103

Independent Living Resources Center
4429 Cabrillo Street
San Francisco, CA 94121

Marin Center for Independent Living
710 Fourth Street
San Rafael, CA 94901

Independent Living Resource Center
423 W. Victoria
Santa Barbara, CA 93101

Adult Independent Development Center
1190 Benton Street
Santa Clara, CA 95050

Cheshire Homes/Santa Cruz Co.
P.O. Box 1334
Santa Cruz, CA 95061

Community Resources for Independence
915 Piner Road, Suite J
Santa Rosa, CA 95401

UCP Adult Activity Center
347 E. Poplar Street, c/o UCPA
Stockton, CA 95203

Blind Disabled Action Center
P.O. Box 882
Ukiah, CA 95482

Darrell McDaniel Independent Living Center
14354 Vescoco
Van Nuys, CA 91401

The Center for Independent Living of San Gabriel Valley
2231 East Garvey Avenue
West Covina, CA 91791

San Luis Center for Independent Living
P.O. Box 1536
Alamosa, CO 81101

Center for People with Disabilities
1450 Fifteenth Street
Boulder, CO 80302

Colorado Springs Independent Living Project
122 South 16th Street
Colorado Springs, CO 80904

Atlantis/Colorado Springs
2340 Robinson, #113
Colorado Springs, CO 80904

Holistic Approaches to Independent Living—HAIL
1249 E. Colfax Avenue
Suite 107
Denver, CO 80218

Atlantis Community, Inc.
2200 W. Alameda, #18
Denver, CO 80219

Independent Living in Home Teaching
524 Social Services Building
1575 Sherman
Denver, CO 80203

The Center on Deafness
2250 Easton Street
Edgewater, CO 80214

Handicapped Information Office
1001 North College
Ft. Collins, CO 80524

Hilltop Independent Living Center
475 28–½ Road
Grand Junction, CO 81501

Camelot
1734 8th Avenue
Greeley, CO 80631

Greeley Resources for Independent People
314 A 25th Avenue Court
Greeley, CO 80631

Center for Independent Living of Greater Bridgeport
P.O. Box 3366
165 Ocean Terrace
Bridgeport, CT 06605

Independence Unlimited
410 Asylum Street
Hartford, CT 06103

New Horizons, Inc.
410 Asylum Street
Hartford, CT 06103

Independent Living for the Handicapped
3841 Calvert Street
Washington, DC 20007

DC Services for Independent Living
1400 Florida Avenue, N.E., #3
Washington, DC 20002

Independent Living, Inc.
Apt. 129, E. Willis Road
Dover, DE 19805

Easter Seal Society of Del Mar—Independent Living Project
2915 Newport Gap Pike
Wilmington, DE 19808

Channel Markers for the Blind
1610 N. Myrtle Avenue
Clearwater, FL 33515

Center for Independent Living Services—DAWN
1001 Northeast 28th Avenue
Gainesville, FL 32609

Cathedral Center for Independent Living/Memorial Regional Rehabilitation Center
3599 University Boulevard South
Jacksonville, FL 32216

Independent Living for Adult Blind
50 E. Second Street
Jacksonville, FL 32206

Center for Survival and Independent Living
1310 N.W. 16th Street, Room 101
Miami, FL 33125

Center for Independent Living in Central Florida
130 West Central Boulevard
Orlando, FL 32801

Center for Independent Training and Education/Blind
215 East New Hampshire
Orlando, FL 32804

Center for Independent Living of NW Florida, Inc.
908 West Lakeview Avenue
Pensacola, FL 32501

Leon Center for Independent Living
1380 Ocala Road, #H-4
Tallahassee, FL 32304

Florida Institute for Independent Living
307 East Seventh Avenue
Tallahassee, FL 32303

Self-Reliance, Inc.
2002 G East Fletcher Avenue
Tampa, FL 33612

Tampa Lighthouse for the Blind
1106 West Platt Street
Tampa, FL 33702

Independent Living Project/Georgia DHR
47 Trinity Avenue
Atlanta, GA 30334

Atlanta Center for Independent Living
1201 Glenwood Avenue, S.E.
Atlanta, GA 30316

Heart of Georgia—Independent Living Project
707 Pine Street
Macon, GA 31208

Independent Living Project—Roosevelt Warm Springs Rehabilitation Institute
P.O. Box 369
Warm Springs, GA 31830

Center for Independent Living
Big Island
60 Keane Street
Hilo, HI 96720

Hawaii Center for Independent Living
677 Ala Moana Boulevard #615
Honolulu, HI 96813

Transitional Living Program
226 N. Kuakini Street
Honolulu, HI 96817

Kauai Center for Independent Living
P.O. Box 3529
Lihue, HI 96766

Maui Center for Independent Living
1446-D Lower Main Street, Room 105
Wailuku, HI 96793

Center for Independent Living Rehabilitation Services/State Commission for the Blind
4th and Keosauqua Way
Des Moines, IA 50309

Independent Living, Inc.
26 East Market
Iowa City, IA 52240

Hope Haven
1800 19th Street
Rock Valley, IA 51247

Cedar Street Living Center
Box 388
Blackfoot, ID 83221

Co-AD, Inc.
1510 West Washington
Boise, ID 83720

Stepping Stones Inc.
408 S. Main
Moscow, ID 83843

Housing Southwest No. 2, Payette ID
1224 First Street, South
Nampa, ID 83651

Center of Resources for Independent People
707 N. 7th Avenue, Suite A
Pocatello, ID 83201

Center for Comprehensive Services, Inc.
306 West Mill, P.O. Box 2825
Carbondale, IL 62901

ALMA
1642 N. Winchester Avenue
Suite 100
Chicago, IL 60622

Center for Disabled Student Services
30 E. Lake Street
Chicago, IL 60601

Access Living of Metro Chicago
505 N. LaSalle
Chicago, IL 60610

Illinois Independent Living Center
512 West Burlington Avenue
LaGrange, IL 60525

Central Illinois Center for Independent Living
320 East Armstrong Avenue
Peoria, IL 61603

Winning Wheels Northwestern Illinois Center for Independent Living Inc.
R.R. 3, Box 12A
Prophetstown, IL 61277

Rockford Access and Mobilization Project (RAMP)
104 Chestnut Street
Rockford, IL 61101

Springfield Center for Independent Living
426 West Jefferson
Springfield, IL 62702

Damar Homes Inc.
6324 Kentucky Avenue, P.O. Box 41
Camby, IN 46113

Allen County League for the Blind
5800 Fairfield, Suite 210
Ft. Wayne, IN 46807

New Hope of Indiana
8450 N. Payne Road
Indianapolis, IN 46268

Project Independence, Inc.
P.O. Box 133
Arkansas City, KS 67005

Operation LINK
Box 1016
Hays, KS 67601

Independence, Inc.
1910 Haskell
Lawrence, KS 66044

Kansas Rehabilitation Center for the Blind
2516 West Sixth Street
Topeka, KS 66606

Mainstream/VA Hospital
2200 Gage Boulevard
Topeka, KS 66622

Topeka Resource Center for the Handicapped
1119 W. 10th Street, Suite 2
Topeka, KS 66604

Project AID Resource Center Inc.
4808 West 9th Street
Wichita, KS 67212

Contact, Inc.
191 Doctors Drive
Wichita, KS 67212

Center for Independent Living—University of Louisville Cancer Center
P.O. Box 35260
Louisville, KY 40232

Independent Living Center for the Blind
1900 Brownsboro Road
Louisville, KY 40206

Center for Accessible Living
835 West Jefferson, Suite 105
Louisville, KY 40202

West End Awareness
402 S. 38th Street, #2
Louisville, KY 40212

New Orleans Center for Independent Living
320 N. Carrollton Avenue
Suite 2C
New Orleans, LA 70119

New Horizons, Inc.
4030 Wallace Avenue
Shreveport, LA 71108

Organization D.E.A.F., Inc.
215 Brighton Avenue
Allston, MA 02154

Stavros, Inc.
691 South East Street
Amherst, MA 01002

Center for Independent Living at Massachusetts for the Blind
110 Tremont Street
Boston, MA 02108

Boston Center for Independent Living
50 New Edgerly Road
Boston, MA 02115

Student Independent Living Experience
3 Randolph Street
Canton, MA 02021

Independence Associates Inc.
693 Bedford Street, P.O. Box 146
Elmwood, MA 02337

Highland Heights Apartments
85 Morgan Street
Fall River, MA 02722

Association of Retarded Citizens—Independent Living Program
38 Hiramar Road
Hyannis, MA 02601

Independent Living Center
Northeast Inc.
190 Hampshire Street, Suite 101B
Lawrence, MA 01842

Renaissance Program
21 Branch Street
Lowell, MA 01851

Berkshire Project
496 Tyler Street
Pittsfield, MA 01201

Vision Foundation Inc.
2 Mt. Auburn Street
Watertown, MA 02172

Rehabilitation Services/Easter Seal Society
37 Harvard Street
Worcester, MA 01608

Center for Living and Working
600 Lincoln Street
Worcester, MA 01605

Maryland Citizens for Housing for the Disabled, Inc.
6305-A Sherwood Road
Baltimore, MD 21239

Motivational Services, Inc.
114 State Street
Augusta, ME 04330

Maine Independent Living Center
74 Winthrop Street
Augusta, ME 04330

Alpha I—Outreach Office
96 Harlow Street, Suite 5
Bangor, ME 04401

Independent Living Center
Bell Dorm, Husson College
Bangor, ME 04401

The Together Place
P.O. Box 1125
Bangor, ME 04401

Southern Maine Association for the Physically Handicapped
32 Thomas Street
Portland, ME 04102

Shalom House, Inc.
90 High Street
Portland, ME 04101

Alpha I—Maine International Living Program
169 Ocean Street
S. Portland, ME 04106

Alpha I—Outreach Office
373 Main Street
Presque Isle, ME 04769

Center for Independent Living Serving Washtenaw County, Inc.
2568 Packard, Georgetown Mall
Ann Arbor, MI 48104

Family Resources Center—Association of Retarded Citizens
51 W. Hancock
Detroit, MI 48201

Rehabilitation Institute Center for Independent Living
3 E. Alexandrine Towers
Suite 104
Detroit, MI 48201

Southeast Michigan Center for Independent Living
1200 6th Avenue, 11th Floor, South Tower
Detroit, MI 48226

Participants Advocate Group
2645 Vail Lane, Rt. 2
Gaylord, MI 49735

Northern Michigan Rural Center for Independent Living
209 1st Street, P.O. Box 246
Gaylord, MI 49735

Grand Rapids Center for Independent Living
3375 Division South
Grand Rapids, MI 49508

Association for Retarded Citizens/Ottowa County
246 S. River Avenue, #65
Holland, MI 49423

Kalamazoo Center for Independent Living
268 East Kilgore
Kalamazoo, MI 49001

Cristo Rey Hispanic Handicapper Program
1314 Ballard Street
Lansing, MI 48906

Center/Handicapper Affairs
316 N. Capital Avenue
Suite C1
Lansing, MI 48933

Association of Retarded Citizens Resource Center/ Independent Living Project
P.O. Box 1491
Midland, MI 48640

Senior Blind Program
310 Johnson Street
Saginaw, MI 48607

Grand Traverse Area Community Living Center
935 Barlow
Traverse City, MI 49684

Vinland National Center
3675 Ihduhapi Road
Loretto, MN 55357

Rural Enterprise for Acceptable Living
244 West Main Street
Marshall, MN 56258

Comprehensive Services for Disabled Citizens, Inc.
1350 Nicollet Mall, East Tower 106
Minneapolis, MN 55403

Courage Residence
3915 Golden Valley Road
Minneapolis, MN 55422

Rochester Center for Independent Living, Inc.
1306 7th Street, N.W.
Rochester, MN 55901

Accessibility Improvement Program
400 Sibley 300
St. Paul, MN 55101

Minnesota State Services for the Blind
1745 University Avenue
St. Paul, MN 55104

Metropolitan Center for Independent Living, Inc.
1821 University Avenue, Suite N350
St. Paul, MN 55104

Opportunities Unlimited
111 South 9th Street, Suite 211
Columbia, MO 65201

Rehabilitation Institute
3011 Baltimore
Kansas City, MO 64131

Paraquad
4397 Laclede Avenue
St. Louis, MO 63108

Places for People, Inc.
4120 Lindell Road
St. Louis, MO 63108

Life Skills Foundation
609 North & South
St. Louis, MO 63108

Disabled Citizens Alliance for Independence, Inc.
Box 675
Viburnum, MO 65566

Alpha Home
P.O. Drawer 30
Hazlehurst, MS 39083

Center for Independent Living
P.O. Box 1698
Jackson, MS 39205

Great Falls Independent Living Project
1812 Tenth Avenue South
Great Falls, MT 59405

Montana Independent Living Project
1215 8th Avenue
Helena, MT 59601

Summit—Independent Living Center
3115 Clark Street
Missoula, MT 59801

Metrolina Independent Living Center
1012 South Kings Drive, Doctors Building G-2
Charlotte, NC 20203

Fraser Hall
711 South University Drive
Fargo, ND 58103

Mandan Center for Independent Living
1007 N.W. 18th Street
Mandan, ND 58554

Handicap Reach Out, Inc.
Box 948, 345 West Third
Chadron, NE 69337

Goodwill Center for Independent Living
1804 S. Eddy Street
Grand Island, NE 68801

League of Human Dignity, Inc.
1423 O Street
Lincoln, NE 68508

League of Human Dignity Independent Living Center
700–½ W. Benjamin
Norfolk, NE 68701

Granite State Independent Living Foundation
105 Loudon Road, Prescott Park, Building 4
Concord, NH 03301

D.I.A.L. for Independent Living
234 Parker Avenue
Clifton, NJ 07011

Handicapped Independent Programs
44 Armory Street
Englewood, NJ 07631

NJ Community for the Blind—Centers for Independent Living
1100 Raymond Boulevard
Newark, NJ 07102

New Vistas Independent Living Center—Outreach Office
1812 Candalaria N.W.
Albuquerque, NM 87107

New Vistas—Independent Living Center
1421 Luisa Street, Suite H-2
Santa Fe, NM 87501

Center for Independent Living of Southern Nevada
P.O. Box 28458, c/o Nevada Association for the Handicapped
Las Vegas, NV 89109

Northern Nevada Center for Independent Living
190 East Liberty Street
Reno, NV 89501

Capitol District Center for Independent Living
22 Colvin Avenue
Albany, NY 12206

Model Approaches for Independent Living Projects
Human Resources Center
Willets Road
Albertson, NY 11507

Southern Tier Independence Center
232 Clinton Street
Binghamton, NY 13905

Bronx Independent Living Center
1268 Stratford Avenue
Bronx, NY 10472

Independent Living for the Handicapped
408 J Street, Room 401
Brooklyn, NY 11201

Western New York Independent Living Project
3108 Main Street
Buffalo, NY 14214

Suffolk County Office of Handicapped Services
65 Jetson Lane
Central Islip, NY 11722

Western New York Independent Living Project
2015 Transit
Elma, NY 14059

Long Island Center for Independent Living/SUNY
Administration Building, Suite 115
Farmingdale, NY 11735

Southwestern Independent Living Center
880 East Second Street
Jamestown, NY 14701

Resource Center for Accessible Living
664 Broadway
Kingston, NY 12401

Long Island Center for Independent Living
3601 Hempstead Turnpike, Room 103
Levittown, NY 11756

Suffolk Independent Living Organization
74 Southaven Avenue, Suite H
Medford, NY 11763

Office of the Executive Services for the Physically Handicapped
240 Old Country Road, Room 610
Mineola, NY 11501

Rockland County Center for the Physically Handicapped
250 Little Tor Road, North
P.O. Box 312
New City, NY 10956

Center for Independent Living, Self-Help Network
318 East 15th Street
New York, NY 10003

Center for Independence of the Disabled of New York
853 Broadway, Room 611
New York, NY 10003

Dutchess Center for Accessible Living
244 Church Street
Poughkeepsie, NY 12601

Rochester Center for Independent Living
464 S. Clinton Avenue
Rochester NY 14620

Independent Living in the Capitol District
2660 Albany Street
Schenectady, NY 12304

Help Me Independent Living Center
5 Hillman Place
Spring Valley, NY 10977

A.R.I.S.E. Inc.
501 E. Fayette Street
Syracuse, NY 13202

Resource Center for Independent Living
401 Columbia Street
Utica, NY 13502

Westchester County Independent Living Center
297 Knollwood Road
White Plains, NY 10607

Yonkers Independent Living Center
201 Palisade Avenue
Yonkers, NY 10703

Total Living Concepts, Inc.
3333 Vine Street, Suite 101
Cincinnati, OH 45220

HELP Six Chimneys, Inc.
3907 Prospect Avenue
Cleveland, OH 44115

Independent Living Program
3774 Eakin Road
Columbus, OH 43228

United Cerebral Palsy of Columbus and Franklin Counties
4133 Karl Road
Columbus, OH 43224

Services for Independent Living
25100 Euclid Avenue, Suite 105
Euclid, OH 44117

Green Country Independent Living Resource Center
P.O. Box 2295
Bartlesville, OK 74005

Cleveland County Independent Living Project
320 S. Crawford, Suite 104
Norman, OK 73069

Total Independent Living Today, Inc.
601 N. Porter
Norman, OK 73071

Tulsa Independent Living Center
1724 East 8th Street
Tulsa, OK 74104

Community Services of Lane County
2621 Augusta Street
Eugene, OR 97403

Columbia Gorge Rehabilitation Center
2940 Thomsen Road
Hood River, OR 97031

Living Opportunities
P.O. Box 1072
Medford, OR 97501

Southern Orange Citizens for Independent Living
P.O. Box 1072
Medford, OR 95701

Volunteer Braille Services, Inc.—Independent Living Project
1105 S.E. Morrison Street
Portland, OR 97214

TriCounty Independent Living Program
8213 S.E. 17th Avenue
Portland, OR 97202

Independent Living Services
4001 N.E. Halsey
Portland, OR 97232

Center for Independent Living—Erie Independence House
956 W. Second Street
Erie, PA 16507

Resources for Living Independently Project
4721 Pine Street
Philadelphia, PA 19143

Center for Independent Living—Nevil Services for the Blind
919 Walnut Street, Room 400
Philadelphia, PA 19107

Three Rivers Center for Independent Living, Inc.
5129 Penn Avenue
Pittsburgh, PA 15224

Allied Services for the Handicapped
475 Morgan Highway
Scranton, PA 18508

Brian's House
Box 802
West Chester, PA 19380

Centro de Vida Independiente
P.O. Box 1681
Hato Rey, PR 00919

PARI Independent Living Services
Independence Square
500 Prospect Street
Pawtucket, RI 02860

Blackstone Valley Center, Independent Living Project
115 Manton Street
Pawtucket, RI 02861

The Providence Center
520 Hope Street
Providence, RI 02906

Independent Living, South Carolina Life Exploration
1400 Boston Avenue
West Columbia, SC 29169

Adjustment Training Center
612 10th Avenue, S.E.
Aberdeen, SD 57401

Independent Living Transitional Program
Box 2104
Rapid City, SD 57709

Prairie Freedom Center for the Disabled Independent
800 West Avenue North
Sioux Falls, SD 57104

Easter Seal Center for Independent Living
1177 Poplar Avenue
Memphis, TN 38105

Educational Support Services Office
Box 19028, University of Texas at Arlington
Arlington, TX 76019

Austin Resource Center for Independent Living
2818 San Gabriel
Austin, TX 78705

Independent Living Rehabilitation Program—Criss Cole Rehabilitation Center
4800 North Lamar
Austin, TX 78756

Texas Rehabilitation Committee—Independent Living Services
118 East Riverside Drive
Austin, TX 78704

Independent Living Rehabilitation Program—State Committee for the Blind
4410 Dillon Lane, Suite 20
Corpus Christi, TX 78415

Dallas Center for Independent Living
8625 King George Drive, Suite 210
Dallas, TX 75235

El Paso Opportunity Center for the Handicapped
8929 Viscount, Suite 101
El Paso, TX 79925

Deville Independent Living Program—Lighthouse of Houston
4039 Bellefontaine
Houston, TX 77025

Independent Living Rehabilitation Program—State Commission for the Blind
8100 Washington Avenue, Suite 119
Houston, TX 77007

Independent Life Styles
7320 Ashcroft, Suite 214
Houston, TX 77074

Houston Center for Independent Living
6910 Fannin, Suite 120
Houston, TX 77030

Independent Living Project for the Retarded
810 Marston, Cullen Residence Hall
Houston, TX 77019

Independent Living Program
2201 Sherwood Way, Suite 118
San Angelo, TX 76901

San Antonio Independent Living Services
416 South Main
San Antonio, TX 78204

Utah Independent Living Center
764 South 200 West
Salt Lake City, UT 84101

Virginia Department for the Visually Handicapped—Independent Living Center
2300 South 9th Street, Suite 203
Arlington, VA 22204

ENDependence Center of North Virginia
4214 9th Street North
Arlington, VA 22203

Crossroads Center, Inc.
215 North Main Street
Bridgewater, VA 22812

Woodrow Wilson Center for Independent Living
Box 37 WWRC
Fishersville, VA 22939

Endependence Center, Inc.
100 W. Plume, Suite 244
Norfolk, VA 23510

Richmond Center for Independent Living
6118 Jahnke Road
Richmond, VA 23225

Independent Living Program—VAMC Richmond
1201 Broad Rock Road—VAMC
Richmond, VA 23249

Independent Living Center Network—Department for the Visually Handicapped
1809 Staples Mill Road, Suite 101
Richmond, VA 23230

Department for the Visually Handicapped
1030 Jefferson Street, Suite 200
Roanoke, VA 24016

Virgin Islands Association for Independent Living
P.O. Box 3305
Charlotte Amalie, St. Thomas VI 00801

Rural Independent Living Project
37 Elmwood Avenue
Burlington, VT 05401

Vermont Center for Independent Living
174 River Street
Montpelier, VT 05602

Independent Lifestyle Services KCAC
115 West Third
Ellensburg, WA 98926

Independent Living Center
407 14th Avenue, S.E., Box 1086
Puyallup, WA 98371

Epilepsy Association of Western Washington
1715 E. Cherry
Seattle, WA 98122

Peer Counseling—Washington Coalition of Citizens with Disabilities
3530 Stoneway North
Seattle, WA 98103

Legal Advocacy Project
914 E. Jefferson, Room 328
Seattle, WA 98122

Independent Living—Easter Seal Society
521–2nd Avenue West
Seattle, WA 98119

Handicapped Services Unit
105 14th Avenue
Seattle, WA 98122

Community Service Center for the Deaf
914 E. Jefferson, Room 329
Seattle, WA 98122

Resource Center for the Handicapped
20150–45th Avenue N.E.
Seattle, WA 98155

Independent Living Program
190 Queen Anne Avenue North
Seattle, WA 98109

Adventures in Independence Development
819 S. Hatch
Spokane, WA 99202

Disabilities Law Project
949 Market Street, Suite 416
Tacoma, WA 98499

Independent Living
9108 Lakewood Drive, S.W.
Tacoma, WA 98402

Northwest Services for Independent Living
702 Broadway
Tacoma, WA 98402

Coalition of Handicapped Organizations
3127 E. Evergreen
Vancouver, WA 98661

Independent Living Project—Curative Workshop Rehabilitation Center
2900 Curry Lane, P.O. Box 8027
Green Bay, WI 54308

Access to Independence, Inc.
1954 East Washington Avenue
Madison, WI 53704

Program for Independent Living
University of Wisconsin—Stout Vocational Development Center
Menomonie, WI 54751

Southeast Wisconsin Center for Independent Living
1545 S. Layton Boulevard
Milwaukee, WI 53215

Society's Assets
720 High Street
Racine, WI 53402

Christian League for the Handicapped
P.O. Box 948
Walworth, WI 53184

Appalachian Center for Independent Living
1427 Lee Street East
Charleston, WV 25301

Huntington Center for Independent Living, Inc.
914–½ Fifth Avenue
Huntington, WV 25701

North Central West Virginia Center for Independent Living—Coordinating Council for Independent Living
P.O. Box 677, 1000 Hospital Drive
Morgantown, WV 26507

Wyoming Independent Living Rehabilitation
104 North Platte Road
Casper, WY 82601

Rehabilitation Enterprises of Northeast Wyoming—Independent Living Program
245 Broadway
Sheridan, WY 82801

International Centers of Independent Living

The Happiness for the Handicapped Organization
P.O. Box 7289
Johannesburg, 2000, South Africa

Independent Living Center of New South Wales
P.O. Box 351
Ryde, New South Wales, Australia

Centre for Independent Living in Toronto
170 Bloor Street, W., Suite 304
Toronto, Ontario MSC 1T9, Canada

Ten Ten Sinclair Housing, Inc.
1010 Sinclair Street
Winnipeg, Manitoba, Canada

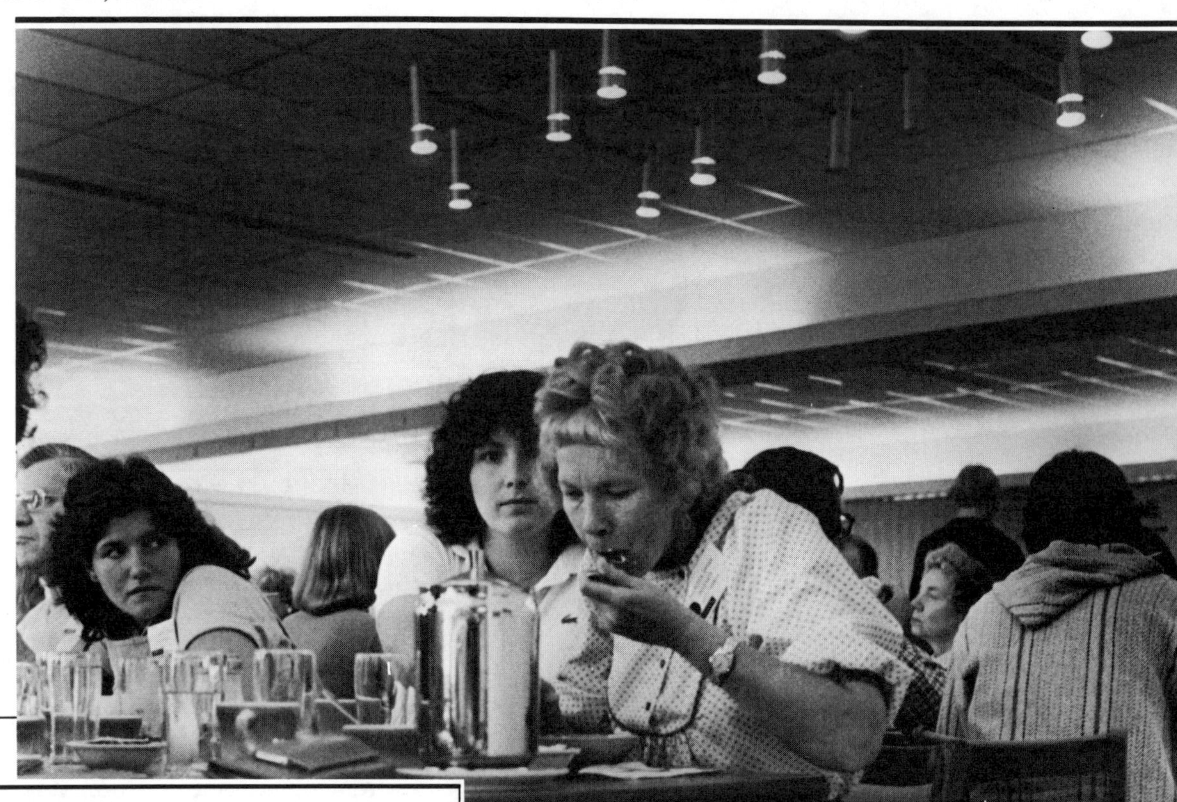

Her Seeing Eye dog waits patiently.

A SHOPPING LIST OF SERVICES

Federal regulations say centers must either offer or "coordinate through referral":

- ***Housing***
- ***Attendant care***
- ***Reader and/or interpreter services***
- ***Information about goods and services relevant to independent living***

Other suggested activities for centers include:

- ***Running a transportation service or a transportation registry***
- ***Peer counseling***
- ***"Independent living skills training"***
- ***Equipment maintenance and repair***
- ***Recreational or socia***
- ***Advocacy or political***

Harriet Bell, Ph.D.

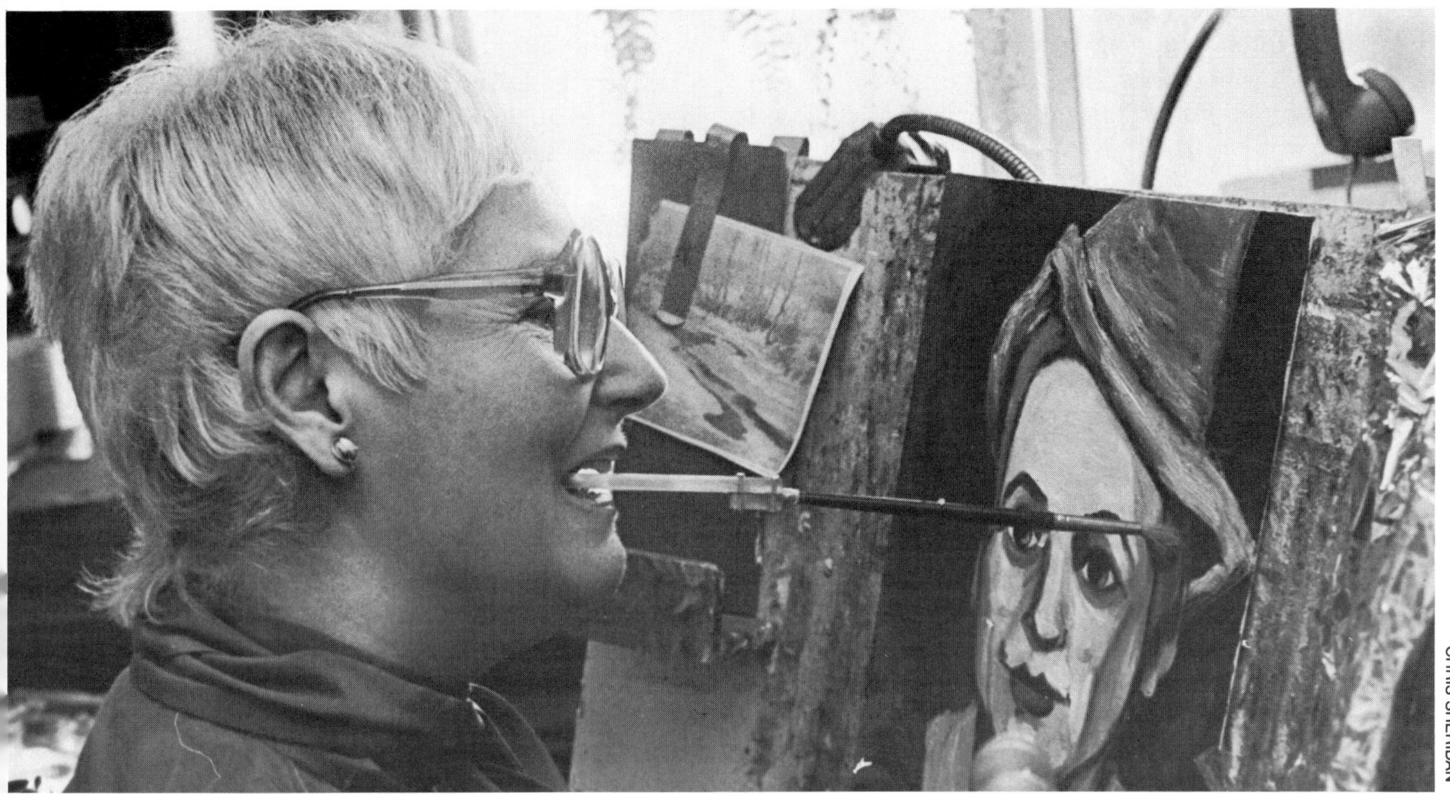
CHRIS SHERIDAN

Harriet Bell paints.

Harriet Bell was one of the first people I interviewed for this book. At the time, she was living at Goldwater Memorial Hospital on Roosevelt Island, New York, where she had lived for twenty-five years.

I placed my tape recorder too close to the stick shift Harriet uses to drive her motorized chair, and Harriet and the tape recorder went flying across the room. Recalling the incident embarrasses her to this day.

In remembering that day, she says, "I knew right away we would be friends." Harriet has a confounding quality of always being right. We are best friends, and we are also colleagues. Together, we established the Polio Information Center and have spoken at conferences in different parts of the country.

A health advocate, a leader in the disability rights community, and a public member of the New York State Board for Nursing, Harriet is a doctoral candidate in family counseling. In 1982, I nominated Harriet to be the recipient of the Wonder Woman award, and she won! To mark the 40th anniversary of Wonder Woman, the comic book heroine, awards and financial grants were given to women for their significant contributions to society. This award is the highest acknowledgment given to a disabled woman.

When she accepted the Wonder Woman award, Harriet said:

> *I am neither a saint nor a heroine as many people think of disabled people. I saw a job to be done and I did it.*

Polio chased me all my life. I was frightened of it, terribly frightened.

I have two sisters; one is my own sister, one is my stepsister. My own sister and I used to go to Atlantic City when we were little girls. One summer, perhaps it was 1931, we drove back to Buffalo at ninety miles an hour because she had contracted polio. Fortunately, it was a mild case.

In 1949, when I was pregnant with my first child, my stepsister had a very severe case of polio. She had just visited me, and this worried me.

I have three children and, like every parent, I worried about the possibility of them getting polio. The summer before I became sick, I asked their pediatrician if there were any precautions I could take to protect them. I was afraid of them playing outdoors, and I didn't know if I should keep them inside, away from everyone.

Then, when I was thirty-one, I became very ill with

polio. It was there and had been chasing me all my life.

I remember the first day I came to the hospital, they said, "We expect great things of you." I took that to mean I would walk out of there. The first winter there, they told me how beautiful it was during the summer. I said, "Don't tell me. I won't be here." I was there for twenty-six summers.

When I arrived at the hospital, my children had to be sent away because they were so small and my husband couldn't take care of them by himself. My oldest was five and the twins were not even two.

Polio was in the prehistoric ages when I was hospitalized. The first polio vaccine wasn't available until April 1955 and I had contracted polio in October 1954. What timing!

The attitude was, if you try, you will get better and you will walk again. That is the way it was supposed to work, but that isn't the way it went. You stayed in bed for one year because they didn't know how to get you up. Physical therapy was done with you in bed. I was confined to an iron lung for a while and still use respiratory aids for up to 16 hours a day. I use a motorized wheelchair because I have very limited use of my hands.

There is a psychological pattern that people go through in becoming adjusted, accepting their condition. The stages are denial, anger, bargaining, depression, and, finally, acceptance. These are the same stages one would go through if faced with a terminal illness, only in the case of polio, it is the loss of your limbs. I went through all of these phases, or feelings, very harshly. When you finally reach acceptance, it need not be passive. It can be a very active acceptance. It's much better to breathe than to have a red nose from crying all the time. It's also very boring to just lie there, roll over, and play dead.

"When you finally reach acceptance, it need not be passive. It can be a very active acceptance. It's much better to breathe than to have a red nose from crying all the time. It's also very boring to just lie there, roll over, and play dead."

From the beginning, my husband came to visit me every day, but we didn't speak to each other for a time because I kept insisting upon going home. Looking back, with three small children and me needing constant care, it was very unrealistic; it would have disrupted the lives of the entire family. But I would make up terrible stories, say outrageous things to him. He'd be visiting and I'd say, "I'll be home Tuesday; my special bed will arrive in the morning. I'll be there later." He'd get so upset, poor man. He'd say, "I'll change the lock on the door; I won't let you in." I'd say, "That's okay. The Scully-Walton ambulance will stay with me until I die in the hall." I was very dramatic!

For a while after you get sick, you are sort of wiped out—too sick to really know what's happening. One of the expressions some of us use is that you "lose control." You've lost your husband because he doesn't live with you. You can't lean on him. You've lost your children. You've lost your home. You've lost control of your life. What do you do? You panic! You say rotten things to your husband when he visits, and you don't treat the nurses very nicely when he leaves.

"The first thing you realize is you can control your life, even if you're quadriplegic and have to depend upon machinery to live. It takes a long time to really believe that you are in control of your life again."

Then, at some point, you look at yourself and say, "What am I doing?" The first thing you realize is you can control your life, even if you're quadriplegic and have to depend upon machinery to live. It takes a long time to really believe that you are in control of your life again.

My husband also had to get control of his life; he was in shock and couldn't work for a year. A turning point for him was when he found out that our son was being abused by the woman he had hired to take care of the children. He packed them up and brought them home. Assuming responsibility for the children forced him to get control of his life very quickly.

I offered to give him a divorce because I didn't feel he should be tied down—he was an extremely attractive man. But he didn't want a divorce, and eventually we were able to start doing things together again. I went to Girl Scout and Boy Scout meetings, just as other parents did; I went to First Communions. I went every place everybody else went—only I went in a wheelchair. I started meeting most of my old friends. From then on, I started getting involved in life again. I also left the hospital for day trips to museums

"I don't think your personality changes due to illness; you're still the same person. What's important is the quality of life you want, not quantity: what you want to do with yourself; how you look at yourself; how you want your family to look at you."

and I went out to dinner. I did whatever I used to enjoy doing.

I don't think your personality changes due to illness; you're still the same person. What's important is the quality of life you want, not quantity: what you want to do with yourself; how you look at yourself; how you want your family to look at you.

My children are extremely independent, self-willed individuals. One daughter has a degree in business administration, owned her own taxi, and is the mother of my two granddaughters.

The other two are twins, a boy and a girl. That's the real jackpot! My son now has a nice job, builds furniture, and is a talented and underdeveloped artist. His twin is a respiratory therapist.

Every Sunday, for years and years, I left the hospital and went home for the day. I taught the children to cook, sew, knit, and crochet. My husband was always there at home to take care of them.

I lost my husband several years ago. The last few years of his life, he was out on the water a lot. He loved it. He had a very exciting job. The big cement barges that go up and down the river sometimes get holes in them and start to sink. His job was directing the operation that took them to a place where they could be repaired, along with getting the tug boats to work properly. Early in his career, he was an insurance agent. He hated it, but it made it possible to raise the children because his hours were flexible.

Both my husband and I made sure we brought the children up together. It really was a whole family. My cubicle in the hospital was an extension of their apartment. If any one of the children wasn't allowed to play outside because of being punished, they could still come and talk to me for the day. As they got older, did rotten things; (like skipping school for 53 consecutive days), my husband would bring the child over, have him or her wait outside my cubicle, and come in and talk it over with me first; then we would all discuss it. I would talk it over with the child alone; then we would all discuss it again. That would put us back on the right track, at least until the next time something happened. It was always like that.

I think that unity in the face of adversity is why the children are so independent and still have a strong sense of family. A good example is when my oldest daughter graduated from college on the rainiest day I've ever seen in my life. I hired transportation at the last minute—my husband had to check out a bad boat and couldn't be everywhere at once. He met me at the graduation with my other daughter and son. When the ceremonies were over, we made rounds

"Both my husband and I made sure we brought the children up together. It really was a whole family. My cubicle in the hospital was an extension of their apartment."

with my husband in the afternoon. Then we had a celebration at the hospital. What a fine day that was, even though we all got soaked!

My husband and I had a very happy marriage. While we were able to live together, it was spectacular. Later, it was much more difficult. It's always hard when you're handling a situation and one person is here and one person is over there somewhere. But for thirty-one years, I always knew where that man was, every minute. Most people don't believe me. I knew where he was, and he knew where I was.

My Daughter Is Leaving Home. What Do I Do Now?

Betty Pendler

After my daughter Lisa was born, and during the first years of her life, if anyone had told me that she would make the statement, "I can hardly wait to move out and get rid of my mother," and that I would get a sick feeling in the pit of my stomach at the prospect of it, I would never have believed it. During the first few difficult years, the prospect of being tied down all the rest of my life loomed heavily over me. Lisa has Down's syndrome.

As time went on, Lisa became more and more independent of me. Since I had successfully travel-trained her, I no longer had to take her to or pick her up from every program. She also began to have a livelier social life than I was having, going to programs three nights and two afternoons a week. I felt that I was successfully letting her out of the nest. So imagine my surprise at my own reaction of really not wanting her to move out when she was ready!

I think it will be helpful to many parents if I share some of my adverse feelings and my anguish and doubts, as well as my firm conviction that I have arrived at the right decision—to support Lisa's getting rid of me!

I should feel very proud of myself for having helped Lisa get to the point where she herself wants to move into an adult residence. So why do I have such mixed emotions when Lisa, like all young men and women in their twenties, wants to be on her own?

I believe that some parents of my generation still may be suffering from unresolved guilt feelings from wanting, at some time or another, to place their child when the days looked dark and difficult, and not having had the courage to do it. And, as independent as I have tried to help my daughter become, I believe that I still do not really want to relinquish my role as the protective, loving mother.

There is absolutely no doubt in my mind that this move for Lisa, at age twenty-three, is the wisest, most correct, and necessary move at this point in both our lives. She is an extremely independent and outgoing young lady. Very early, perhaps for selfish reasons as well as for her own good, I began to teach Lisa how to be on her own—to prepare her own lunch and to get her clothes ready for the next day. When she entered the workshop run by the New York City Chapter of the Association for Retarded Citizens she learned to travel the maze of the New York subways. And she learned to travel other specified routes for the various recreational activities she attended. She learned to go to the bank and cash her own checks. I was not really aware that I was preparing her for "independent living" all this while.

I am very active in the local chapter of the Association for Retarded Citizens. As a committee chairperson, I frequently attended meetings. Naturally, Lisa came with me. After the second visit, my ego was quite deflated when Lisa announced that she preferred staying over with her friends and not coming home with me. I was not prepared to accept that my need to be needed was being undermined.

As the movement toward group homes and independent apartment clusters grew, I saw firsthand the growth and development of the young men and women away from their protective parents. I knew that I owed it to Lisa to file an application. I felt that I was a sophisticated, active, and far-sighted parent and immediately requested applications from several facilities. I had soul-searched my feelings and knew this was the right thing. I knew that I was doing it for her. I knew that I wanted Lisa settled during my lifetime so I could help her make the adjustment.

Yet I confess to the world that those applications sat

on my desk at home for one whole year! Here I was, an involved parent, giving advice to other parents about the need to help sons and daughters become independent. And I was immobile for a whole year! Perhaps I should have started to think about the positive aspects of moving out when Lisa was as young as fifteen or sixteen so that the ambivalent feelings might have been resolved much sooner.

Finally, I did file all the applications. I was so relieved when I was told that there was at least a whole year's waiting list. I could tell myself, and everyone else, that I had "taken the step," but there was no room. Actually, that year's waiting period was extremely helpful. As my emotions seesawed each time I mentioned the subject to friends, neighbors, and coworkers, I was forced to think about it very seriously.

"I had soul-searched my feelings and knew this was the right thing. I knew that I was doing it for her. I knew that I wanted Lisa settled during my lifetime so I could help her make the adjustment. Yet I confess to the world that those applications sat on my desk at home for one whole year!"

At last, Lisa was officially accepted at one of the facilities. She began visiting the group home once a week to get acquainted with the routine. (She moved in five months ago.) It was during this period that I realized that the comments of many parents, whenever the discussion of group homes came up, were really cop-outs—"I'm not sure I want to have my son share a room with another person because at home he has such a lovely, comfortable room for himself"; "I don't like the location of this particular group home"; "Why should I rock the boat at this time?"

I realized that these parents are not seeing the other important, albeit less tangible needs—to grow and develop, to become independent, and to learn to be on one's own, even if under some supervision; and, most important, like every other young person, to eventually make the transition of separating from the parents. These parents need to learn that a group home is not simulating a "family" situation but is an "adult" situation. Certainly, regardless of the person's disability, at the age of twenty-three, an "adult" situation is appropriate.

For most parents, I think the stigma of "putting our child away" remains. We still seem to view a group home as "placement." This became evident to me from the various comments made to me by other parents when I announced my decision, and particularly when it became definite. I heard such remarks as, "Why do you have to place her now since life is easier for you, and she is happy at home and does so much for herself?" or "How will she manage without you?" or "She'll miss you." These comments showed me that these parents have not made the transition to today's thinking of "normalization" and community and independent living. Needless to say, these comments did not help my own already ambivalent feelings about whether I was doing the right thing.

When I forced myself to do further soul-searching, I realized that my decision was based on what was good for Lisa. I am not aware of how many times I had to remind myself of that fact. During the period from the time that she was definitely accepted to the time she moved in, I constantly had butterflies in my stomach. As she and her brother and I sat down at dinner together, when she came out with one of her delightfully humorous statements, teasing me over my morning coffee before I went off to work, or when I saw her and her brother still having those good-natured, childish jousts as they did when they were small, the pit of my stomach sank. Again I would say to myself, "Why do you want to spoil this wonderful family togetherness? It gives them pleasure and surely gives you such pleasure and joy." For one minute, I would be tempted to go to the phone, call the agency, and say, "Let's wait for another opening." Again, I would do more soul-searching and say to myself, "Wait a minute. Whose comfort and happiness are you really concerned with—yours or your daughter's?" Once I got off that unbalanced end of the seesaw, I told myself that I am absolutely convinced that it is my duty at this stage in my life (past sixty years of age) and at this stage in Lisa's life to evaluate what is important to her.

I realized that learning to be on her own, under supervision, is far more important than the material comfort she would have at home. Some gains cannot be truly measured except in an intangible manner. Furthermore, her family structure will always remain, surely as long as both her brother and I are alive. Since we would be visiting her and she would be making periodic visits back home, we would continue our birthday and holiday celebrations in much the same manner as a college son or daughter does when he or she returns home, or a married child, with spouse, making periodic visits. It is just the next step in her normal development of growing up.

When I told the neighbors about my decision, some of them commented incredulously, "How could you let this sweet, darling child leave such a warm, loving home?" I had to remind myself that they were the same ones who were incredulous when I first began to let her go to the basement to put the clothes in the washing machine. When I permitted her to go across the street to learn to make small purchases, such as milk and bread, and when I let her travel the subways a few years later, the comments of these neighbors were, "Aren't you pushing your luck—how can you let her do those things?" If I had listened to them all along and hadn't done what I knew was right to make Lisa's life happier, she never would have reached this stage.

When I stop to analyze the variety of reactions I received from neighbors, friends, and other parents, I think, sad to say, it indicates that many of us still do not view persons who are retarded as whole human beings entitled to as full a life as is possible for them to achieve. Many of the comments seem to be a reflection of attitudes that still prevail, and this saddens me.

If I were asked what advice I could give to parents as a result of my experience and mixed emotions over these few years, I would say that one should begin very early preparing one's son or daughter for eventual independence. As I look back, I did that without realizing it. I think I was taking the advice that Sol Gordon has given to parents in his "Bill of Rights for Parents." Dr. Gordon tells us that martyred parents are seldom appreciated by anybody, least of all their disabled child, and that we should enjoy life as intensely as possible even though we have a child who is disabled.

Because I have the need to be busy and be active in organizations as well as to seek a cultural and social life, it was imperative for me to make Lisa as independent as possible as early as possible. At the same time, it was helping her toward maturity. When she was very young, I had permitted her to use a knife and prepare the salad before I got home from work. I confess that when I taught her to travel by herself, it was as much to give me freedom as it was to give her more mobility and independence. Therefore, for the sake of your child's future, begin very early to teach independent living skills. This starts with permitting your child to do things without your help.

When Lisa was only nine years old, I sent her to the local grocery with a note to buy one or two items. I didn't know then that I was getting her ready to be able to do this once she moved into a group home. Fortunately, today parents can begin this type of training and realize that it is the start of a long-range plan to aid their child when he or she is ready to move away from the loving, protective home environment. It is crucial for parents to recognize all along that just as their other sons or daughters are going to move away from home eventually—off to college or marriage or their own apartments—so, too, this son or daughter who happens to be disabled can move away at the comparable stage of his or her development. As group homes are being developed for more severely disabled people, there have been tremendous advances made in teaching independent living skills. I am convinced that the more we truly love our children, the more we should be willing to let them go.

Life is full of changes. Everyone must learn to adjust. We and our children are adjusting constantly to new programs, to new teachers, to new locations. While we have qualms about exposing our children to a new environment and begin to get negative thoughts about it, let us be honest and admit that it is *we* who are afraid of the change. Therefore, when we say that the group home won't have as many material comforts or the location is not as convenient compared to our own home or that our son or daughter is giving up a parent's love, let us be honest and admit that we are not yet willing to let our sons or daughters go on to their next rightful step for independent growth. We are depriving our children of the opportunity of experiencing an alternative life-style.

As I look back at the twenty-three years of my life with Lisa and her brother Paul, the fact that she is "dying to get rid of her mother" is proof that I did something right. I am very proud that she is going to her new environment so well prepared. I am not insulted at her comment but am thrilled at her ability to want to be on her own.

I felt this thrill and pride especially tonight, when she kissed me, and I inadvertently said, "I'll miss you, darling." Lisa replied, "But Mommy, you know I love you—and besides, I'll come visit you once in a while if you are not out at a meeting or a concert!"

"My Daughter Is Leaving Home. What Do I Do Now?" first appeared in *The Exceptional Parent*. Betty Pendler, a frequent contributor to that magazine, serves on its board of directors, and is a parent chairperson of the New York State Association for Retarded Citizens. Lisa is successfully living on her own, in an apartment, with some support services.

Deprived, Exhibited

Albert Davidson

For reasons beyond my parents' control, I entered a large New York facility for the care of the handicapped at the age of eight. I was thirty when I left. Since I am a quadriplegic, I must be assisted with such daily needs as grooming, dressing, getting into and out of bed, and going to the bathroom. For people like me, the institution becomes the real world. On my infrequent outings, I was a visitor in my parents' home.

In my experience, a child's institutional life is controlled by many adults who often give conflicting commands. He must quickly learn who has the most authority and obey that person. Failure to obey can mean punishment, such as being put to bed for the night in the middle of the day. Conformity is the key to getting along, but the price is high: submergence of one's personality and loss of self. The staff emphasized physical care; the need for affection was ignored.

"Usually good behavior was rewarded by a loveless kind of tolerance and bad behavior was punished as a warning to others. But sometimes attendants did not react at all, and this was the most damaging response because it meant the child could make no impression on his surrogate parents. If his peers also ignored him, he was seriously impaired emotionally."

Children competed for attention in ways that ranged from "very good" to "very bad." "Very good" children helped make beds, placed laundry for collection, or ran errands. "Very bad" children soiled their clothes, hit other kids, or threw things out of windows.

Usually good behavior was rewarded by a loveless kind of tolerance and bad behavior was punished as a warning to others. But sometimes attendants did not react at all, and this was the most damaging response because it meant the child could make no impression on his surrogate parents. If his peers also ignored him, he was seriously impaired emotionally.

In the institution, anticipation of physical and emotional maturity became another burden. Most of what a boy learned about sex came from other boys (whose information was also skimpy) and from *Playboy*-type magazines.

Since there were no secluded areas, necking with a girl was a stealthy, awkward, and embarrassing series of gropes and grabs. The results were mixed: a thrilling sense of achievement at having been able to do it at all, and a depressing feeling of having participated in something you'd been taught was "dirty." The staff denigrated any sign of sexuality, and a boy awakening with an erection could expect teasing by the attendants.

Many factors reinforced the patient's sense of insecurity. Constant rotation of staff members made it nearly impossible for meaningful relationships to develop between attendants and patients. Transfer of patients from one section to another could end years-long friendships.

When one needs help to keep a dental appointment or make a phone call, these tasks assume a meaning out of all proportion to their true importance. One is forced to live strictly in the present. The past doesn't count and the future never comes.

There was little solidarity among the patients. I saw friendships dissolve in bitterness over such trivialities as two patients wanting one remaining portion of lunch meat. Material possessions proved one did exist and were, therefore, zealously guarded. Some patients spent 90 percent of their time near their beds protecting their things.

Few deep relationships could develop because each person was absorbed in meeting his own needs.

The "normal" child can, at times, get away from watchful adults. From childhood through young manhood, I was on public display while I ate, slept, or defecated, and there was no means for me to have sexual experience. It is humiliating to be called "a nice boy" at the age of twenty-seven.

Responsibility is a concomitant of maturity. In my institution, patients were given no personal responsibility. All decisions, even the most insignificant, were made for us. These circumstances perpetuate the unhappy phenomenon I call "the elderly adolescent."

I still remember vividly the day in 1962 I received a motorized wheelchair. It was March 23 at 2:30 in the afternoon. It meant I could move any time I wanted to. The chair represented freedom from dependence on others to take me from place to place. It was my first taste of freedom, and I was nearly twenty-two years old.

Albert Davidson lived for twenty-two years in a large city facility. This article was published in *The New York Times*, October 11, 1975. Reprinted with permission.

(opposite page)
Bernard Carabello says, "This is how I get into my coat, I'm not embarrassed, I want people to see what a struggle it is for a person with a disability."

Bernard Carabello

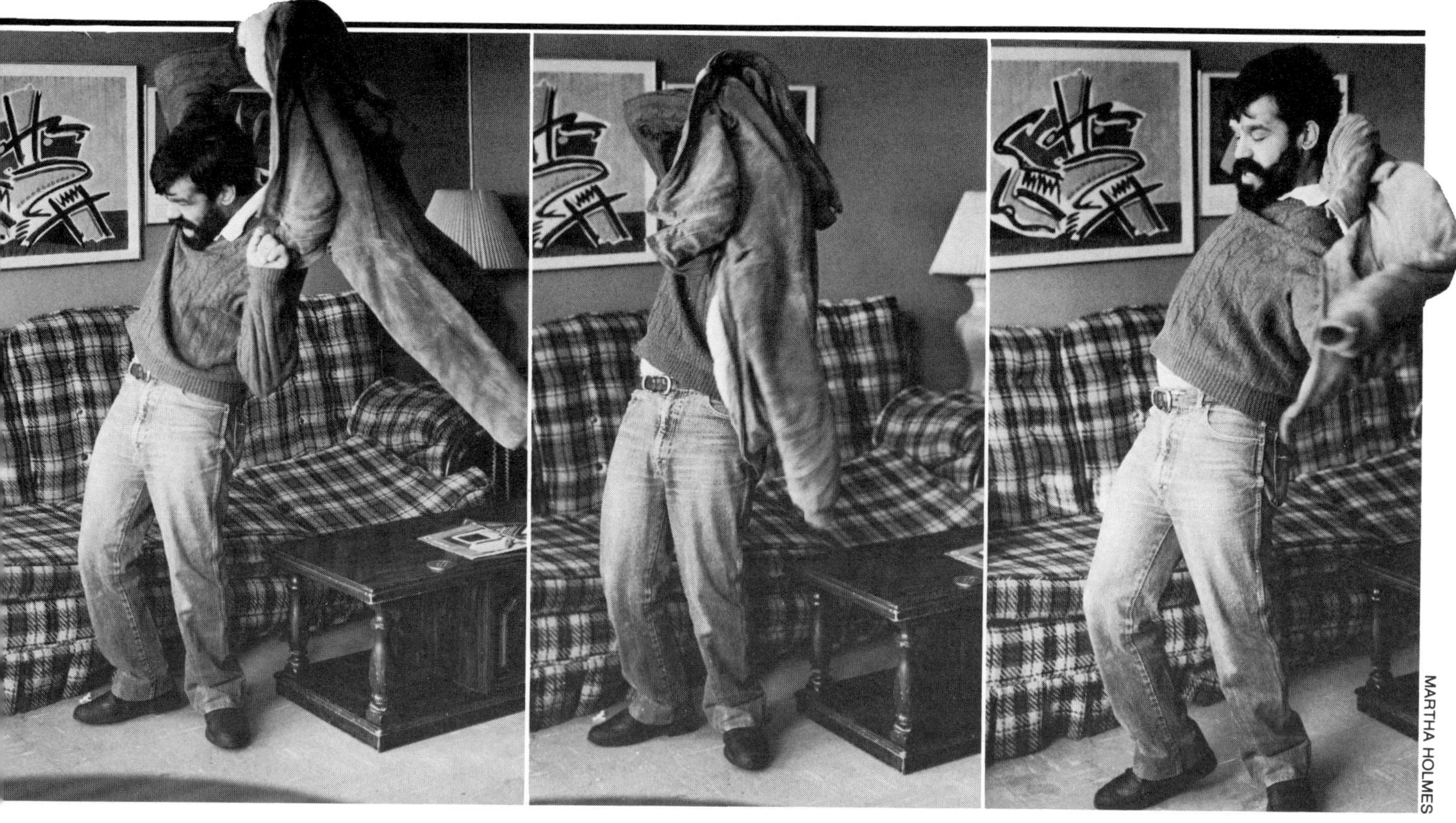

MARTHA HOLMES

By now, Bernard is a family member. We first met during a march in Washington, D.C., and served together as founding members of the New York City League of Disabled Voters. Bernard, with reporter Geraldo Rivera, broke the story of the inhuman treatment of residents at Willowbrook, a state institution in New York.

Bernard is a self-advocate for the Resource Center for Developmental Disabilities.

I felt freer sometimes when I was living in the institution then when I got out. Society shuts you out. Because you're disabled, they don't want you in their world.

I lived on a ward with eighty people. My family put me there when I was three or four, and I stayed until I was nineteen. It was a state institution for the mentally retarded. I have cerebral palsy.

You wake up at five in the morning. It's dark outside. Then you get dressed and eat. You go to school for two and a half hours a day then you sit on the ward for the rest of the day looking at TV. I sat on the ward until I turned eighteen, and then I walked the grounds. Someone would visit me once a year, sometimes not for four or five years. Other people had visitors every Sunday. I'd stand by the window because my family promised they would come. But they didn't.

When I was eighteen, two attendants made me a birthday cake. They were good friends. There were a few good people, but the only outstanding person was Michael. He was a doctor who came to work at the institution. He took an interest in me and was the first person in my life to tell me I was not retarded, that I was very intelligent.

I finally got out of there when I was nineteen. But I didn't want anybody to see me walk or anything like that. I was ashamed. Mike forced me. He was teaching me to be independent on the outside. Sometimes I got really mad at him. He would show me how to get places and then leave me on my own, and I had to find my own way back.

That first year out was a nightmare. I didn't know who was going to cook or clean for me. I had a roommate, but we used to fight like cats and dogs. Then I took an apartment on my own.

I started out with a mattress on the floor and a couple of dishes. I have a nice place—a color TV, a stereo, posters, a job, friends, the whole works. I've come a long way. And I earned it. And I'd do it again. I could. Everything gave me strength.

The Right to Travel

One day I asked Evelyn Pierce, who started riding the new, accessible public buses currently in use on some routes in New York City, what she said to people who showed impatience toward her because it took time for the driver to lower the lift at the rear of the bus so she could board the bus in her wheelchair. "I often have to wait for six buses, thirteen buses—whatever the number of buses that have passed me that have nonfunctioning lifts. And if I am going to get to my destination, I have to do this. I have to hold up the bus."

There's a whole socialization that has to take place within a community. There are people who never get out

We often forget about people who have really been isolated and who have great difficulty looking at the post signs on corners, trying to figure out what bus to use if one happens to come by.

and don't feel safe enough to be on their own. We often forget about people who have really been isolated and who have great difficulty looking at the post signs on corners, trying to figure out what bus to use if one happens to come by.

Pierce requires the use of special lifts to board a bus. Apparently, they are not cycling these lifts at the beginning of every day as they should. Like the brakes on the bus, if the lifts are not cycled every day, the mechanisms often break down. That was her experience on two new routes that were opened up in March. One night on the way home,

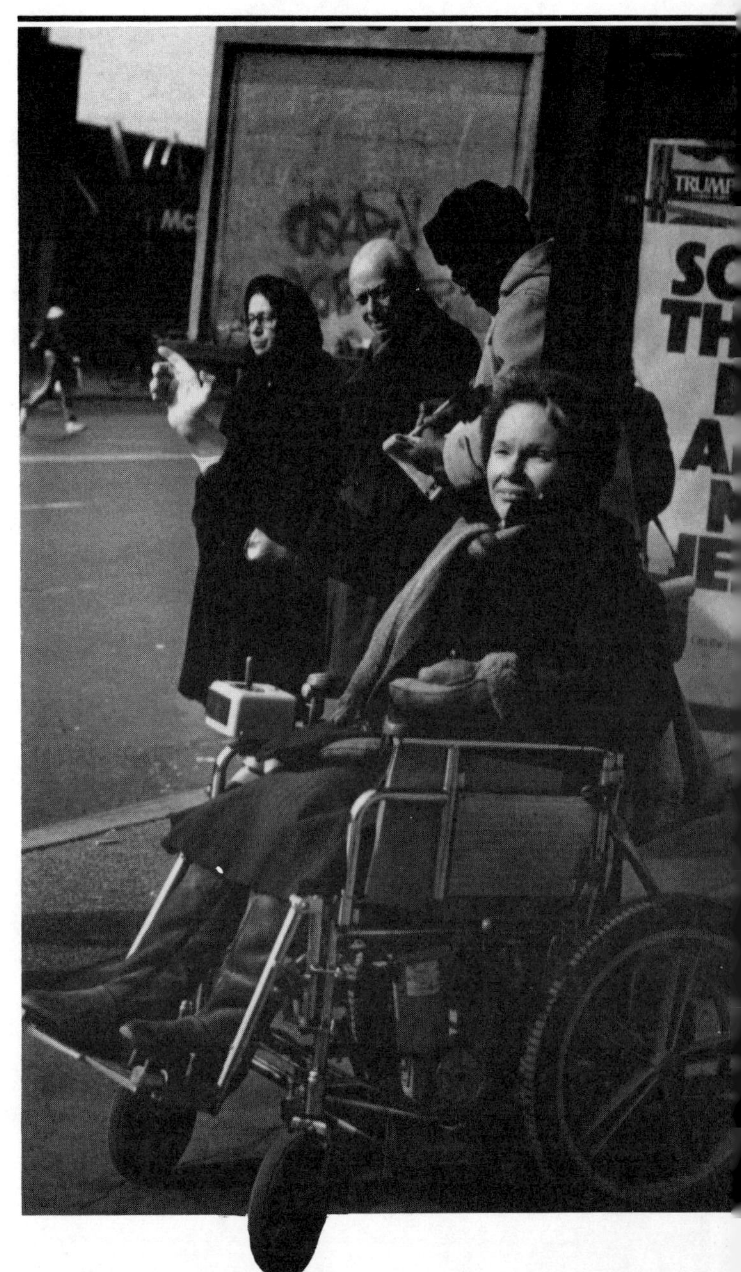

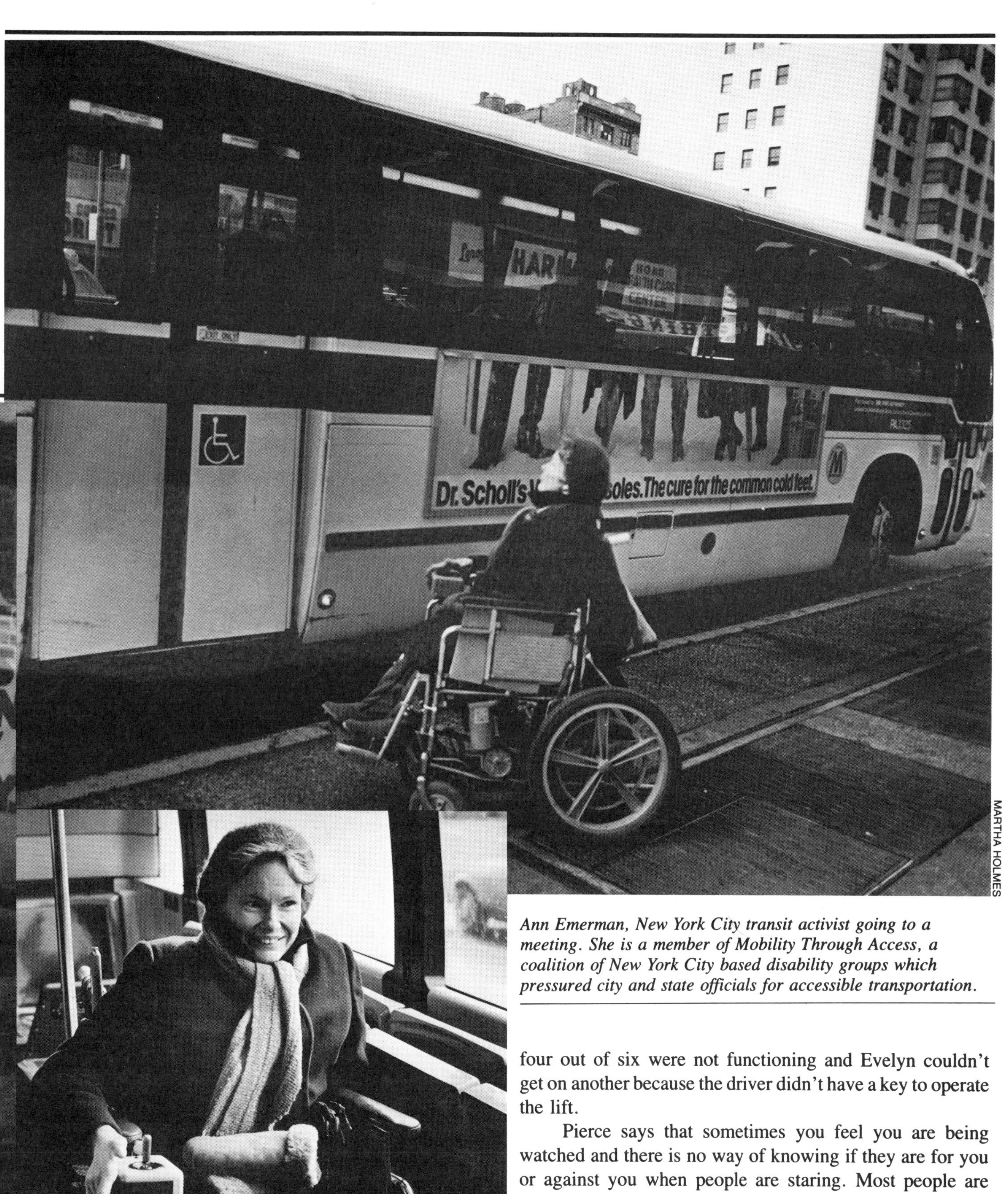

MARTHA HOLMES

Ann Emerman, New York City transit activist going to a meeting. She is a member of Mobility Through Access, a coalition of New York City based disability groups which pressured city and state officials for accessible transportation.

four out of six were not functioning and Evelyn couldn't get on another because the driver didn't have a key to operate the lift.

Pierce says that sometimes you feel you are being watched and there is no way of knowing if they are for you or against you when people are staring. Most people are supportive. And, in fact, some people come over and say, "I'm with you." There are always one or two who make a

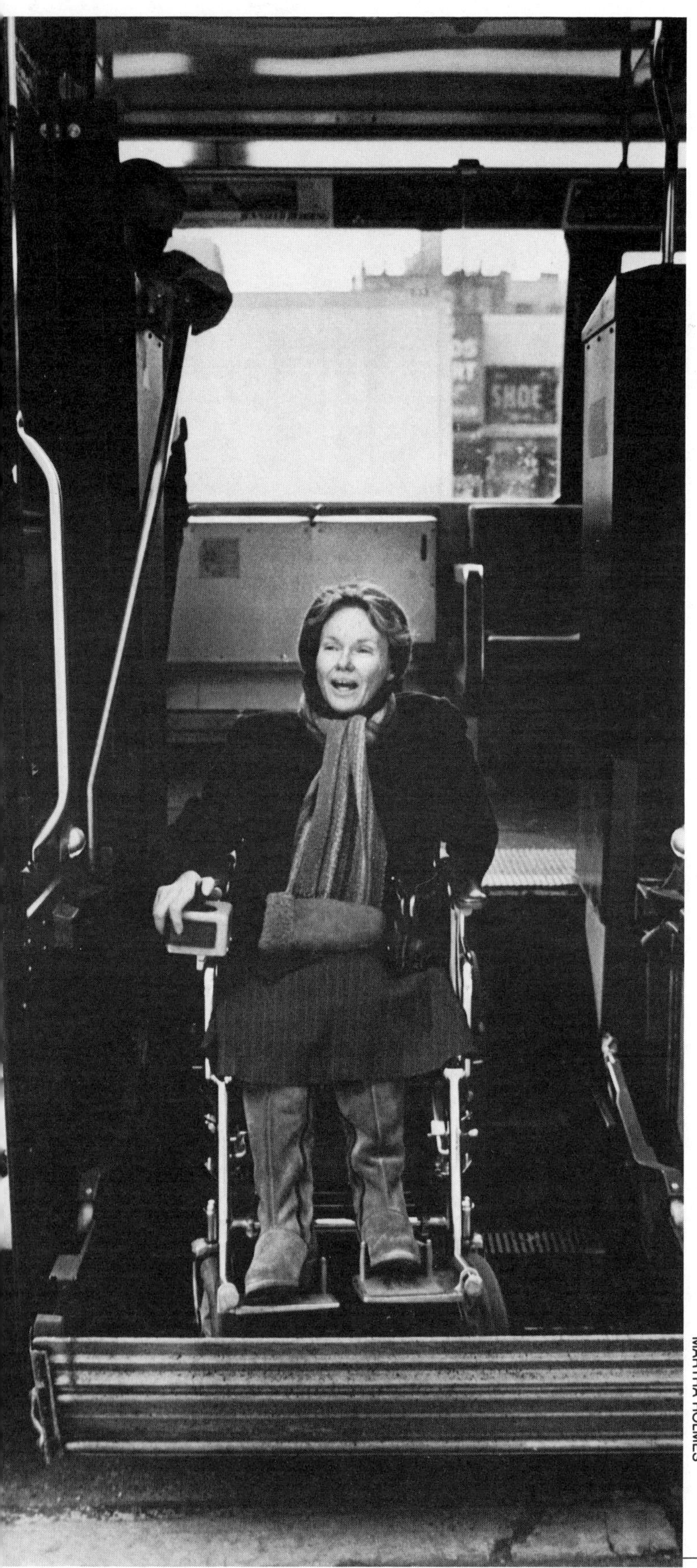

MARTHA HOLMES

lot of noise. They ask why can't you take a cab, why do you have to hold up a bus and hold up all these people? "I say that I, too, would like to ride the bus and I don't like having to wait, either," Pierce said, "and, then I tell them the number of buses that have passed me that did not have functioning lifts."

Accessible transportation for the disabled was never an issue until Congress passed the Rehabilitation Act of 1973. Until the passage of this law, civil rights for disabled citizens were largely ignored. It was assumed that disabled people did not need public transportation since they were rarely seen on the streets.

On December 1, 1955, when Rosa Parks, a black woman in Montgomery, Alabama, refused to get up and give her seat to a white man and was arrested, the consciousness of the American people was triggered. The Bus Segregation Ordinance was declared unconstitutional by a federal court following a protest and boycott. The subsequent publicity embarrassed people, and the indignities that had seemed acceptable were no longer tenable.

When we talk of Rosa Parks, we are talking about rights.

And when most physically disabled citizens cannot use buses, trains, subways or get into toilets on planes or have the equal right to travel, we are talking about not upholding the Constitution of the United States.

Although certain cities around the country access their buses, making it possible for individuals with mobility limitations to use public transportation, anyone traveling around the United States would soon realize that accessible transportation is no certainty.

The American Disabled for Accessible Public Transit, the Eastern Paralyzed Veterans Association, Disabled in Action, members of independent living centers, parents groups, and transit activists, have challenged the segregation of disabled passengers.

The coming year promises to be a watershed in the disability rights movement's push for accessibility to the nation's buses, subways, and airlines.

Ann Emerman rides a lift on an accessible bus.

The Friendly Skies Are Not Always So

Simon & Schuster published Frommer's *A Guide for the Disabled Traveler,* written by Frances Barish. A number of significant things set this book apart from books that are sometimes thought of as "disability books."

For openers, Frances Barish, an avowed globe-trotter for both professional and personal reasons, is paraplegic, uses a wheelchair, and shares with readers her point of view that freedom to travel is almost a part of the Bill of Rights. She holds that just as in education, employment, and housing, travel is an area where today's disabled population should be determined not to be left out.

The guide is written for travelers who use special equipment—a wheelchair, crutches, a cane, an ileostomy bag, a pacemaker, a respirator, a need for oxygen, a Seeing Eye dog, or a hearing aid.

People with disabilities have places to go, things to see, and need to use the toilets, too.

Arthur Frommer is aware of the many millions of travelers with special needs who increasingly bring in large revenue. It is no longer unusual to see a porter waiting at the arrival gate with a wheelchair for a passenger who finds the miles of airport corridors overwhelming.

Imagine now boarding a plane in New York bound for Los Angeles or Paris and being unable to use the inaccessible toilet. People with disabilities have places to go, things to see, and need to use the toilets, too. It comes close to home if one experiences it firsthand or travels with a colleague, as I did.

We almost didn't make it to St. Louis for the second International Post-Polio Conference. Harriet Bell was asked to deliver a paper on the Polio Information Center she had established on Roosevelt Island, in New York, and we were determined to get there.

For the better part of two weeks, we were on the phone to a few travel agents who claimed to be experts but seemed to make things worse. Then we spoke to the customer relations representatives of close to a dozen airlines, whose job it is to handle any extraordinary services. True, we were not presenting them with something simple.

Harriet's motorized chair weighs in at a little less than 400 pounds. On the back of it, there are two wet cell batteries, which power the respirator, and two more to run the chair. There are few nonstop flights to St. Louis and our requirements would mean not only changing planes but changing airlines. Connecting flights would allow us a little more than a half hour to unload the chair, transfer, get our baggage, and make a dash across the terminal. At best, it was unrealistic.

"One new budget-fare airline, anxious for passengers, offered first-class service for tourist fare. When we called, they sounded eager until we outlined our needs. They then suggested a few of their competitors."

Some airlines turned us down flat, saying they didn't have personnel experienced in connecting the respirator to their electrical system. One airline could handle it without any problems, was experienced, but they had a rule that the plane had to have no further destination when we deplaned. The plane we needed was heading out to the coast.

One new budget-fare airline, anxious for passengers, offered first-class service for tourist fare. When we called, they sounded eager until we outlined our needs. They then suggested a few of their competitors.

When we seemed to have an obstacle course keeping us from getting to St. Louis, we decided to figure out what more we could do. Sealed gel batteries that could be charged the night before, last two hours, did not need to be wired into the electrical system, seemed like a good beginning in simplifying things. We would still have to take the other batteries with us, but they could be stowed with the chair during the flight.

Harriet is an experienced traveler, and when airline personnel listen she can tell them exactly what she needs and how they can help. "I am usually boarded a half hour before anyone else, so that all the passengers are not looking down the aisle at me transferring," she says. "It is a courtesy, a necessity, because it involves my dignity."

An hour and a half before takeoff, we are in front of the checkout counter. The personnel are unfamiliar with transferring procedures and say to us that they have never handled anything like this before. We tell one airline representative assigned to assist us that it will take at least a half hour to get us on board and stow the chair, and we suggest we go through security check and meet at the gate. He becomes petulant but agrees that would be a good idea.

Not until all passengers are in the plane are we boarded. The transfer chair is not at the gate, which means Harriet needs to enter the plane in her motorized chair, not giving room to maneuver the transfer.

It takes ten minutes to clear the galley, where one steward says to the other, "They shouldn't have allowed them on in the first place."

Passengers lean over in their seats to see Harriet being lifted and placed in her seat. The plane is now 15 minutes behind schedule.

The stewards, seeing that we are determined to remain, assist us with our luggage and place things in the overhead compartments. The passengers are, for the most part, hostile. Several are supportive, and we exchange smiles.

When we are airborne, the pilot gets on the intercom and apologizes for the delay, explaining that we had to wait our turn on the runway and "accommodate a 'handicapped' passenger."

We are met in St. Louis by two capable gentlemen who come aboard after everyone has deplaned, come up to Harriet and say, "We're here. How can we be of help?"

The skies have not been friendly to passengers with disabilities. But no more have buses, trains, subways, ships, or anything else that allows people to get to work, shop or go on vacation.

Resources: TRAVEL

Travel Information Center, Moss Rehabilitation Hospital, 12th Street and Tabor Road, Philadelphia, PA 19141, provides free information on accessibility of national and international cities, hotels, motels, cruise ships, and airlines.

The Society for the Advancement of Travel for the Handicapped, 26 Court Street, Brooklyn, NY 11242, is an organization established to assist members of the travel industry to better serve travelers with disabilities. They will provide, free of charge, a list of experienced travel agents.

Airports, ***published by Airport Operators Council International Inc., lists design features, facilities, and services at 472 airport terminals in forty-six countries. Available from Consumer Information Center, Pueblo, CO 81009.***

Rehabilitation International U.S.A. (RIUSA), 20 West 40th Street, New York, NY 10018, has published **"Travel Tips for the Handicapped."** ***This is also available from Consumer Information Center.***

Fire!

Two recent tragedies involving the death of disabled veterans by fire and the growing concern for the safety of many others prompted the publication of "Wheeling to Fire Safety," a booklet about fire emergency procedures for paralyzed and disabled people.

Details on the death of the first veteran, who was paralyzed, were never clear—he lived alone and died in his bed, possibly when a cigarette set fire to the sheets.

The second individual, who used an electric wheelchair and was dependent on the assistance of an aide, died in a fire caused by faulty wiring on the Christmas tree. The smoke alarm in his apartment had been dismantled, a small fire extinguisher was inoperable, there were too few accessible exits, and there was no emergency plan to follow. Panic set in.

The information in the booklet, carefully compiled and published by staff members of the Eastern Paralyzed Veterans Association, addresses the aspects of fire prevention and safety for individuals with mobility limitations, as well as for those with visual and hearing impairments. The guide is invaluable for any person needing special assistance in an emergency.

Sprinkled throughout the booklet are cartoons with the character Beetle Bailey. My favorite shows him smoking a cigar in the bathtub, his head resting on an oversized pillow. The captions reads: "If you must smoke in bed sleep in the bathtub!"

There is good, sound fire prevention advice that should be read and shared with others.

Basic guidelines for "fireproofing" your home and work environments are:

- Contact your local fire department and let their representative know exactly where you live and what your disability is. This is important in case special equipment or rescue procedures might be necessary. If it would be difficult for you to exit on your own, your fire department must know about it.
- Request that a representative from the fire department visit your home or apartment to discuss fire safety procedures with you. He will need the following information: the type of house you live in—one-story house, apartment building, trailer; the floor on which living quarters and bedroom are located; your doctor's name, address, and telephone number.
- In an emergency, the elevator in your apartment house or office cannot be used in exiting. Make a mental note of fire exits and plan two alternative exit routes.

Develop an escape strategy taking into account the extent of your disability. Be aware of your capabilities and limitations.

- Develop an escape strategy taking into account the extent of your disability. Be aware of your capabilities and limitations. For example, if you can lift yourself through a window, check that the windows are designed so that your body will fit through them easily. If you can crawl, practice sliding down the stairs. If you can use your arms, a mechanic's crawler that grasps the ground provides greater mobility.
- Have your employer designate coworkers who will assist you in an emergency and familiarize you with the building's alarm system, available exits, and existing fire emer-

gency procedures. Be sure coworkers are aware of your special needs.

- If you have a hearing impairment, ask your employer or apartment building owner to install a fire alarm system that contains a visual alarm, such as a flashing light.
- The fire department can advise you on the types of smoke detectors that are available, how they operate, and where to place them.
- Home care attendants or aides should be thoroughly familiar with your exit plan and understand what they should do in case of fire. Practice your plan together.
- Memorize the fire department's telephone number. Post it on or near your phone(s).

The unattended cooking fire is one of the leading causes of fires. Some of the suggestions made to prevent or, if necessary, handle this type of fire are:

- Do NOT start cooking and then leave the room for any length of time.
- When cooking, wear close-fitting clothing so that sleeves cannot come in contact with burners. Keep clothes and flammable objects away from the stove.
- If a fire starts when you are cooking, turn off the stove. If you, your aide, or someone in your family can operate a fire extinguisher, keep one near the stove in an easily accessible spot.
- Never move a pan fire—either to the sink or outdoors. Smother a pan fire with a large lid. Baking soda can be used on a grease fire. NEVER use water on a grease fire.
- Arrange cooking and eating areas to allow maximum mobility. Be especially careful to prevent burns when transferring food from stove to serving areas. A direct route from stove to table is best.

Some additional basic safety guidelines are:

- Portable space heaters should not be placed near curtains, bedding, or clothes. Standard safety practice discourages placing space heaters in bedrooms.
- Check all electric cords and make sure they are not worn. Electric cords should not be run under rugs, over hooks, or through doorways.
- If your clothing catches fire, drop to the floor and roll to put the flames out. If you cannot do that, keep a blanket or rug nearby to smother the flames.

To obtain copy of "Wheeling to Fire Safety," send a self-addressed, stamped envelope to:

Eastern Paralyzed Veterans Association
432 Park Avenue South
New York, New York 10016

For additional information, nine publications dealing with fire safety, prevention, and fire aid are available from:

National Fire Protection Association
470 Atlantic Avenue
Boston, Massachusetts 02210

SOME SAFETY TIPS

Depending upon a person's disability, an evaluation of safety needs and equipment must be made.

- *Every household should have one or two fire extinguishers. At least one should be in the kitchen. A good place for a fire extinguisher is the bedroom, particularly if there are smokers in the house.*
- *Smoke alarms are required in multiple dwellings in an increasing number of states and are suggested in individual homes. Smoke alarm batteries should be checked monthly to make sure they are working. Smoke alarms with flashing lights rather than a siren are available for hearing impaired individuals.*
- *Lamps and other appliances should be checked for worn wiring and overloading of electric outlets eliminated.*
- *Users of motorized chairs and respirators need filled and charged batteries, especially in the event of a power failure. Utility companies often have auxiliary power resources and will assist in an emergency.*
- *Utility companies often maintain a listing of the names, addresses, and apartment numbers of individuals with a disability who may need assistance in the event of a power failure. Call them for charging of batteries or electric power for other equipment.*

Closed-Captioning: Accessing Television

We had made a commitment not to speak; instead, we would use sign language to communicate. No radios or alarm clocks were allowed. The telephone could be used, only if necessary, by signing to an interpreter, who would speak and then sign the message back.

Fifty of us enrolled in an intensive total immersion program created to teach American sign language. Some of us were parents of children who are deaf or had a hearing impairment ourselves, some were teachers or social workers or actors interested in interpreting or performing in companies such as the Theatre of the Deaf.

Then there were others of us who came to this suburban college campus, a growing number of people who wanted to learn the language for a variety of reasons—perhaps we knew someone who was hearing impaired and who signed. Lawyers, teachers, and nurses, indeed, all of us, wanted to learn sign language to communicate with our hearing impaired clients and friends who sign.

It was a challenge to live in this environment. Once a young man in the cafeteria began taunting me, pretending not to understand what I was ordering, and I burst out crying.

During the evening, we were shocked to find how few television programs were captioned. We were told that only forty hours a week of programs are captioned—less than 5 percent of prime network television hours. The airwaves were not to be taken for granted.

Numbers are important to networks. Advertisers are interested in how many customers see their commercials and buy their products. Captioning accesses television for the estimated fourteen million individuals who identify themselves as hearing impaired and an undetermined number of viewers who benefit from the support of written captions. Yet there are only 80,000 homes in the United States equipped to receive closed-captioning, which translates into a viewing audience of approximately 300,000.

A one-time investment buys a decoder that, when hooked up to any television set, receives and displays closed-captioned programs. Captions do not obstruct the picture and are easily visible. Sears, J.C. Penney, VideoConcept (a nationwide chain of video outlets), a number of hearing impaired interest organizations, and the National Captioning Institute, 5203 Leesburg Pike, Falls Church, Virginia 22041, sell decoders. Sears also sells a 19-inch portable color television with built-in decoding circuitry. They also repair all decoders, no matter where they have been purchased.

In addition to the major networks, a number of cable programs are being captioned. A growing number of home video movies are captioned and are available at video outlets.

- ***Fire departments often maintain a listing of names, addresses, and apartment numbers of people who need special assistance in the event of a fire. For identification in case of emergency, some fire companies place a sticker of a firefighter on the door of residents in apartment houses who require this service. In the event of a power failure, fire departments can also be of assistance.***

- ***Sinks, stove, and cupboards should be at a safe level. Long, loose-fitting sleeves should not be worn while cooking at the stove, since this can cause serious burns.***

- ***It is essential for visually impaired individuals to mark—in large letters or in Braille—containers, medicines, and cleaning substances that are harmful if ingested.***

- ***Safety belts must be worn by the driver and all passengers at all times while in a moving car. One of the major causes of epilepsy in children is head injury sustained in automobile accidents.***

- ***Smooth walkways, with properly sloped and textured curb cuts and handrails on sloped areas, are essential for access as well as accident prevention.***

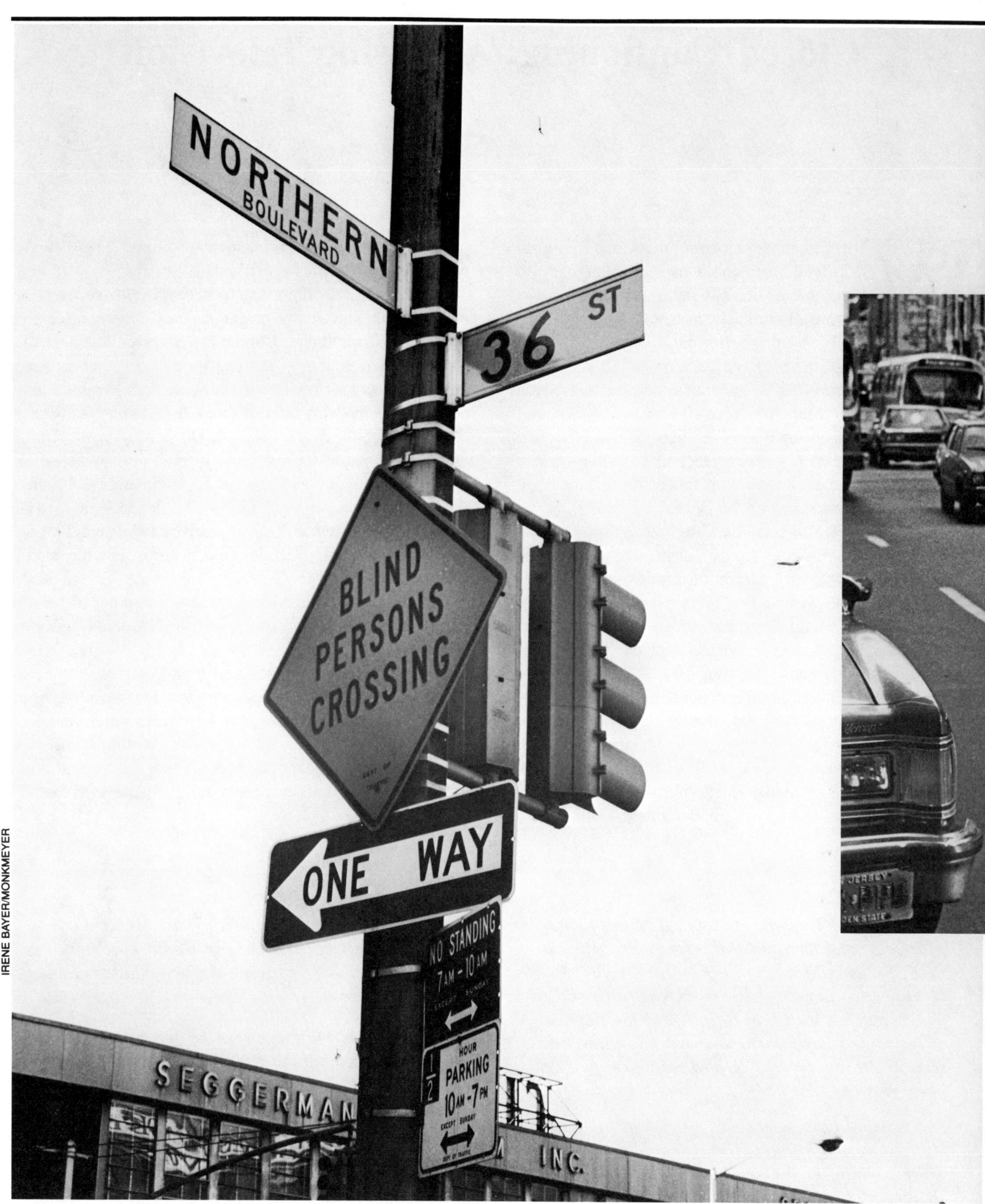

IRENE BAYER/MONKMEYER

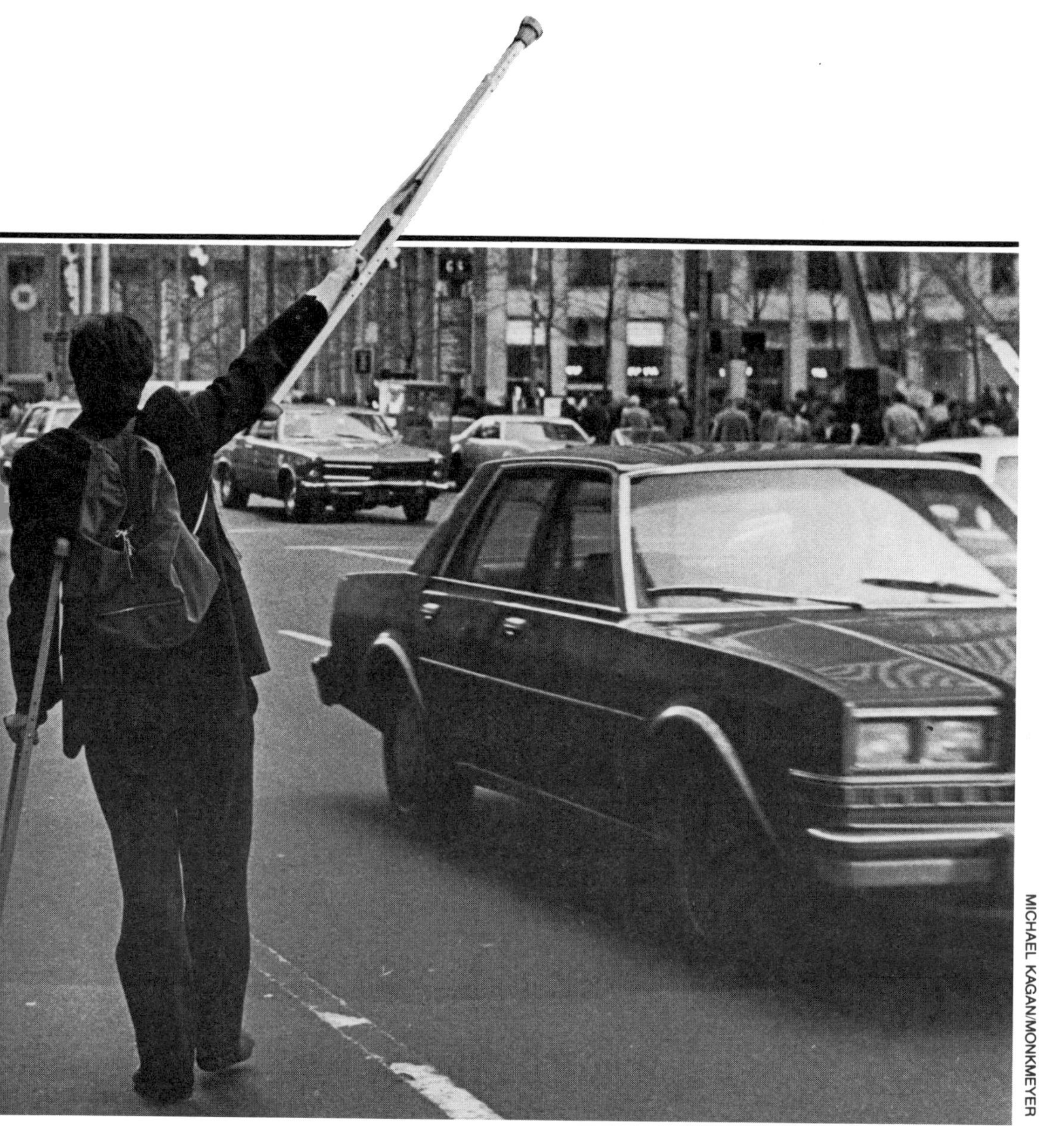

MICHAEL KAGAN/MONKMEYER

Chapter 3
Who Wouldn't Want Me?

AGNES ZELLIN

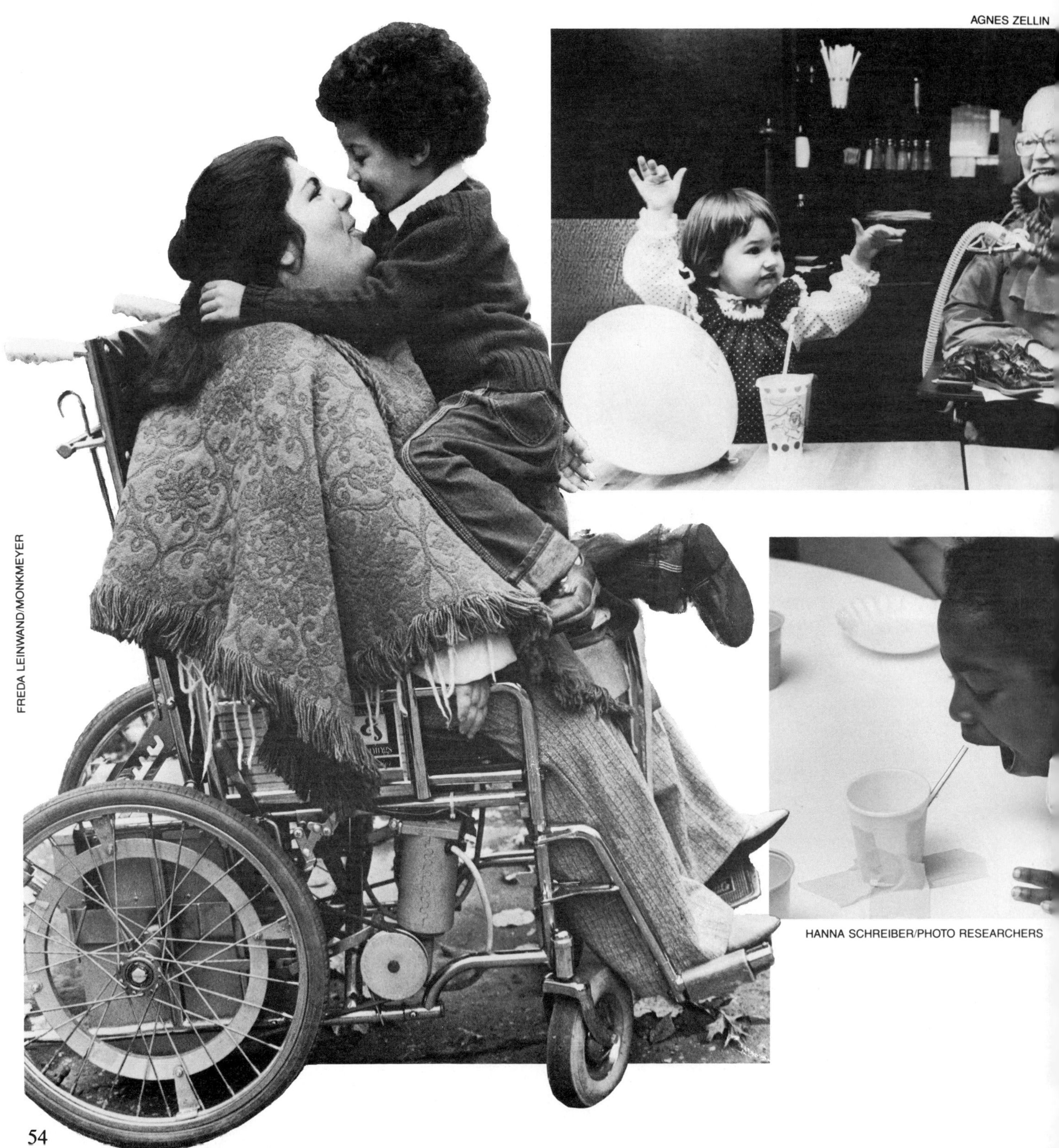

FREDA LEINWAND/MONKMEYER

HANNA SCHREIBER/PHOTO RESEARCHERS

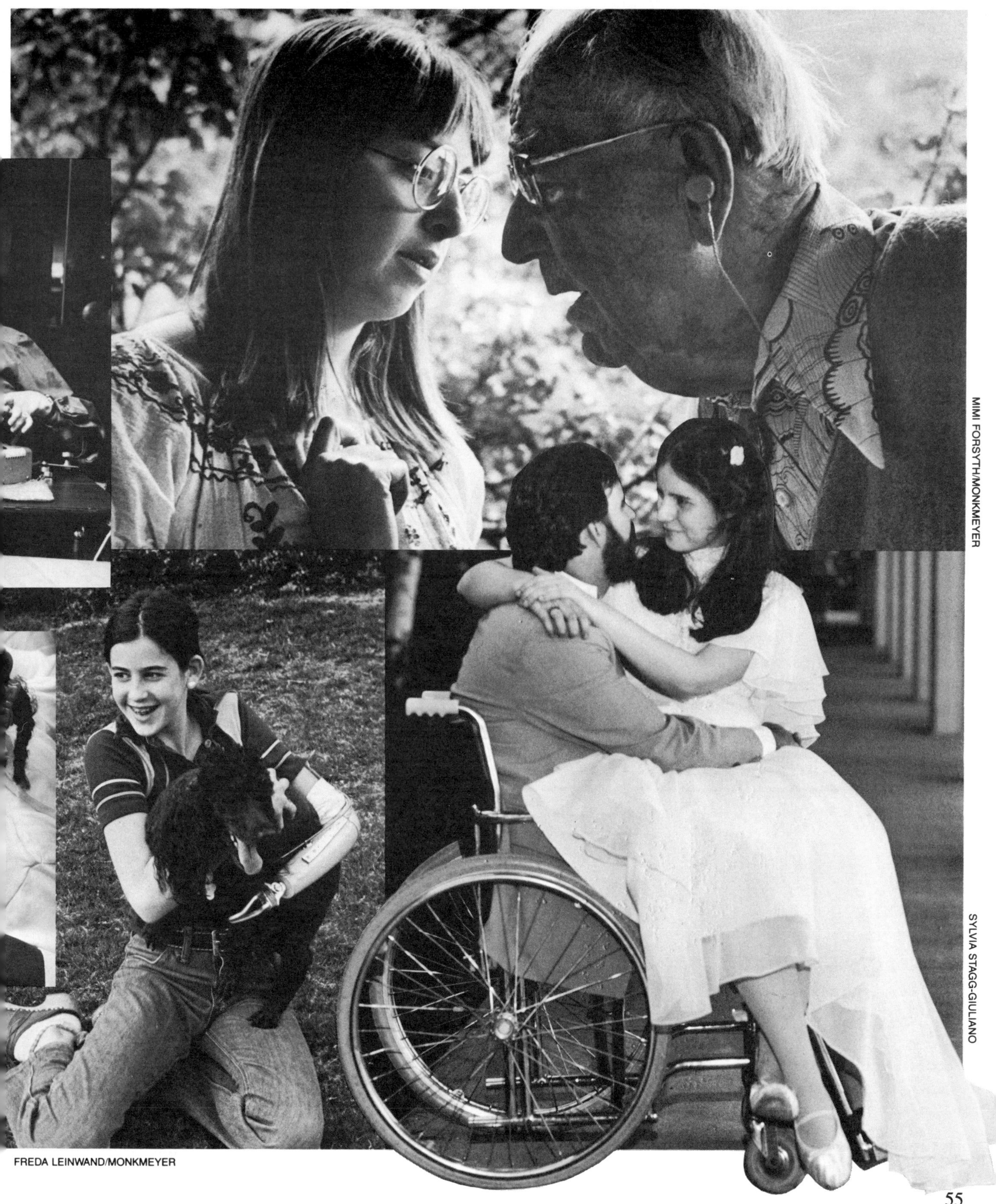

MIMI FORSYTH/MONKMEYER

SYLVIA STAGG-GIULIANO

FREDA LEINWAND/MONKMEYER

Personal Theory

William Roth, Ph.D.

Love by my family was mediated by my disability. I interpreted some love as pity, some as unbelievable, some as warped, and some, by a curiously circular logic, as love existing only because I was loved in the first place.

Frankly, I did not realize the social consequences of my disability as a child, and the main consequences of my disability were that I used a typewriter at school, walked strangely, could not cut my meat, and had a certain distance from my own body. But the greatest consequence of my disability was that I was always designated to play right field in school softball games. Never was a ball hit my way. It was a long trek back and forth to right field, where I did nothing except follow the ball with my eyes, nurturing the faint possibility that it might be hit my way. What I enjoyed most was recess, talking with the girls.

"I had decided that the feeling necessary for love was simply too painful. With time, I became hard, sarcastic, supercilious, and, in general, a pathetic human being except to those who loved me sufficiently to excuse my behavior."

At the very start of high school, I started to cry on the way home from an orthopedist who had wrapped me up in a body cast. My mother cried with me. By the time we reached home, I had decided that the feeling necessary for love was simply too painful. With time, I became hard, sarcastic, supercilious, and, in general, a pathetic human being except to those who loved me sufficiently to excuse my behavior. Past crying at certain stories, I had quite put out of my mind what feeling was. It was not that feeling could sometimes hurt; rather, it usually did. It was less painful to cut it out. I went through high school and the first two years of college as an unfeeling rock. A hollow man—rather, boy. So I had read.

I went to an elite, independent school from grades seven to twelve, or, as the school called them, forms one through six. This was not out of a desire for class or a classy education. I went to a school where I had to wear a tie (which my mother had to tie) because in the sixth grade, I was invited to a birthday party by a girl named Susan Chess.

Her menstruation had started during the previous year. Because my mother was a gynecologist, I was, of course, the class sage in such matters. Indeed, my first teaching had been to explain to Susan what menstruation was. My wide readings in the field, from Havelock Ellis to Magnus Hirshfield to the *American Journal of Obstetrics and Gynecology*, had made me an expert in questions of sex.

My sixth grade teacher, a rouge-cheeked aspirant to the Daughters of the American Revolution, had, because of my disability, prohibited me from participating in a class square dance. When Susan Chess invited me to her birthday party, and when Bobby Allison confided that Spin-the-Bottle would be played when Susan's parents went out for ice cream, I knew, as my teacher had told me, that I did not belong.

The excuse I contrived for not going to the birthday

party was medical. So there I was, my pediatrician sticking tongue depressors down into my mouth, looking deeply into my ears, feeling glands, and being far more intimate overall than a kiss in a game of Spin-the-Bottle. However, I knew enough about excuses to know that this sort of thing could not be kept up indefinitely. And I had learned in school that an ounce of prevention was worth a pound of cure. So I went to an all-boys prep school. After that, I went to Yale, an all-men's college.

I lived in a dormitory. I had many acquaintances and, in my junior year, formed my first strong friendships, some of which last to this day. Like Adam or Golem, the prep school rock became sentient.

I knew about mixers, so I usually spent weekends at home with my parents. At school when a woman was at a table, I would choose another. I ignored my sister. I ignored her friends, especially those who, had I not been what I was, should have attracted me. I knew that something was missing and knew that it involved half the people in the world. The absence became more painful as I grew in other ways.

In my junior year, a friend fixed me up with Chris, a friend of his future wife at Oberlin. Oberlin was choreographed to music, which seemed to come out of every window. Chris played the harp. It was a very simple weekend, really. We just went on a walk and studied the rest of the time. I fell in love with her. I did not know the things that could build in such a weekend. I was too ignorant even to write her, let alone go back for another visit. By now Chris is two people, whoever she is for herself and a memory for me. The two will never meet.

I thought deeply into the matter. I wondered what had gone wrong. I did not have the tools to think, much less act. It was apparent to me that love had changed from the family to the larger world. Too, it was beginning to occur to me that love had an inevitably erotic component. Bluntly, knowing sex was a prerequisite to knowing love. And knowing both were prerequisites to growing up. The able-bodied have years to learn: the disabled (at least in my case) learn virtually nothing. Unlike Adam, I had not been created an adult.

I tried again. My sister fixed me up with Audrey. We met in New York, in Cinema I, the first movie without a curtain, and watched a foreign film. I have no recollection of it because I was thinking of how to touch Audrey.

Where do you touch a woman? On the arm? Perhaps a leg? Maybe you put your arm around her shoulder? Or do you try to hold her hand? But that would be too dangerous; she might not hold yours. Perhaps a breast? What about a pat on the head? Or a tweak of the ear lobe—did Audrey have ear lobes? Or a light caress on the nose? I settled on a grip of her closest shoulder. Audrey concentrated on the film. So there we were in Cinema I, Audrey watching, me clutching, afraid to let go. The end of the movie was a welcome relief to both of us.

Before the episode with Audrey, while contemplating what was to be done, I had formulated a dazzlingly simple strategy. An easy change in words would magically simplify matters with women. GO OUT. MAKE OUT. MAKE IT. But when I set about making the first of the transformations with Audrey from GO OUT to MAKE OUT, I failed utterly. I knew nothing about making out except that I was afraid. My physics teacher, Beringer, had said, "When force doesn't work, you're not using enough." I decided to reverse the order. MAKE IT. MAKE OUT. GO OUT. Maybe that was a viable progression.

"My theory went something like this. If you do the hardest thing first, everything else will be child's play. It was one of those personal theories whose function, no doubt, was linked to my disability."

My theory went something like this. If you do the hardest thing first, everything else will be child's play. It was one of those personal theories whose formation, no doubt, was linked to my disability. If the truth be known, there had been aspects of my life that had been difficult, and it had frequently been wise to tackle the hardest obstacles first.

How best to MAKE IT? Back then, there were no woman at Yale, which, as I have said before, was why I chose it in the first place. There were my sister's friends, but, as I have said, I was not on speaking terms with them.

"The plan, as it began to develop, was that Gene, Frank, and I would drive to New York, find a prostitute, and MAKE IT."

I thought of speaking to a rather dashing cousin, but I didn't know how to bring up the topic. Every route seemed a dead end, and I had no cognitive map.

Eight of us occupied single rooms on either side of a bathroom in Eero Saarinen's successful experiment in dormitory design. The plan, as it began to develop, was that Gene, Frank, and I would drive to New York, find a prostitute, and MAKE IT. It was, in part, a group effort. But we also had our individual, pressing reasons.

We left New Haven one Friday evening in my uncle's 310 horsepower, fuel-injected, two-tone Oldsmobile compact. Frank drove. (I can't drive so I took my accustomed place in the suicide seat.) Gene stretched out in the back seat. The jet-propelled hockey puck, as Gene liked to call it, averaged ninety miles an hour on its journey into New York.

I had been there but rarely. I did not know it, as I later would, to be an intimate cluster of microcosms—villages, occupations, languages, nations, worlds, ideas. That was for much later. I knew about as much about Manhattan as a teenager from Long Island. We were foreigners in New York City looking for a prostitute.

We cruised down 72nd Street. The number of people was staggering. The Olds went slowly. Traffic ran by on our sides and nudged us from the rear. I had not heard about male prostitution at the time, so I figured that the prostitutes would be female. I knew nothing about kiddie porn or runaways, so I figured that the prostitutes would be adults. I knew nothing about the life expectancy of the profession and, therefore, nothing about upper age limits. I was pretty much stuck with the possibility that half the people out there—the female half—walking the streets were, to use a word that I then thought meant just that and no more, "streetwalkers." Imagine such a rudimentary personal theory of the social world that four million New Yorkers were likely to be prostitutes!

A blonde in her early thirties walked in front of the car, smiling. Is that prostitute behavior, a blonde walking in front of a car and smiling at three college kids? Maybe there was more to it than being female.

The blonde woman got into a cab. If she was a prostitute, we had failed to make our interest in her obvious. A double problem. First, you have to figure out who the prostitute is; then you have to figure out how to make it clear to her that you're interested in her.

Women were walking quickly up and down the sidewalks. Did that mean you had to catch a prostitute? How do you catch a prostitute? Only one thing was clear; what New Haven lacked, New York had in abundance.

Gene's knowledge of the social world was, in large measure, far more extensive than mine, yet it turned out that he didn't know how to identify a prostitute either. I tried to ask a question that would not be embarrassing. "Which way should we turn?"

As we got further down Broadway, it became the Great White Way. Movie marquees. Theater marquees. Broadway at midtown is New York to many non-New Yorkers.

We slunk into Times Square, well known to all by its yearly television appearance on New Year's Eve. The traffic was starting to ease. Forty-second Street was dazzling, with movie marquee after movie marquee. Throngs, masses, hordes of people marched up and down the streets, crossing over and back, going in and out of movies and shops.

"Too many people," Frank said.

"Isn't it amazing that they don't bump into each other?" I said.

"Too many people for whores, I meant," Frank said, and he accelerated toward 34th Street.

Off to the left was a person. The person was lying down. That seemed a good bet to me. Since prostitutes practiced their profession lying down, perhaps they advertised their presence the same way. It was an attractive thought. All we would have to do is stop the car, get out, walk up; she would get up, wink at us, we would wink back, and she would lead us to her resplendent loft. Probably it would have a wall-to-wall bed, crimson drapes, and a Victorian coat rack. It occurred to me that we would have to get undressed. There would be three dressing rooms. There would be a high-fidelity system, its Fletcher Munson Curve adjusted for low-volume listening. The music would probably be Bach or maybe Byrd. Perhaps she would have partners. Then there would be three sections of wall-to-wall bed, one prostitute in charge of each. We would go upstairs and choose our prostitute from a menu. Doubtless, there would be provisions for spending the night. I, of course, would reciprocate by inviting her to Yale for the Harvard game. We would fall madly in love. I would spend many weekends in New York. She would have accepted my handicap from the outset, knowing that her love could cure me of it. After college, we would go to Europe. Then we would return to New York. I would be Dwight McDonald, she Susan Sontag. Her palace would become a salon—the Salon of the Garment District. We would have Halston in our coterie. The garment district would become the social hub of the world. The once-crippled Yalie and the one-time prostitute. What a team we would make!

Frank stopped the car and I insisted that we get out. The person on the sidewalk had an empty bottle of muscatel next to him. He also had a beard and a scruffy coat. He was snoring. There was an ulcer on his leg. A small puddle of blood oozed through a cut on his lip. "Can we be of assistance, sir?" Gene asked. The man continued snoring.

Without touching him, Gene bent over and said loudly above the man's ear, "Sir?"

The man was startled from his sleep. He looked up at us and said, "I don't have any money. Leave me be. Don't hurt me. Let me sleep." We looked at each other and returned to the car. Frank put it into drive and we continued prowling. We prowled up and down, all the way to Chelsea.

"Let's go down to the Village," Gene directed.

The Village was not as crowded as midtown. And, unlike the garment district, there were women. Definitely a place of promise. Frank shifted from prowl to cruise. Most of the women were with men. Then we saw one by herself. She was walking down Bleecker Street. "This is it," Frank said.

We followed her for a short distance, waiting for a sign. Her hand went into her purse. Perhaps this was a sign, an advertisement. She stopped abruptly and looked behind her. Her eyes stopped on the Oldsmobile. Frank was right, this was it. Then she turned around, inserted keys into a door, and disappeared.

The problem of how to approach a prostitute was academic by now. We simply couldn't find one. The truth was we didn't know how to go about it and it was getting late. We headed downtown past Houston Street, through the empty loft buildings of SoHo, through Little Italy and Chinatown. We ended up at the South Street Seaport and saw the Brooklyn Bridge.

It was 2:00 A.M. as we headed up Park Avenue toward 125th Street. Here in Harlem, our social maps were even less adequate. Harlem was not home. But searching for a prostitute at 2:30 A.M. in New York City had stretched any concept of the familiar hopelessly past our attempts to make sense of fact. The streets were just about bare. The Apollo was closed. At this hour, even the bars were closed.

Frank hung a left off 125th and went south down Lenox. The avenue was almost empty. Like the garment district after working hours, this was Lenox asleep. A young black woman in a fly-front trenchcoat was leaning against a doorway at 116th Street. She was reading. She looked up as we passed. Frank stopped the car.

"This is the place," he said.

"What place?" I asked.

"Back there, that woman," Frank answered. At 2:30 in the morning, anything was plausible.

"That woman must be out there for some reason," Gene said. By now, we surely had eliminated every other possibility in the city.

We got out of the car and walked over to her. She said, "Hello."

Frank said, "Hello." The book she was reading was *The Fall* by Albert Camus. I had just read it for a French literature course taught by Henri Peyre. Peyre was for existential leaps and had a sufficiently advanced view of courage to have dismissed Hemingway as a coward.

My heart leaping, I took an existential leap. "How do you like the book?" I asked.

"Compelling," the woman answered. "What do you boys want?" It was true, of course, that the book was compelling, as it was true that we were boys.

"Do you want to come upstairs? We have a kind of club."

She led. Frank followed. Gene next. Me last. My legs were shaking, not the tremor characteristic of my disability but a new kind of weak shake that started in my stomach. "Baby, you're scared," I thought.

I was. It was one long flight until she opened a door and we all walked into a large, dim room painted pea green. There was a small bar along one wall. "This is the palace, boys," she laughed. "It's late. All the other girls have gone home."

An old man was tending bar. "We got bourbon, rye, and Bud. Sit down and make yourselves at home." On a small radio, James Brown sang softly. "Yep, would have been a clean sweep for New York. Yankees won. Dodgers won. Giants won." Frank and Gene had Buds. I asked the man for a double bourbon. He looked at me and laughed. "You sure ready for a party!"

The woman sat at the bar. "Can I have some ginger ale, Fred?" She quickly finished it and slowly turned to us. "You get thirsty standing down there under the moon."

"At least it ain't summer," Fred said, and he laughed again.

It was not my garment district fantasy palace, but it was a warm, friendly place.

"I'm in no hurry. I sleep late Saturdays. My name is Carol."

We introduced ourselves.

"How do you want to do this?" Carol asked.

Gene and I were silent. Frank said, "I'll go first."

"All right, come right along." Carol put down her glass and she and Frank walked to a door at the back of the room. Carol opened it. She and Frank went in. The door closed.

I picked up the glass of bourbon. The shakiness spread from my stomach, through my palpitating heart, and into my arms and hands, which trembled around the glass, and mingled with the tremor of my disability. My eyes were getting used to the dim light. There were four doors off the room, two at either end. I guessed that must be where other woman conducted their business at more reasonable hours. It occurred to me that I had no concept of what the business involved. What would I do when it was my turn? The question had no answer. I pushed it away to the back of my brain and put a padlock on it.

Doubtless Gene was thinking his own thoughts. He did not speak them to me and I did not speak mine to him. We were alone, together. I asked Fred for another bourbon.

"Single or double?"

"Double." There was no saying anything, no thinking anything. I entered a glazed hibernation, a meditation, a nothingness that has left no memories. I don't know how much time passed, but Frank came out of the door and sat down at the bar.

"Who's next?" he asked, looking at Gene and me. I was no more ready than I had been when we first came upstairs.

"Why don't you go?" I said to Gene, trying to make it sound like a gracious offer.

Gene got up. He walked over to the open door. It closed behind him.

Frank was loquacious. He radiated contentment. He had accomplished what he came to do. Driving to New York, around New York for seven hours, then ending up at 116th Street and Lenox Avenue. It was all an enjoyable excursion. Now he was ready to savor it.

He asked Fred for another Bud. Frank made some joke at which Fred laughed and returned another one. Laughter had left my repertory, never mind joking. I asked Fred for another double bourbon. Frank leaned over to me and said something about it not being a good idea to drink too much at such times. I followed his advice and sipped slowly. I felt as distant from him as before from after. I returned to my state of suspension. Frank and Fred bantered somewhere distant. Again, I have no recollection of what happened or how long it was before Gene came out of the room and sat at the bar.

Gene did not have to ask me. It was obvious who was next. Gene asked for a Bud and I swallowed the last of my bourbon.

I slid off my stool and walked endless steps to the open door. Carol closed it behind me. She had on a satin robe. The room was small and the same color as the big room. There was a small dresser on one wall, coat hooks on the other, and a sink in the corner. Along the wall opposite the door was a bed. Carol walked over to the bed and sat down.

I stood still near the closed door. Carol looked at me. "Why don't you come sit here?" she asked, patting the bed. "I want to talk with you." The situation controlled me. I walked over and sat on the bed.

"I want to talk, too," I said in a voice that was not yet my own.

"This is your first time, isn't it?"

"Yes."

"Don't worry. We'll take it nice and easy. Carol put her hand on mine. "I won't rush you or anything. Tell me what you like to do."

"Read, for one."

"Me, too."

"I noticed." The voice was becoming my own.

"It gets me out of their weird life into something that makes sense."

I looked up at her. "That's why I'm here."

"How do you mean?"

"I mean, there are weird things, too many, in my life. That's why I'm here," I repeated.

"You come to Lenox Avenue and I read." We both laughed.

"You got a handicap."
"Yes," I said.
"Is that why it's your first time?"

"You got a handicap."

"Yes," I said.

"Is that why it's your first time?"

I had to think about it. "I don't know. Probably."

"Is there anything special you can't do?" she asked.

"I don't know."

"Is there anything special you want me to do?" Carol asked.

"Please go easy."

"Don't worry. I usually ask for twenty dollars up front, but you can pay me after. You want to take your clothes off? You make yourself at home," she laughed.

"Sure," I said and got undressed.

"You can hang your clothes on the hooks."

I sat down on the bed, naked. Carol took off her robe.

Once, in a city called New York, a boy, toward the end of his childhood, after a ludicrously long search, a year before he was to leave for California and France, was on Lenox Avenue and 116th Street. He met a woman named Carol. He hardly became a man overnight. But he did start a belated adolescence that, like other adolescences, lasted for many years.

I think back to then. The boy was very lucky.

Dr. Miguel Ortiz

Seated in his wheelchair when he makes rounds, Dr. Miguel Ortiz has an easy way about him, somewhat less formal than his colleagues in the spinal injury unit of this venerable English hospital. In his early thirties, he looks much younger. Two more months remain of the year he has to study rehab medicine here. As he looks at the flurries falling this spring day, he laughs gently about the less than ideal climate of England and speaks wistfully about his country, Costa Rica.

We eat a quick lunch in the buffet; he then goes up in the lift, I take the stairs, and we meet on the first floor and find an empty classroom where we can talk.

"Perhaps looking at me making my rounds encourages someone with a new spinal injury. Lying in that bed, that person knows I have been in the exact place, but now I am here, living my life."

There are incredible difficulties for people with spinal injuries to produce a child. So it was some time after being married that my wife and I really began to say we wanted a child. That doesn't mean that I never wanted one. I always wanted not one, but many, because I really love children, and I always have. We tried different things. Sometimes it worked, sometimes it didn't. Anyway, it was a long struggle for my wife to get pregnant. Both of us had to go through a great deal. I am paraplegic, my wife is able-bodied.

We were in Oxford when Anne became pregnant. It was an incredible experience knowing that Anne was pregnant; we absolutely didn't know what to say, we were so overwhelmed with happiness. My wife complained that I didn't express what I was feeling. I tried to, but all my feelings were within me, and at night, I couldn't keep from sobbing with happiness when I thought about the baby we were going to have. I think we were both worried whether the baby was going to be healthy, although I didn't talk about it. This seems to be something that everybody thinks about. Perhaps, because I am a physician, I thought of all the possibilities even more.

Anne wanted to be awake when the baby was delivered, hold the baby immediately, and breast-feed the baby. Unfortunately, she had to have a Caesarean and could not be awake for the delivery. On that day, I was glad it was a Caesarean because I didn't have to wait so long. I was so nervous waiting, it is impossible to describe it. Anne went to the operating theater at nine o'clock; I waited downstairs. I was told the baby was going to be brought down in the lift by the nurse or pediatrician. I saw that lift door open at least seven times before the baby was brought down. Finally, I saw the pediatrician; he said, "Congratulations, Doctor, you have a baby boy."

The pediatrician quickly examined the baby and gave him to me before he was even washed and cleaned. I held him in my arms and kissed him. I remember him opening his eyes. I cried for joy.

I sometimes wonder what my son's reaction to having a disabled parent will be. Hardly anything has been written about children's reactions to disabled parents. It doesn't worry me, but I wonder what his friends at school will think.

Every morning he is awake very early—five or six o'clock—and that is playtime for him. I usually get up with him, take him with me when I have breakfast. He is a very active boy who likes to be with people. Sometimes when I take a bath or shower, I sit him in his chair and take him right in with me. He doesn't like to be alone.

"My wife complained that I didn't express what I was feeling. I tried to, but all my feelings were within me, and at night, I couldn't keep from sobbing with happiness when I thought about the baby we were going to have."

I like basketball a lot; I will teach my son to play. But I know I will not be able to play football with him.

Recently, some good papers have been written about sexuality and people with spinal injury. If a physician is interested, he or she ought to give the patient information.

But if the physician is uncomfortable, for whatever reason, another person should be found to give the support that is needed. In most instances, I think the person who can give some advice will have to be paraplegic or quadriplegic himself. It is a delicate and a vast topic; there are so many things to be understood. We first have to fully understand "normal" sexual function. When giving sexual information, people can be the most effective if they do not put their own sexuality into play. In a way, the physician, or the one who is helping, should forget his or her own sexuality and prejudices.

One problem is that the ignorance about sex is so widespread. Very few medical schools in the world have sex education. Often those that do include this in their curriculum are archaic. Physicians really do not know about sex, not any more than the person on the street. Nondisabled people have so many sexual problems. If a person has sexual problem, becomes quadriplegic, and the doctors themselves have sexual problems, we are not going to get anywhere!

Just today, a friend who is taking a course in urology was told by his professor that all persons with spinal injury are completely impotent! If a professor of urology can say that, you can imagine the amount of misinformation that surrounds this subject.

I think there is a myth surrounding anyone with a disability. Because you're in a wheelchair, or have any defect whatever, most physicians think you will not need information regarding sex. Doctors are surprised when disabled women ask for contraception or ask how they should take precautions against becoming pregnant. These same doctors would never go to bed with any woman with a disability and, therefore, really cannot be objective.

I wouldn't want to make a big problem of it; it has its complications, but often it can be rather simple. People need additional advice and encouragement and often find their own way.

I have lived through all the stages the patients I take care of will experience. I want to do many things for the paralyzed people of my country. Maybe when they see our little boy and the happiness I have found, it will show that there are great possibilities for us all.

David

When people are disabled, the questions they ask most often, even before discussing their bowel and bladder function, relate to their sexuality. "Am I still a man?" "Will someone still want me?" The neurosurgeons at the clinic told me a few things, but they didn't tell me much. On Tuesday afternoons, there was an "education" session. They brought out an old-fashioned skeleton and went through a lot of the medical details of what all of us had suffered. The first session was six weeks after my accident. I was twenty-five.

Then I took part in an experiment called S.A.R., Sexual Attitude Reassessment. They probably made it more difficult, made us more self-conscious, because they showed a bunch of dirty movies. Even if I were not in a wheelchair, I think I would have felt uncomfortable because I do not like voyeurism. I was conscious of the fact that there were several women in the session, the nurses, and I was embarrassed; we all were embarrassed to different degrees.

They didn't talk about sex very much. They said you won't really know until you get back with your wife or your girlfriend, so don't worry about it. Sex certainly was important to me, but I wanted to walk more than I wanted to have intercourse.

Basically, they told us that we could do all kinds of cunnilingus but forget it as far as our phallus was concerned. On an intellectual level, that made sense, but on a gut level, I felt, okay, I can be some kind of pervert but forget it as far as straight sex is concerned. Everyone was kind of embarrassed when the lights came on, including the doctor.

One of the first questions I asked him, and it is one of the questions I am still asking, had to do with reactions and feelings. I was interested in a loving relationship with a woman that didn't seem to involve just the mechanics. It is hard to produce a porno film that portrays feelings because it has so much to do with mechanics. It is like something out of *Mechanics Illustrated*—a how-to—but it has nothing to do with feelings. That was something that made the doctor very uncomfortable, too.

There was something almost bizarre about the fact that we were being shown porno flicks while at the same time we were being told we probably couldn't have an erection. There was a lot of silence in the room. A lot of people were really shocked but would not admit it. Of course, so much depends on your orientation before your injury. There were those who were perhaps trying to figure out what they were going to do about all this, but nobody wanted to talk about it.

I had a girlfriend while I was in rehab. We did a lot of petting in the hospital, in corridors, at the end of halls. She did a lot of sitting on my lap. She waited for me until I finally got out of rehab and then dumped me for a lion tamer. She followed me from the beginning, then she dumped me.

I had a catheter but I never worried about it too much. In my initial relationships after the accident, most sex was above the waist. I didn't think too much about the catheter; I guess I figured I'd get rid of it eventually.

At the clinic recently, I was talking to a young intern. He asked me what I was "trained" to do sexually, and I told him what I was "trained" to do in 1971 and he quite defensively said, "Well, yes, but we've come a long way since then." This doctor offered me nothing, but he talked big—he talked penile implants. There was another doctor who was a very decent man. He talked to me, but I never got any conclusive answers.

"There was something almost bizarre about the fact that we were being shown porno flicks while at the same time we were being told we probably couldn't have an erection."

One very interesting thing he said—I sound so matter of fact about this, though I don't feel matter of fact about it—is that most spinal cord injured men who are in wheelchairs are infertile because they sit on wheelchair cushions a lot and the heat changes the temperature of the scrotum. Not many people know about this. If the doctors do know, they very often don't remember to tell you. In some hospitals, freezing sperm immediately after a man sustains a spinal cord injury has become routine. Too bad they didn't do it in 1971.

I've had a lot of building up of sexual urge, blood pressure increase, but no catharsis. If I ever had a catharsis at all, it was only cerebral. Since my injury, I have not been able to have any real sexual satisfaction as I knew it before. I am not sure if I felt confident that I could please a woman, and to this day, I am not sure. If the woman were satisfied with love and some mechanics, then yes, but if she wanted vaginal orgasm, perhaps with some adaptations, I would go to that extent. But I'm not sure of the pleasure I'd get out of it myself. Since the accident, I have never had an erection that I know of.

One thing I still cannot understand has to do with the fact that as much as things have changed in the 1980s and as much as there have been textbooks and sex is now permissible, there seems to be a lack of alignment. They are still showing porno films, and they are still kind of gung ho on sexuality training, almost to the point of it being extreme. I think that it has to do with sexuality, with sex. We have the professionals in one corner and the spinal cord injured in another corner. Whether they lied to you or whether they just didn't know, they were uncomfortable discussing sexuality. I believe they have the medical books written now—on everything from saving sperm to having intercourse. Now they immediately counsel the wife, the girlfriend, as well as the disabled person.

"Whether they lied to you or whether they just didn't know, they were uncomfortable discussing sexuality. I believe they have the medical books written now—on everything from saving sperm to having intercourse. Now they immediately counsel the wife, the girlfriend, as well as the disabled person."

Physicians are still defining disabled people to society. Disabled people are seen as patients by physicians. I think there is a lot of confusion about sexual training, permission-giving, and love. People have gone from one extreme to another, from no talk on sexuality, sex, to encouraging everybody to get into bed and somehow make it. People have gone from ignoring the subject, from a Victorian type of ignorance and ignoring, to a professional, mechanical, technological presentation of sex to help us turn on our ladies so that we can hold on to them. On the one hand, it is realistic and practical. If I were married and one day had an accident that rendered me a paraplegic, I would hope that my wife would be with me, that our marriage was built on more than just sexual performance.

"Who would want me? I cannot answer the question; perhaps I cannot yet deal with it."

I would like to have a sensitive psychologist-type person talk to me about my sexuality. It really doesn't matter to me whether they are sitting or standing; what really matters is competence. And empathy. That is an added dimension, though sometimes, just because people are disabled, they are not as a result necessarily more understanding, more competent, and more able to work with other disabled people. They, too, have their own problems, do a lot of denying, and may come on as being superior and indignant and aloof in the face of another's lesser proficiency.

Who would want me? I cannot answer the question; perhaps I cannot yet deal with it. There were women before my injury, and there were women after.

I want information and help, not sympathy. Sympathy—I can't eat it, I can't wear it, I can't spend it, and I can damn well do without it.

I am a loving human being, and it is a strong dream, a strong wish of mine to be with a woman. My ability to love hasn't changed. I may have a heightened awareness of love. It is within me, I know. If I found the right woman, I wouldn't hesitate to marry.

Am I a man? Deep down inside me, I am the same, but on the surface, I am not. But still, I am a man.

TIPS ON FINDING A SEXUALITY COUNSELOR

Pamela Boyle, a sexuality counselor certified by the American Association of Sex Educators, Counselors, and Therapists, is coordinator of the Reproductive Health Care and Disability Program at the Margaret Sanger Center of Planned Parenthood of New York City.

Boyle shares these thoughts regarding sexuality and disability:

- ***One sexual attitude reassessment (S.A.R.) doth not a sexuality and disability counselor make! The best of all possible worlds would be to find a counselor who has experience and knowledge in disability as well as sexuality, who can put the two areas together.***

- ***Look for a counselor with experience—it isn't impossible to find someone who has five or six years of counseling/therapy experience these days. There are some good professionals around.***

- ***Don't assume just because someone calls him or herself a sex counselor that the individual has particular training or expertise.***

- ***Don't assume that a person who knows about spinal cord injury will know about mental retardation or that the person who knows about sexuality and cerebral palsy will know about sexuality and people with ostomies, etc.***

- ***Sexuality and relationships are very emotional topics for many people—especially when they are causing you difficulties. Seek out the best for yourself when looking for a counselor!***

- ***There are many family planning/reproductive health care clinics that would welcome people with disabilities but that know very little about serving a person with unique needs. Individuals with a disability can be very helpful to health care providers by making their needs known and by patiently assisting them to understand what is needed in terms of help in transferring, dressing/undressing, etc. Most providers will be very appreciative to receive this information and will do their best to make a visit the very best that it can be.***

- ***Disabled women should educate themselves about the various methods of contraception, trying to find out as much as possible about the possible contraindications related to one's own disability. Many doctors are not aware of special contraceptive needs of individuals with disabilities.***

Sources of Information

Independent living centers, rehab centers, and United Cerebral Palsy chapters in some places have sexuality counseling available.

In addition, Planned Parenthood, listed in the telephone book and with affiliates throughout the country, provides reproductive health care services to men and women, with great emphasis placed on counseling and education.

Not all Planned Parenthood affiliates have a stated commitment to working with people who have disabilities nor are all centers accessible.

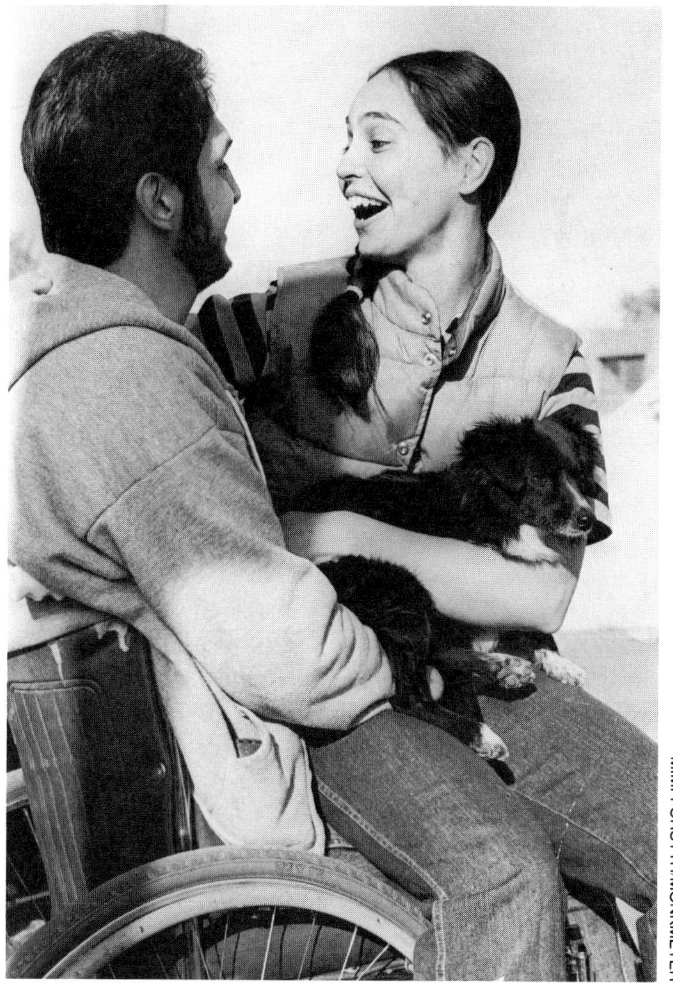

MIMI FORSYTH/MONKMEYER

Jim Weisman

Jim Weisman understands the civil rights laws for disabled citizens, and he is willing to explain them in understandable words.

Jim approached several questions put to him about a law this way: there is should, could, and are. In this way, it was simple to see what the law stated (should); what could be done to fulfill it; and what actions are actually taking place.

There is a law in the state of New York that makes it an illegal discriminatory practice to refuse admission to people with disabilities at a place of public accommodation. Not meant to be exhaustive, it then lists public places, every place you could think of where people go.

Four or five years ago, we had a case of a woman who was a former Olympic medalist in swimming, who went to a public place and wanted to use the pool. She was now disabled and required the use of a wheelchair. The only criterion for admission was residency, and she met that. She was told, "You cannot come in; you can only use the pool between the hours of two and four on weekday afternoons if you are orthopedically disabled because those are lower use times. Then you may only use the facilities if you pass a special test administered by the lifeguard."

The woman said, "This is baloney; you only test people in wheelchairs and in braces and on crutches?" And they said yes. She had the gumption to say, "Nonsense," but they still wouldn't let her in. Since she could swim better than most people who used the pool, she seemed like the ideal plaintiff. We called the parks commissioner. He was immovable. So we sued. Their position was that disabled people would be dangerous to themselves and to everyone else in a public pool.

I asked them to explain. They said disabled people would jump in water they couldn't swim in. As if physical disability means you are so stupid you are likely to jump into water you can't swim in! As if amputation of a leg removes a degree of intellect! Strange as it seems, the man I spoke with had that belief. He also said disabled people would be dangerous to the safety of everyone else because the lifeguard would pay more attention to them to the detriment of others. I asked him wouldn't the lifeguard pay more attention to a woman in a bikini? He answered that he supposed the lifeguard would. The effect is the same: the lifeguard's attention would be somewhat diverted, yet they were only prohibiting women in wheelchairs and not women in tiny bathing suits. He said if they were *really* tiny bikinis, they didn't let them in. We walked out of there laughing, thinking we were going to win the case.

But we lost! The judge's decision said that disabled people would be dangerous to themselves and dangerous to everyone else. The law says you can't discriminate in this manner—it is a place of public accommodation—but that is exactly what they did!

"The effect is the same: the lifeguard's attention would be somewhat diverted, yet they were only prohibiting women in wheelchairs and not women in tiny bathing suits. He said if they were really *tiny bikinis, they didn't let them in. We walked out of there laughing, thinking we were going to win the case. But we lost!"*

This proves that judges and politicians don't make public opinion, they reflect it. If the judge's opinion was unpopular, he wouldn't have the public's support. This issue was a popular notion, which is why he supported it. The other point I think it proves is worse, and I would like to think it is subconscious on the part of the court. Somewhere in this man was the thought, "I'm not getting in the pool with that woman." And he squirmed and he twisted and he contorted his legal opinion and legal reasoning to make it consistent with his desire not to swim in a pool with this disabled woman. I don't know how much of an element that was, but I think it was there, at least subconsciously.

That type of attitude is not innate, it is acquired. Children go up to disabled people and talk to them. It is only when their mothers drag them away that they think something is wrong. Perhaps the judge acquired this attitude in his childhood and behaves that way as an adult. But I think this attitude can be changed.

"If disabled people keep asserting themselves over and over again, the same thing will happen. Activism is the farthest thing from protectionism and patronization. Most able-bodied people patronize and most disabled people accept patronization."

There are some things that people just logically differ on. Should an epileptic be a policeman?; should he work with caustic chemicals?; should someone with a hearing disability drive a bus? You might say yes, others might say no, and some people might be annoyed with the ultimate decision, but the fact that there is even an issue is a positive step. It is possible that as people more and more often bring cases to the courts, perhaps, in a sense, this can take on positive symbolism.

The women's movement is a good example. I was a teenager when women marched down Fifth Avenue and burned their bras. A lot of people thought it was a joke. Of course, bra burning was symbolic. The whole women's movement was kind of laughed off. However, fifteen years later, the world is a different place. Even if you are a sexist, you are a different sexist than you were.

If disabled people keep asserting themselves over and over again, the same thing will happen. Activism is the farthest thing from protectionism and patronization. Most able-bodied people patronize and most disabled people accept patronization.

The present economic situation is slowing up the movement substantially. When you take food off people's tables, they worry more about eating than how other people feel about them. We used to be able to call on different organizations for support. Now when we call them, they say, "Are you kidding? We're drowning. We're losing this. We're losing that!" Everyone has his own problems now because the government is pulling out of funding a lot of programs. A lot of new obstacles are in the way, and people are going to have to start over again. But they won't be starting from square one.

There are many more educated people out there. The effect of this is that disabled people have been educated. There are people who know things and want to do things and have abilities and desires. And their disabilities won't stop them from implementing those things. The perception that disabled people have of themselves has changed. I think able-bodied people still think of disabled people as either heroic or pathetic. What they don't realize is that disabled people are just people and, if educated and given a skill, they can do something. It is the same with everybody else; it is not heroic, it is human nature. What you want to do, what I want to do, what anybody else wants to do is basically to be needed. It is a question of being a contributing member of society.

Susan Lo Tempio

Susan Lo Tempio comes into a favorite coffeehouse on Telegraph Avenue in Berkeley, and a number of young men look up and acknowledge her loveliness. Things are going just right—some good friends, a job she likes, and a nice place to live.

It is obvious California agrees with her, and we talk about it. "I guess I am another Easterner who has made the trip out here, and it feels right," she says, "but I could live in any number of places. Probably, it has to do with feeling at home first with yourself, and the rest falls into place.

"Life is very exciting. I am just beginning to realize what is going on for me now. It is a pulling together of a lot of things; moving to a place that I like and feel comfortable in. I have a good job, new friends, good friends, new male relationships, and I am learning to take care of myself. If my car breaks down, I don't panic. I can take care of it. My life is together now."

In college, I dated both disabled and nondisabled men. I cannot remember a time when I dated a nondisabled man that was a really good relationship. It took me until now to get all that straightened out—the differences. When I first came to California, I dated a disabled man for nearly a year. But he could not accept *my* disability, and I later learned from other disabled women that he never had dated a disabled woman before me and they were absolutely shocked that we had dated. That kind of awakened me. Now I don't even know any disabled men in this town, to really know them.

I have finally come through a crucial issue. It is about security. I think people sometimes date disabled people because they feel secure; they don't have to prove themselves. That security is what I have developed. I don't feel that I have any prejudice against either. I just feel I like some disabled men because I like them—it has nothing to do with the chair particularly—and some I don't. I think a man is a man is a man is a man.

They are all alike, in a lot of ways, I think. The whole liberation issue gets to me. You have to be on your guard all the time, especially a woman facing the disability issue as well as the feminism issue. It is double messages, double cues. I don't know if a lot of women with disabilities have really plugged in to how they feel about this.

We were brought up to feel—to be—dependent, to want to be dependent. Mom wanted to take care of us. Dad wanted to take care of us. And then you read about feminism, where you are independent, you can do what you want. First of all, you have to incorporate that into yourself and believe in yourself. When you finally believe that you are an independent, liberated woman, the rest of the world still treats you like you are a disabled, dependent woman, and it drives you nuts!

"When you finally believe that you are an independent, liberated woman, the rest of the world still treats you like you are a disabled, dependent woman, and it drives you nuts!"

According to certain feminist doctrines, to be whistled at is very gauche, you don't want that kind of crap, and yet you love it. Why not, especially if you've never been whistled at, were the only person in your high school with a disability, and haven't gone through these things?

I struggle with that constantly. I love to be whistled at, and I love to have goo-goo eyes made at me, and I'm not supposed to! I just reject that part of the feminist doctrine. But the other side of it is that I am free to ask a man out. I am free to be equal to a man. That has helped me because I don't have to sit around waiting for some guy to call me, who may be kind of taken over by the disability and is uncomfortable. And so, I can make the first move.

There is something that is going on, and that is using feminism to be neuter: not dressing up, being nonsexual, being nonsensuous. One would be taking a risk putting on mascara at this point. In some places, you are a traitor to the feminist movement if you start putting on makeup again. The woman with a disability has a foot in both worlds—

"I feel very liberated at this point. It took me ten years to get where I am. I have recently come to the realization that for the first time in my life, I am really happy and content."

and is standing on stilts. How does she balance it?

When I was working in Washington, D.C., two years ago, I got really involved in the disabled rights movement. That, for me, was more important than the women's movement, mostly because I was in it. But what that taught me was that we are all in the same boat. We are all into human rights, so that is why I reject some of the tenets of the women's movement that I feel are stupid. I just ignore those things, and yet I don't feel that I am rejecting the women's movement. I am for people's rights, whether disabled, women, or blacks. I don't have to get involved in the way-out stuff, though we still get involved with the coalition of lesbian rights.

And, though I don't work with some of the way-out stuff, I still support it. It is a struggle, struggle, struggle. Women are letting go of the marriage dream. I would marry; I am not for it, and I am not against it. I don't want to be married right now. I have a hope that eventually I will, but not yet.

I feel very liberated at this point. It took me ten years to get where I am. I have recently come to the realization that for the first time in my life, I am really happy and content. I can go with whatever happens now because I have reached a point that I have wanted to reach.

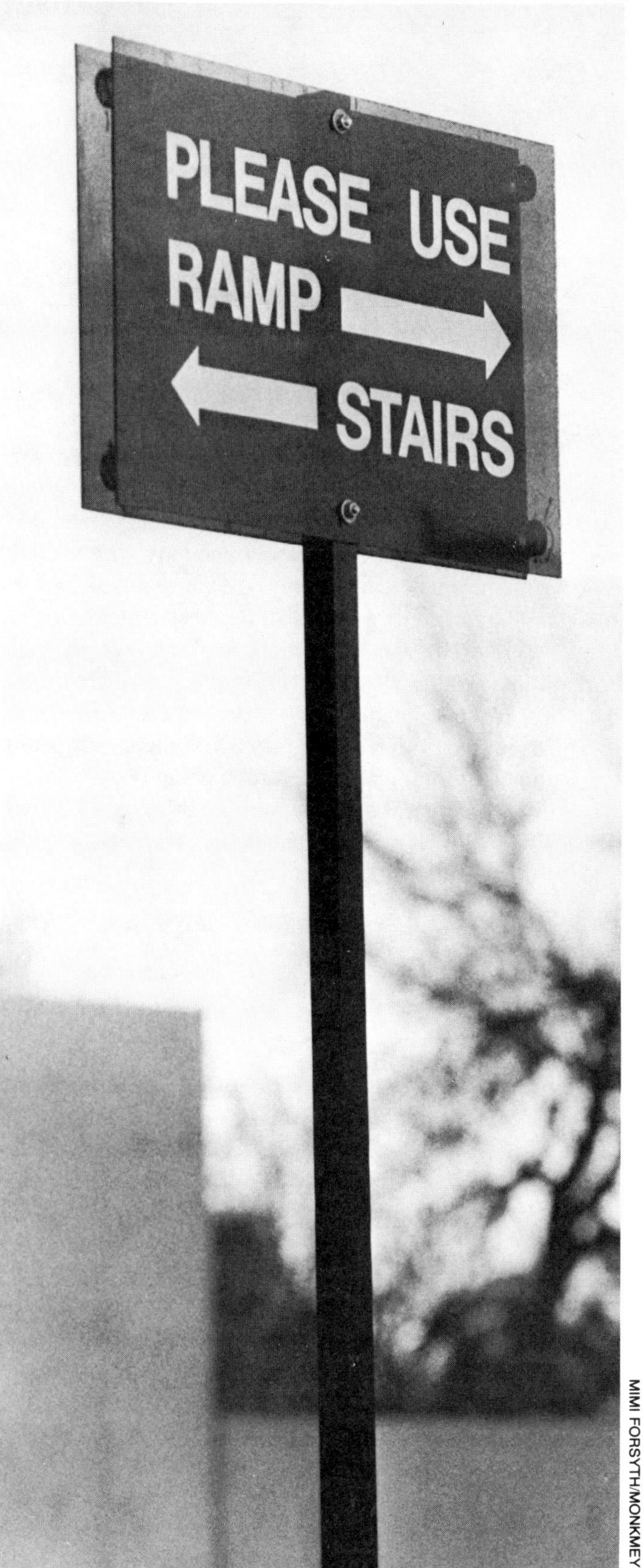

MIMI FORSYTH/MONKMEYER

John Kurlowicz

My wife would come to visit me—we were young married people—and we had the same desires that most young married couples have.

The fact that one is incarcerated in a hospital does not remove the desires that you've got.

When my wife was around, two or three nurses would make absolutely certain that the curtains around my bed were all open. But there was one particular nurse who asked me if I wanted the curtains closed when my wife visited; I said yes. She made damn sure they were closed, and she also stood guard. Obviously, that nurse became our friend!

I've often thought about this attitude and society's need to look upon physically disabled people as sexually neuter. Part of it is the assumption that everybody must perform in the missionary position and, if they don't, there is something very unusual, pornographic, or dirty going on.

Consequently, it's not possible to think of a man who can't lift up his arm or a woman who can't walk getting pleasure in another position or way.

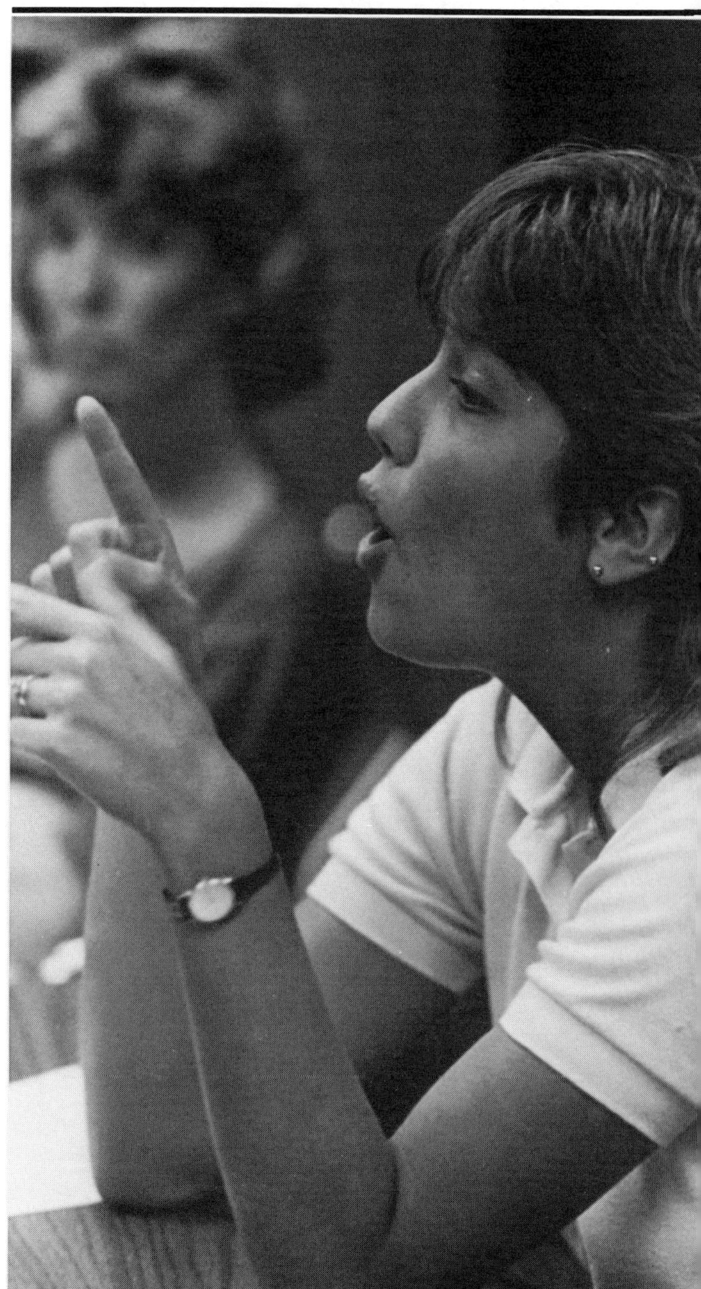

At Gallaudet University class participation is conducted in Total Communication—sign language, speech, and sign spelling.

Nina Myers

Without my hearing aids, I don't hear much of anything—a truck going by or a dog barking, maybe. Hearing aids only amplify sound a person already has. They can't give you hearing that you do not have.

To hear, I have to concentrate very hard and at the same time read lips for the sounds I don't hear, the words I miss. When I talk, I know the lip movements and how it feels. That's how I can talk.

It's hard for me on a first date. I'm nervous, I guess, like anyone else, and if we go into a dark restaurant, I can't read my date's lips. If I can't see, I can't hear, so sometimes I've said yes when what I meant was no. It can get pretty embarrassing! A lot of people don't know I'm hearing impaired because my speech is pretty good. I went out with a guy in college—I never told him. I went out with him for two months, and he started getting really serious about me. Then I told him that I had a hearing loss, that I wore hearing aids. I never heard from him after that—never! I knew it had to be that because he had already told me how he felt about me.

But with some people, I just can't talk about it because I feel they won't understand; they don't have the empathy to deal with the situation. I feel if I met someone, a man with normal hearing, and he asked me out a couple of times, then I would tell him. But it depends. If the person is open-minded, I would talk about it.

"I'm between two worlds . . . I was brought up in the hearing world, but because I am deaf, I am not part of the hearing world. I am deaf, but I didn't grow up in the deaf world, so I don't belong there, either."

Sometime ago, the TV show "60 Minutes" interviewed a young woman from Gallaudet College. She was deaf, and she talked about her boyfriend, who was also deaf. Mike Wallace asked her, "How does it make it different—loving someone who's deaf?" I really liked her answer. "What difference can it make if you love someone?"

But, you see, I'm in a different position altogether. I'm between two worlds. I really am. I've gone out with a couple of deaf men, but I don't feel comfortable with them. Yet I don't really feel comfortable among hearing people. I was brought up in the hearing world, but because I am deaf, I am not part of the hearing world. I am deaf, but I didn't grow up in the deaf world, so I don't belong there, either. Very often, I'm tired—maybe confused is a better word—sometimes I'm both tired and confused.

When I was younger, I don't think it affected me as much. I remember wearing my hair pulled back and having my hearing aids exposed. Everyone saw them. When I got to be an adolescent, I became very self-conscious about the way I looked. I wore my hair covering my hearing aids. Even now, I won't wear my hair back.

"I wonder if, down deep, I'm not apologizing because I feel like damaged merchandise."

I am the only teacher who is deaf in a school for the deaf, and I had to fight for that teaching position. I can speak and make myself understood; this probably gives parents some hope. I always speak, but throughout the day, I sign; and I teach the children signing.

When I'm not teaching, I'm physically very active. I love to go camping, play tennis, jog. I belong to a tennis club, mostly singles. I've met a lot of nice people, and my social life is not too bad (it's not too great, either). Some experiences have been very disappointing; that goes for everyone, I guess. Maybe I take it a little harder. I wonder if, down deep, I'm not apologizing because I feel like damaged merchandise.

Karen Malkin

Socially, the most painful time for me was when I was a teenager. As a young adolescent, even when I was feeling kind of good about myself, looking nice, I'd still walk out and think, "No matter how nice I look, I still walk funny. Well, that's life." Or if I was walking down the street, feeling good, and someone laughed at me, that was a real downer. It is very painful, particularly when you are a teenager, struggling so much with how you feel about yourself, your desirability, your attractiveness.

My family was always supportive of me academically. But I don't think they thought I had much social potential; not that they discouraged me . . . but just that they never encouraged me. I remember one day I said something like, "Mom, I'm never going to get married." My mother said, "You never can tell," not, "What do you mean, you'll never get married? Of course, you will!" She herself was not too sure. Very often, the message was not so explicit, but it

"Some people assume that if you are disabled, you can't have a social life or a sex life. This reflects one's own fears that unless one looks terrific physically, he or she will not be wanted. This is very potent stuff."

was, nonetheless, implied. I was never pushed to go out to social affairs. My mother never asked me questions about boyfriends or asked me why I wasn't going out. Kids who went out complained, "How come my mother asks me all these questions?" In some ways, you need those questions. I needed them to validate the fact that I was a woman, a female, and that I was desirable. I think now, in a way, some women with disabilities are flattered by sexism because when someone acts toward you in a sexist manner, the message you get is, "I am a woman." It stinks, but at least it is a validation of one's sexuality, and that is very important.

Some people assume that if you are disabled, you can't have a social life or a sex life. This reflects one's own fears that unless one looks terrific physically, he or she will not be wanted. This is very potent stuff.

"You've heard the old cliché that says, 'If you take yourself seriously, other people will, too.' There is a grand, grand truth in that."

We are all desirable; each of us has sexual potential. It is part of us someplace, somewhere. There is opportunity—it is not easy, but there is potential—if you look for it. We are all sexual by definition; it is part of our existence. Unless people are in a bad state psychologically, the sexual feelings are there waiting to be discovered.

It is damn hard the first time you go out on a date; you get scared to death! I am thirty-three years old, and I guess it is only in the past six or seven years that I've had anything resembling a social life. I was really amazed how easy my first date was. I had an image of dating being the most impossible situation, the "How can *I* ever go out on a date?" type of attitude. Yet it's not so hard. I imagined immediate rejection—"Hello, how are you? Goodbye!" Sometimes that did happen; fortunately, not on the first date. But a number of men didn't reject me and, of course, you discover men who want you and whom you don't choose. There is nothing sacred about "catching a man" or touching a partner. It is a matter of finding someone who can satisfy you.

You've heard the old chiché that says, "If you take yourself seriously, other people will, too." There is a grand, grand truth in that."

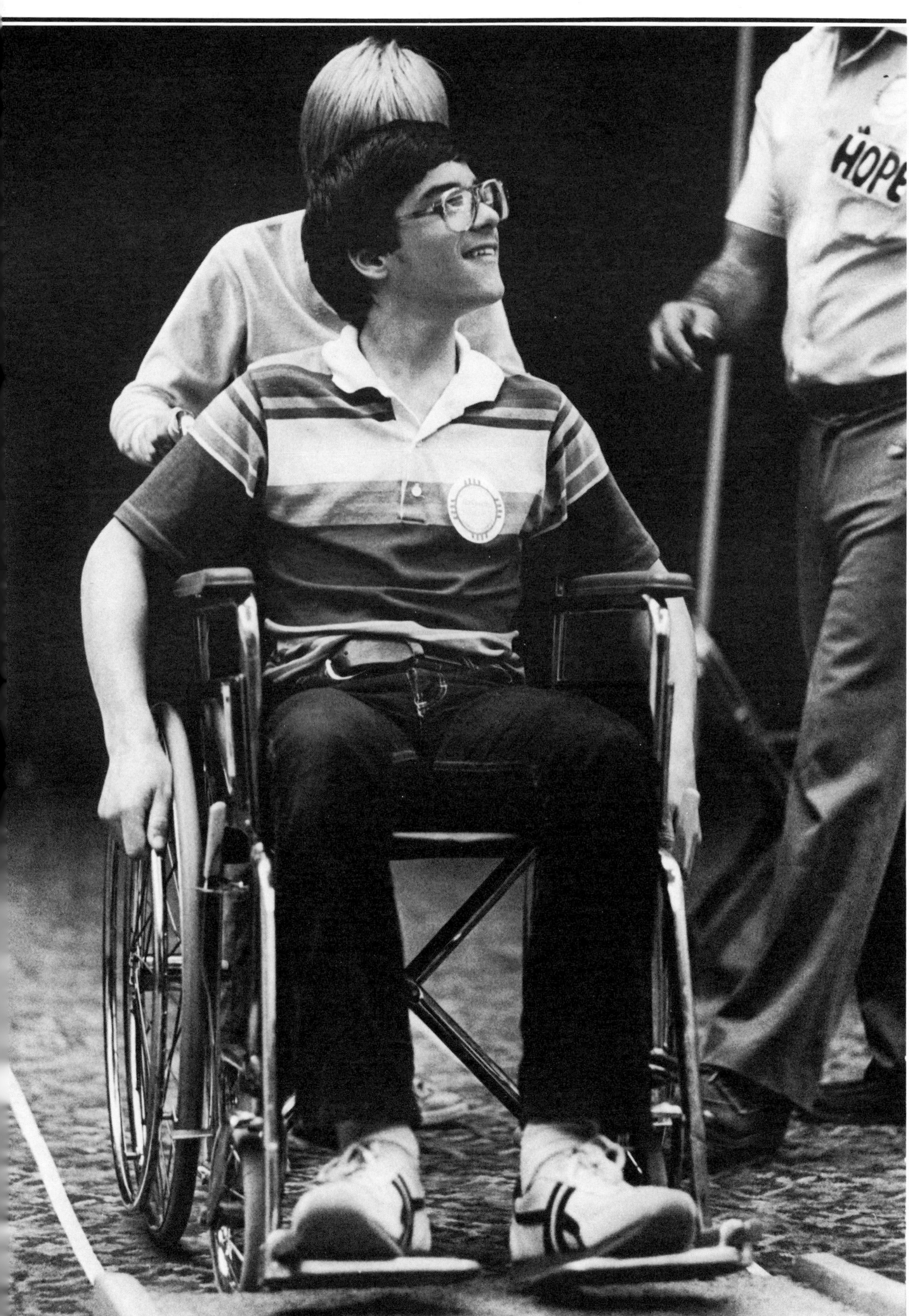

MIMI FORSYTH/MONKMEYER

In Albuquerque, this student participates in a sensitivity training workshop where he helps people without disabilities learn how to better understand people with disabilities.

Joanne Juarequi

The sun floods the space set aside for deaf services at the Center of Independent Living (CIL) in Berkeley, California. Three women sit enjoying the direct eye contact rarely experienced by people new to one another outside the deaf community.

The interpreter translates for Joanne Juarequi and me. After a few minutes of looking almost simultaneously at my lips and at the interpreter's signs, she asks me if I have a New York accent. "Sure!" I answer, laughing. "I thought so; I could tell," she says, a little proudly.

She is the director of deaf services. Her friendliness, quick humor, and eagerness to be a part of this work is so exciting that I lose track of time and miss my plane back to New York. We are friends; of that, there is no doubt. Our determination to share transcends any obstacle. When I leave, we hug each other, and my eyes fill with tears. We both sign, "I love you."

My hearing family went through bad times because of my deafness. I pitied them—my mother and father, my brother—I have given them a hard time. I remember my mother would tell me not to do something and I rejected her authority. My poor mother had a pretty bad time growing up with me. I was so stubborn and rebellious. I didn't listen because I had a hearing problem, I guess.

When I was growing up, my family would discuss things at dinner time and they would leave me out. I would say, "What are you talking about?" and they would answer, "Oh, never mind. It is not important." They never really explained. They treated me like a little girl. So I decided to read a book. I read a lot. I read for communication; I read for company, companionship. I felt left out of the hearing group. I'd love to have had an interpreter with me to explain what they were saying so I would not have felt so left out.

My mother said that you must fight to be involved but must first accept being alone. I accepted the idea that I would always be left out anyway. When I came home with a bloody nose or with a black eye, my mother would know that a kid from my neighborhood had made fun of me and had jumped me, beaten me up. She would run and tell the mothers of those children to leave me alone. She was protecting me. At the time, I didn't understand why they beat me up, so I became a fighter. And when they wanted to jump on me, I found ways to protect myself.

But my family jumped me in their own way, by excluding me from their conversation. They felt they had no time to communicate with me about what was happening at the dinner table. I felt that they had lots of important things to talk about. And I did, too. But we were in poor communication. So I read. I could pick up a lot of stories that were better than my family's stories.

A person gets mixed up if he or she can't count on the people who are close. My mother and brother were very close; I was closer to my father. I felt isolated a lot, but my father gave me a lot of strong support. I could hear a little, and he was the one I could understand best because I could hear the sound of his voice. It was a very strong, loud voice. It helped a lot. We played games together.

I remember my father was concerned about my learning ability and worried that I was a slow learner or something. So he decided to see how much I could learn by teaching me to play chess. When I was about seven, he taught me the rules and then challenged me to a game. I gave him a hard time. He told my mother they didn't have to worry about my learning abilities. He said, "She can learn real fast!"

Somebody grows up in a family and then decides they are going to do it very differently in their own family when they have one. So I chose to marry a deaf man because of the communication and also because I loved him very much. Ninety-five percent of deaf people marry others who are deaf because of the language barrier. Because I cannot communicate as well with hearing people, they leave me flat. Hearing people talk and communicate with one another, and I stand and hear nothing. I can't follow anything, so many times I feel left out. I can lip read, but I can't lip read everybody. And I get lost so easily in a large group.

Since both my husband and I are deaf, we have to look at each other a lot, and that is one of the good things about communicating in sign language. Our life is both hectic and calm. It depends upon the situation.

I first met him in the Haight Ashbury area in San Francisco. He told me he was deaf, but I couldn't believe it because he could talk so well and hearing people were always talking with him. He could follow what they said. I asked him if he was hard of hearing, and he said, "Oh, yeah. I am severely hard of hearing . . . I am deaf." I became attracted to him and his stories and different ideas. We decided to get married and have a baby. That scared me because I married pretty late and I didn't think that I would have children. I thought it would take me a long time to figure out what I wanted. Then I found myself pregnant.

I was scared at first. I didn't know if I would be a good mother. That was the big question. But I had worked with deaf kids for many years, as a teacher, and I had always liked kids. I worried about the baby being deaf and having to move back East, where they had better schools for the deaf.

We have two daughters. One is twelve and the other is eleven. When the girls were babies, I was a teacher of deaf children and my husband was a bum. So I gave him the babies to raise himself. I figured if he got a job, he wouldn't have as good a salary as mine teaching, plus three months vacation in the summer, two weeks at Christmas, and a week at Easter. We decided it would be best for me to stay with my teaching job and he could stay at home and bring up the kids for the first six years. Imagine, he was a househusband! He was very proud of that because it was a new idea.

"A person gets mixed up if he or she can't count on the people who are close."

Meanwhile, he was thinking of what type of work he would like to do when the girls were older. I was offered a better teaching job, paying about $400 more a month, so we moved from San Francisco to San Mateo and bought a little house not too far from the school where I was teaching. My husband was still considering what type of job he wanted to do. I remember that in March I came home from work one day and told him that I had lost my job—I had been laid off. My husband jumped up and said, "Who is going to feed this family?" I told him that he would have to go out and find a job because I wanted to stay home for a while myself. He saw many listings under "Job Placement Agencies," and he looked for one that might serve deaf people. I was teasing him and said, "Why don't you set up one yourself?" And he said, "Yes. That's right; that's the right idea." And he did that. He went to his church in San Francisco and asked for office space, and his office has been expanding ever since. He now has two branch offices, one in Oakland and one in Fremont.

It's great because we can work together and discuss how to develop the kinds of programs badly needed by deaf people who are looking for jobs but who are unsure of how to go about it and who need someone who understands their problems from firsthand experience. My husband takes care of their needs. He can make phone calls with an amplifier on the receiver (he has a very small amount of hearing) but, at the same time, he needs an interpreter to pick up an extension. His hearing, limited to start with, is dropping; it is going down with age. People very often think he hears for himself, but it is not true. He speaks for himself on the phone, and he can convince employers to hire deaf people. So far, in the five years that it has been going on, it has been a very good program.

He was not born deaf and I was born deaf from unknown causes, so I was not really surprised to have hearing babies. When they were growing up, for perhaps the first three years, there was a little bit of confusion. When Jewel was two years old, she would say to me, "I have big ears and you have small ears." I would reply, "Yes, that's right. You can hear all the noises and I can't hear the noises. You do have big ears." It was cute. If I had grown up in a family where I wasn't the only deaf member, maybe I would feel differently, maybe I would say, "I am proud to be deaf. I want deaf children."

Even though their parents are deaf, the girls don't feel very different from other kids. They are used to seeing disabled people around, and that helps them. Their friends want to communicate in sign language, and so my girls teach them. The girls are bilingual—they talk and sign. They feel good about that. I am glad for them because I understand that sometimes in other parts of the country, not just where I grew up, hearing children from deaf families suffer.

As the girls grow up, I see they are learning fast, compared with my experience as an adolescent; their language is amazing, and they pick things up so fast. Now in their teens, both talk on the phone for the longest time. I never did that myself. When I was eleven, twelve, thirteen, no one could ever call me. Maybe I am jealous. Now I call my friends on a TTY [teletypewriter]; we type our messages to one another.

I guess I don't have to be jealous anymore. I now have many friends. The girls keep telling me I have lots of my own friends—we just communicate differently.

Penny and Greg

When you talk about success, I guess you want to talk about overcoming a disability, mine being my emotional disability and the larger one being my epilepsy.

To begin with, I was all by myself until I found someone in a similar position, Penny. She had strong ties to her family, but she was trying to be independent, trying to learn how to work and be on her own. Penny and I met five years ago at the workshop, and we started dating. We went to the movies, and we talked; mostly, we talked. At one point, I was having a series of seizures and got really depressed and couldn't get out of bed. The last thing I needed was a girlfriend; it was just too much for me, so we broke up for a while. Later, Penny and I got back together, and that's when very positive things started happening for both of us. We decided to live together. We found an apartment, and we borrowed some money from Penny's dad and then we called her mother. I loved it when she said she had never told Penny about sex because we had been working on that for several months. Penny's sister was very important in our relationship because she was very serious about us. She loved to talk to us and give us ideas about how to get started.

Then I started seeing a doctor in Albuquerque. He gave me some instructions to follow, and Penny made me follow them. If I started to move too fast, she would say, "Slow down," and I would pay attention and slow my pace down. I began to take my medicine regularly, and Penny kept after me to eat three meals a day. My health started to improve.

Penny and I had lots to overcome. She had a lot of growing up to do, and I had a lot of settling down to do. Putting our feet on the ground in our simple little apartment helped a lot and, most importantly, we had each other. There were two objectives in our lives: to work and to be able to live a "normal" life. Those have been our objectives ever since.

At first, our whole life was very structured: going to work, going to the movies, out to dinner once a week, doing the laundry, and cleaning the apartment. We never over-extended ourselves at all, and we learned how to do the basic things first. And we learned how to make love; that is important. There never was Penny without Greg or Greg without Penny. We've done everything together since the beginning. We lived together for about a year before we spent a night apart. I think in all the time we've been with each other, we've only slept apart twice.

I had a job outside the workshop, and it caused a lot of problems. Depression still set in, and Penny always knew when I was depressed. One thing I love about Penny is how well she knows me. She knows when I am depressed, and she stands off and waits for things to ease up.

Both of us were very frightened that first year. I didn't know whether or not I could handle a permanent job. The pay was low, I was off Supplementary Security Income, and we didn't have any security. I had a lot of fears, but I knew that when I came home, there would be someone to

"Penny and I had lots to overcome. She had a lot of growing up to do, and I had a lot of settling down to do. . . . There were two objectives in our lives: to work and to be able to live a 'normal' life. Those have been our objectives ever since."

comfort and reassure me. Penny wasn't actually trying to find a job; she was sticking to the workshop and she became one of their best workers. A year ago, Penny got a job on the "outside," and now she is trying to establish herself as a worker. We don't have our "handicaps" anymore to the degree that we have to work in a workshop. Her coworkers respect her now, more than they did when she first started there. Initially, they were kind of standoffish. You know, "Well, she's a little slow, makes a lot of mistakes." Now they depend on Penny to do everything, and she catches them in mistakes that they make.

I guess Penny and I could give tips to other disabled

individuals about how to "make it." First, you have to find a community where you're comfortable. Then you have to take advantage of all opportunities. You work hard, pay your bills, cook your food, do your laundry, keep your apartment clean, get to bed early, get up early—that's the whole thing. It's very simple. It might sound silly that I say "do your laundry," but it's true; do your laundry, clean your apartment. If you're disabled, you might not be able to do it all by yourself; you may need another person. If it's another disabled person, which was true of Penny and me, that's fine. Keep it all very simple, very basic. Never complicate your life with foolish things like complicated trips; never extend yourself to late hours; never get wrapped up in petty gossip in your community. Just stick to the gossip between the two of you because you'll discover, as we did, that what the two of you know about each other is the only thing that is important and all the gossip around you won't help you achieve independence.

"Always important was to enjoy life as much as to struggle. Work was number one, our home was number two, and to enjoy ourselves was number three."

I could go on and on about when people have helped us and when Penny and I have just done it on our own. I love saying that a person has to go out and handle it himself, you know, take the bumps. Well, damn it, you do have to take the bumps. Penny and I haven't taken the bumps, not really. We struggled and we wanted to most of the time. Always important was to enjoy life as much as to struggle. Work was number one, our home was number two, and to enjoy ourselves was number three.

I guess if you want to write about independent living for disabled people, everything we've done is right. But so much is commitment, love, and the breaks. And it will still work for a long, long, time, I think, as long as there's a Penny.

Katherine Corbett

There was never any push for me to have a boyfriend, get married, have relationships. I was also in the unique position of having a sister one year younger than me who was not disabled and who was dating from about the age of fourteen (she was sneaking around going steady at eleven.) My parents had a conflict about her going too fast, so they were not in any way going to push me to do it, too. They already had their hands full. One of my other sisters went at a slower pace than you might expect, too. My parents pretty much dealt with her the same way they dealt with me, so I didn't think it was my disability, I just felt that was the way my family was, and it was more okay to go slow than fast. My mother was always saying that people grow up too fast anyway.

Because we never talked about the feelings people might have about me or about how other people might see me, I didn't develop the skills I needed socially. Sometimes, if people were reticent with me, I wouldn't realize that they were feeling uncomfortable with my disability. I would miss things—maybe it was a social opportunity, maybe it was dating—but because I didn't know that they were uncomfortable, I didn't compensate for that.

I didn't date much, even in college. I really felt that people wouldn't notice my disability so much if I had a boyfriend who was not disabled. Then I would be a "couple" and I would show how "normal" and desirable I was, and it would be more okay. It is very funny that I selected a man not very different from myself. I had more social skills than he did. He was very smart, very introverted but didn't have "social behavior" at all. We were very well matched, and one of my frustrations was how well matched we were. We were first lovers with each other, and I always wished afterward that we had done it differently, that we had not been lovers, because we were too insecure and it carried into other parts of our relationship. We never knew if we were going in the right direction or what steps to take next. My desire to be "normal" interfered with my patience. I would rush because I couldn't wait any longer to be "normal." I felt having a relationship would make me "normal." It didn't buy me a lot of acceptability in New England, but it did in California.

My parents never really talked about marriage and children with us. They never asked when we were going to get married. Even now, they do not talk about this. My siblings are married now, but I have one male cousin, my age, who is not married either. Neither my parents nor the rest of my family questions him or me about when or if we will marry.

Whenever I complained about something, my father would say, "Wait until you have your own children," not, "Wait until you are married." I have a much stronger need for family than for marriage. That is why I have foster kids. When I was five years old, there were already four kids in my family, so I grew up with children all the time. I have never quite left children, both in terms of staying in education and when going home. As soon as I moved to California, I went out and found kids; I baby-sat for single mothers who needed free baby-sitting in exchange for my seeing their children. If I didn't live with children or have foster kids, I always adopted families whom I would go and see once a month. When I worked in a nursery school for three years, I thought of those kids as mine. The children are mixed, disabled and nondisabled.

I want to raise my own children, probably disabled kids, adopted. When I think about adopting children as a single parent, I think only about adopting disabled children. Years ago, I think my attitude would have been more of Miss Goody-Two-Shoes—I have to help them. I am better than they are. I have made it out of this ghetto, and I have to go back and help them. Now I feel that there are very few people around who see what I have been able to see, all the possibilities. You can take a kid and say, "You can be anything."

I don't think there are many people out there who believe, or have that attitude, that you can be whatever you want to be.

Paul Pendler

Paul Pendler, the brother of Lisa, talks about growing up with his sister. Betty Pendler earlier told the story from her point of view in "My Daughter Is Leaving Home. What Will I Do Now?"

I used being Lisa's brother to get to know people. From being with Lisa and her friends, I think I have a way with retarded children and young children. Living with Lisa, I had to learn how to deal with someone who is different.

We think we are helping somebody who is disabled but, in a way, they are helping us. There is a sensitivity that disabled people have that others do not. There are many abstract things I have learned, and, basically, my awareness has changed. I have always been aware of people staring, and I have different ways of stopping them. When I was younger, I was more violent. Now I usually just stare back. My mother would confront starers: "I noticed you were staring. Would you like to know more?" That puts people on the spot, and usually they listen. I don't mind if they just stare, but if they try to do something physical, like teasing, then I want to retaliate. Taunting would force me to decide if I would do something about it or just move away. Sometimes people would try to push her on purpose because she was retarded. I once hit somebody for that kind of teasing.

At times, I guess I was ashamed, particularly when I brought friends to my house. I eventually learned that if someone is going to be a friend of mine, he or she has to accept different aspects of my life. Usually when friends were coming to the house for the first time, I would tell them about my sister and I would give her lectures about toning down her act. Sometimes Lisa would sleep over someplace else if I brought home someone who I didn't think would deal well with her. Mother made sure I had my privacy. At times, I didn't want my sister around.

At a meeting I went to recently, there was a sibling panel, but I don't think people were really talking enough about what it really is like to be a sibling of someone disabled. I said that life wasn't just a piece of cake all the time and that there were some pains and a lot of times there is really resentment. Finally, the other four people on the panel really started expressing their feelings about it. It puts a lot of pressure on the healthy sibling to take care of his or her disabled sibling. There is always the question of embarrassment; you go to the park with your sister and more than half of the people get up and move away.

I went to a farmer's market in Holland, and I was just sitting, taking in the sights and sounds. I noticed a group of seven or eight retarded children. After a while, I realized that nobody had stared at them. I asked a friend of mine why no one was staring. I expected people to stare! She said that at a young age, Dutch parents teach their children that disabled children or retarded children sometimes look different but that they are basically the same as other people, not different. Americans are not like that.

"I asked a friend of mine why no one was staring. I expected people to stare! She said that at a young age, Dutch parents teach their children that disabled children or retarded children sometimes look different but that they are basically the same as other people, not different. Americans are not like that."

Tom Clancy

Tom Clancy is Manager of Administrative Systems, for New York University Computer Center and heads a department with ten people reporting to him. Any conversation with Tom is a full course meal. His friendship is one of the dividends of writing this book.

All the time I was in the hospital, I never thought that was the end of things. You had to keep your cool, keep yourself organized—I felt I had to do something to keep things running because I was there. First, we established the residents' counsel. We spoke to reporters when there were problems at the hospital. We dealt with voter rights, running a recreation program from a certain point of view, managing money, fighting for more money for the patients, fighting for patients' rights. In a certain way, it was make-work, but it came to me naturally.

My sole purpose was to keep it going, to keep myself ready because someday there was going to be something more than living in a hospital ward.

"My sole purpose was to keep it going, to keep myself ready because someday there was going to be something more than living in a hospital ward."

One of the problems was that you couldn't get out of the hospital unless you had a partnership of some sort. I chose to get married, and I chose very positively. I didn't do it as an alternative. But others did. There was no attendant care then. A man went and lived with a woman, and the woman was expected to take care of him seven days a week—get up in the morning, get him up, get him to work, meet him on the way home 'cause he couldn't get home with those damn wheelchairs at that time, and know that when he got home from work, she still had this problem to take care of. There's no emotional value to it. The impersonal demands of a human being destroy any kind of emotional value. Yeah, impersonal.

You're out of the hospital, goodbye. You've got a sucker to take care of you, goodbye. The end of the saga. And you pay for it in the relationship because what type of woman decides to undertake a thing like physically taking care of a man seven days a week? The person who undertakes this role wants a dependent individual as a partner. But what never occurred to me was that all the way along, I was not the dependent partner. I was the dominant one. The dependency was what I could generate to accommodate the situation. A woman I know said that I liked my dependent relationships, and there's a truth to it. I cultivate wounded birds, but I told her that I'd like to see those wounded birds fly again.

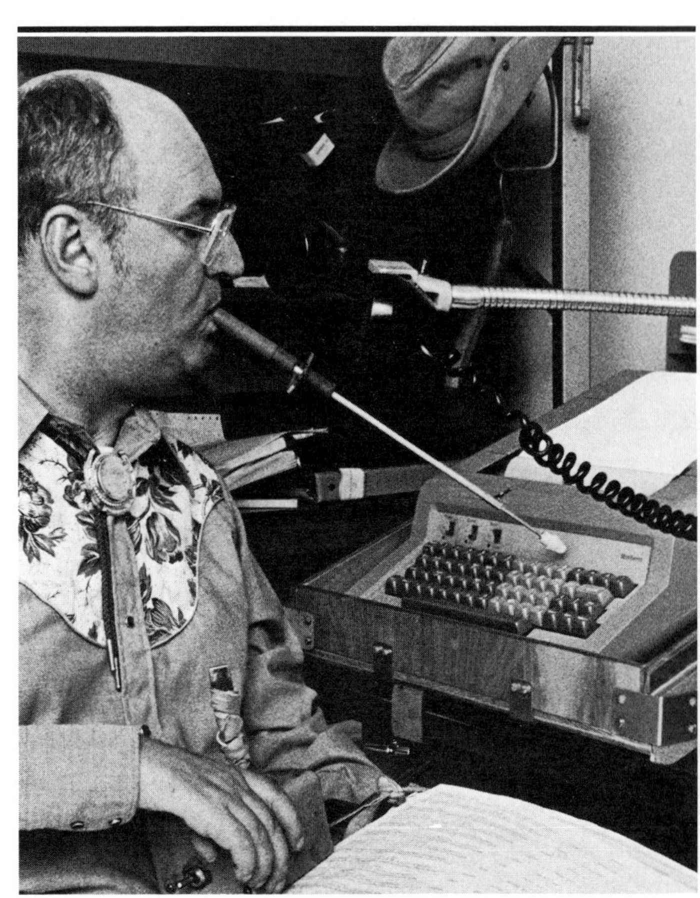

Mark Miller

I'm homosexual and disabled, and that seems more than most people can handle in this society. You need to be perfect, meet all the qualifications, before people think you have the same needs, desires, entitlements as everyone else.

They beat the hell out of us in the group home if we touched ourselves. I remember one attendant pulled a boy all around the room by his penis because he was masturbating. It was terrible. That, and people's reactions to me, have left me with a lot of confusion about my sexuality.

I am an advocate for paralyzed veterans. They were all able-bodied until they became adults; they know what able-bodied people feel and think because they thought it, too. It is harder to pull the wool over their eyes. As an organization, they have the wherewithal to say, "No. That is not the way things should be done."

The thing that struck me when I was working for Legal Services and read all that literature—a lot was about barrier-free design and accessibility—was that I thought they didn't know what they were talking about. I thought, "Once you change attitudes, all the barriers will come down—once people understand what disabled people are all about." It took me three years to realize that I was right and that the literature was right. You can't change people's attitudes if you can't let them meet disabled people. And to meet disabled people is to change your attitude.

"You can't change people's attitudes if you can't let them meet disabled people. And to meet disabled people is *to change your attitude."*

I realized that you are never going to win hearts and minds unless you get disabled people out there. If you can't get disabled people out there, nothing is going to change. So that accessibility—barrier-free design—becomes as important as attitude. You can't have one without the other.

I don't know if there is a better attitude toward blind people, but I think they are at least considered. They are part of people's consciousness, the public's consciousness. And I don't think the blind are abused as much as orthopedically disabled people. The blind people are also better organized, though some of their benefits are questionable. For example, it's not a coincidence that there are a lot of blind newsdealers. If you are blind, you get a preference to be a newsdealer in a federal building. This is a questionable benefit because what is achieved? It simply serves to keep people in their place. Who is really benefiting by that?

I am not a big believer in the law as accomplishing a lot for disabled people. I believe it is a necessary component, that's all. It might even lead the way, but it can't do it alone. It is grass roots. It is disabled people themselves, their families and their friends, who are going to change things if anybody is going to change them.

Jim Weisman

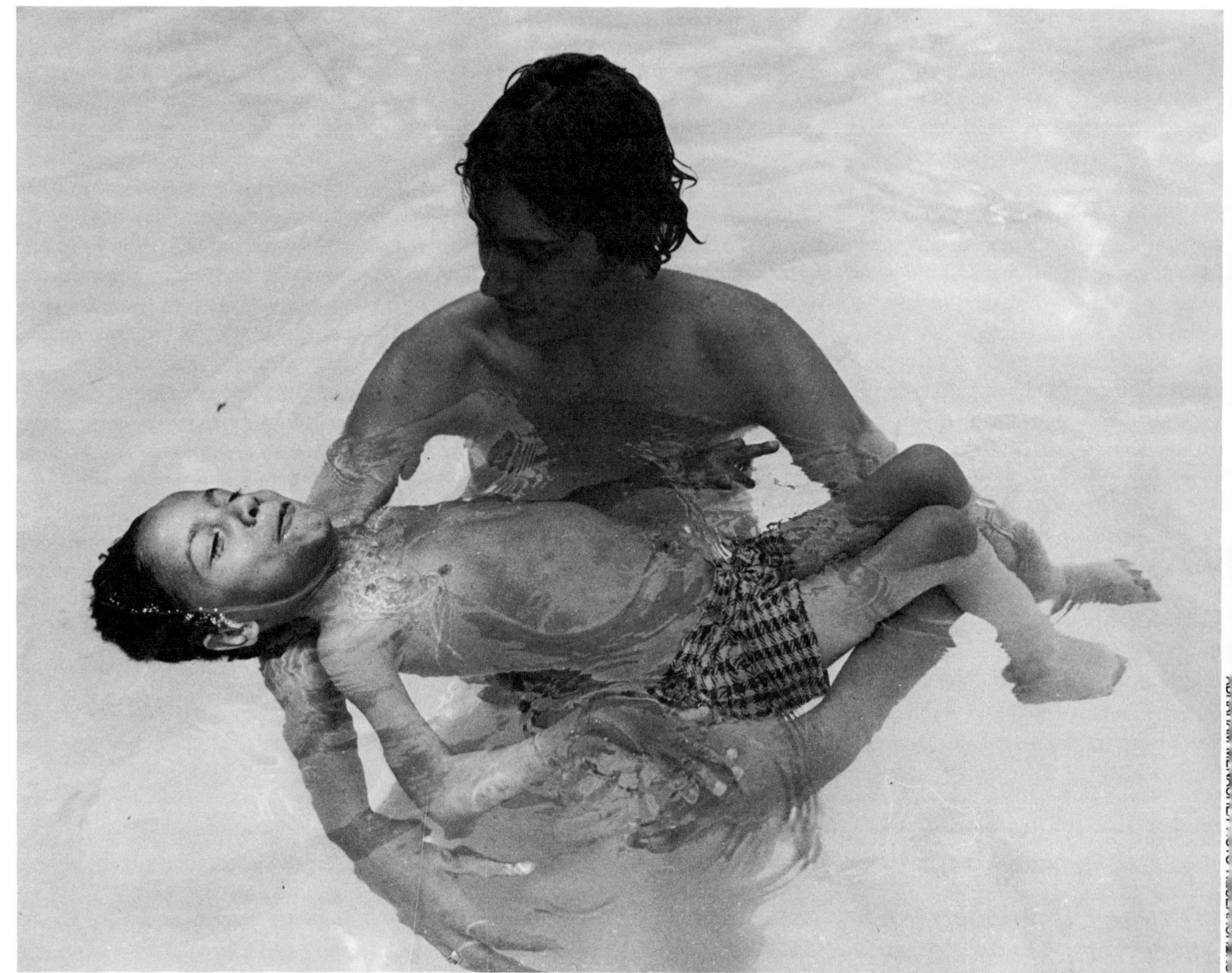

At a summer camp for youngsters with disabilities, this boy with cerebral palsy is encouraged to float by his counselor.

As a teenager, I worked in a day camp for disabled children and through that made friends with some disabled people who remained my friends as we grew older. That was my only contact with disability. Years later, I graduated from law school and, right before I graduated, Joseph Califano [former Secretary of Health, Education, and Welfare] signed Section 504 of the Rehabilitation Act of 1973. I ran into one of my disabled friends, who was also a lawyer. I made the mistake of saying to him, "Oh, I guess you're pretty happy. Everything is terrific. Califano signed." This triggered his response: "It is just a piece of paper. There is a lot of work to do."

We began talking about disability, and I realized that my feelings were that essentially it didn't matter; disabled people were like everyone else. They were either jerks or they weren't, and you dealt with them accordingly. I had never given it much thought, but I realized after talking with my friend that most able-bodied people don't feel that way, that dealing with disabled people was a tremendous problem for them.

I was looking for a job, and when I got one at Legal Services, my friend and I wrote a proposal together and got a project funded. We were viewed as more of a threat to the Legal Services system than as friends because we would be out there advocating for appropriate placements for disabled schoolchildren and transportation and access. At the same time, we had to fight with our own management about the system. They would use the same arguments as the enemy—the enemy being everyone who has run the system at the expense of the disabled: "It costs too much."

"When I first began, it was like the ground floor of the civil rights movement. Wherever you turned was a golden opportunity because disabled citizens were being discriminated against on a wholesale level."

When I first began, it was like the ground floor of the civil rights movement. Wherever you turned was a golden opportunity because disabled citizens were being discriminated against on a wholesale level. It didn't matter what the law said. This is the way people have always behaved in relation to disabled people. When I was working at Legal Services, we began to receive publications from disabled citizens' organizations everywhere, and I got a crash course in the public's perceptions of disability and also in disabled people's perceptions of themselves. I feel I know a lot more about it now than I did then.

I now think there is a difference between catastrophically acquired disabilities and congenital disabilities or disabilities that affect people in childhood. I don't think it is a rule—there are exceptions—but I do think that catastrophically disabled people, young adults in particular, seem much more aggressive, assertive, not afraid to bite the hand that feeds them if that hand is government. Of course, an argument for the opposite could also be true. A large percentage of the leadership in the disability rights movement had polio as young children, were blind, or had had some other disability since birth.

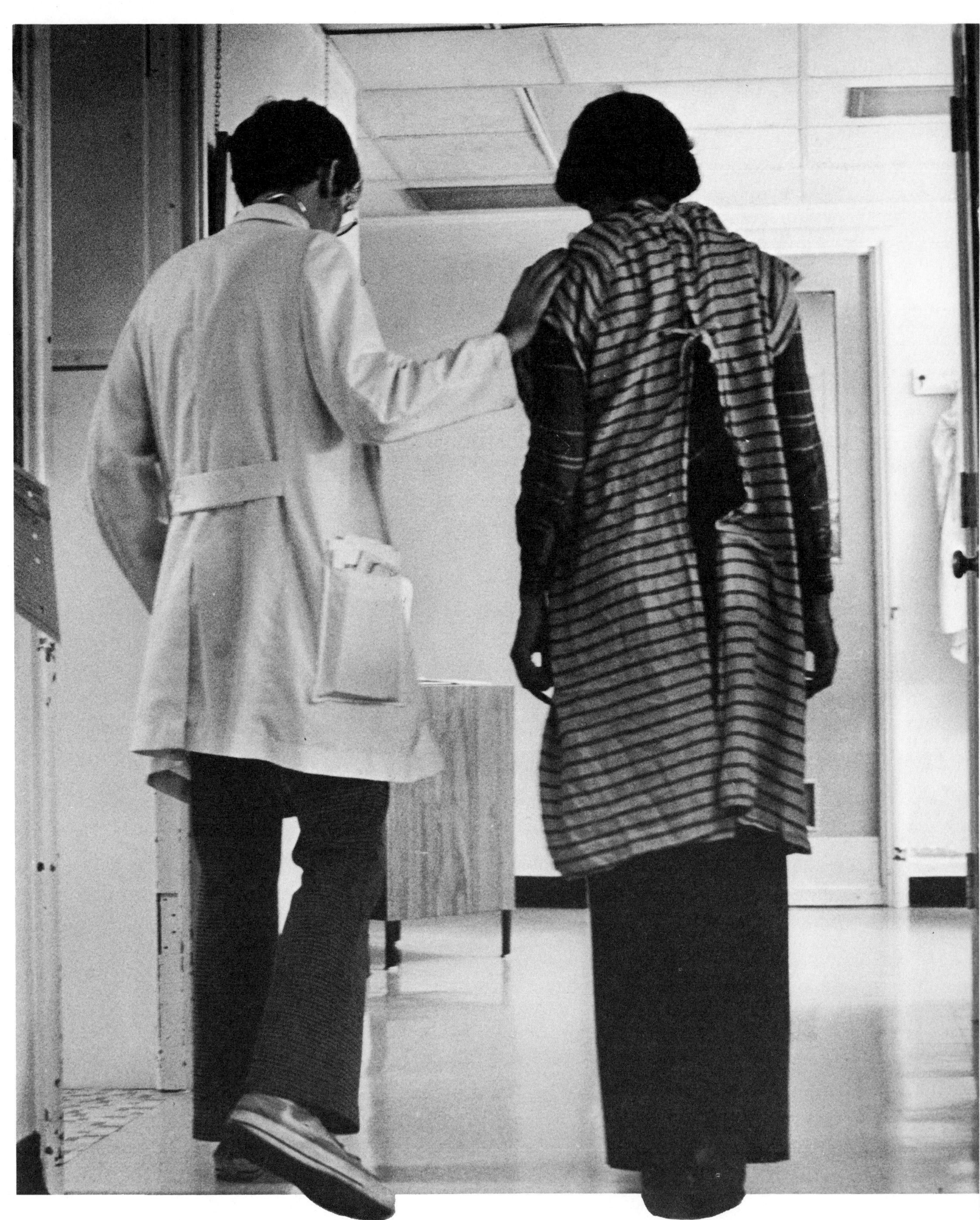

Chapter 4

Doctors, Hospitals, Helping Professions

Into The Land of the Myths

S. L. Rosen

Their voices trailed in from the hall. My good hearing served me well. Perhaps they didn't think I could hear them. But it's more likely, though, I've come to realize, that they simply didn't consider whether I could hear them from the distance spanning a room. Once I was seen as a "handicapped person" rather than a real person, it was as though I wasn't really there. Frequently, they would talk about me, even at the foot of my bed, as though I wasn't there at all.

"Stephen is in a very serious condition, as you all know," the typical hallway discussion would begin. "We're doing all the medical profession knows how, but it's hard to mend bodies." At this point, frequently, Dr. Espin's voice would be replaced by my mother's. "Oh, why did he do this to us? Why? He'd come so far . . . and now he's a hopeless cripple. Just a shadow of what he was, you know."

This I would soon come to recognize as one of a series of little speeches Mother evolved to berate me for my misfortune and, at the same time, assuage a guilt that emerged in her from somewhere I could never determine.

Others in the series were heard from the hall on other days, whispered in hushed tones to friends that had come along to support her on her daily visit to her now "crippled" son. The hushed tone, I came to realize, came from deference to the delicate nature of the subject matter rather than from any real concern that I might hear them. "Cripples," I learned from their lexicon, cannot hear.

"And you know, he had such a future!" The voices droned on, snatching my future from me. "What good is it now?"

"Well, you know, Kate," another voice would rise (I knowing it to be Mother's religious friend, Molly Biven). "It's all for a reason. All for a reason. Even though Steve is an invalid now, and will undoubtedly be a burden to you, there is a plan in this for us. God did not permit Steve to die, did he, Kate? He gave him back to us as an invalid. God has his reasons, Kate. We must pray to know what God has meant for us by making Steve an invalid."

Again, I looked at the word and turned it over in my mind. I began to see through this line of thinking that I had fallen into (by what I sensed to be the most natural of thinking processes) how it was that people came to believe that God has chosen people to survive and that their surviving was of God's choosing. If one was not permitted to die, then, surely, to a caring God, one's surviving was for a purpose. So ran one of the many myths I had grow up with. The myth told us that cripples are a message sent by God. Cripples do God's work. Cripples suffer as God wills, for others, for the world. All childhood teachings. I remembered it all, startled to realize I had known all these

"The hushed tone, I came to realize, came from deference to the delicate nature of the subject matter rather than from any real concern that I might hear them. 'Cripples,' I learned from their lexicon, cannot hear."

myths about "cripples" all along. I realized then that we all know these myths, but we never look at them. I now found myself focusing on these Christian approaches to "cripples" both because I was, to my dismay, one of the "cripples" and because I couldn't help analyzing it as a social construct. It was my training. I began to see things hidden in darkness, things I had never explored before. I knew, with a sureness born out of memories of learned behavior stored up in childhood, that I was now and forever a "cripple" and "different."

"One of them," I would realize, bitterly, as I watched others like myself being wheeled to and from therapy. I had become the Other. In a split second that night, I had moved from the world of the "normal" to the world of the abnormal, the invalid. I ached in an embarrassment at myself.

I discovered the myths, now, in floods of remembering that would wash over me at any and all small incidents that could serve to jar my memory or in images conjured up at will, as I lay in darkness—the myths of disability that lie in the past and are a part of all our unremembered lives.

They would spill out: events I did not remember having participated in, memories heretofore locked safely away, pieces of knowledge, scraps of myths and beliefs, that until they flowed out, I had had no recollection of ever thinking at all.

Such are the deeply rooted beliefs about "cripples" that we store up unconsciously. They are our beliefs about the deformed, the Other; their existence beneath the surface, forming the basis of our attitudes and actions. We do not know yet that our attitudes and actions toward "cripples" can all be traced to these myths. They have seeped into our subconscious in childhood without our knowing. The myths we have never discussed. They are not a part of our spoken and known heritage.

The myths came forth now, jolted by my entry into the land of the myths themselves.

I saw Jeffrey Stone, the man with cerebral palsy, "Rebecca's boy." Conjuring up again from childhood, I watched. What I saw fascinated me. I watched not only Jeffrey, but myself, a boy of eight or nine, uncomfortable, itching in a too-hot wool blazer, sunk back as far as it was possible to sink into Mrs. Stone's electric blue overstuffed armchair as a fire spat in a maroon tile fireplace in the Stones' too-tight living room on a wet December Sunday.

No one, least of all I, saw him as a person. What then? I wondered now. As an object? As an animal? No. I did not know, then, as I bored my eyes into the enormous, overblown roses on the drapes, seeking out any vision other than Jeffrey's boring stare. I could not define it, finally, and had to accept it at that. My understanding of Jeffrey Stone never formalized itself, even, into an understanding of what it was about him that I feared. Only that he was very, very unlike me, as unlike me as one could get and still be a person—no, a human, and that the least of our differences was age. It wasn't his mind. Even I did not deal with Jeffrey directly enough to have known with any certainty whether he had a mind or not.

What was this, then, that I was seeing? A very terrified little boy, confronting another, older boy, who surely must have had emotions and, at that age, the sexuality of a man—consigned to a couch on a Sunday evening to be the object of sidelong glances from a child half his age—on an evening when he should have been out with friends, listening to records, dating, anything but this!

I did not see Jeffrey as anybody at all.

What I saw was . . . nothing. I had then, and still have now, no words for it. All I knew was that he was unlike me by a difference that I wanted nothing to do with and less to know about. As I pushed back farther and farther into the blueness of the chair, I tried to escape from Jeffrey's brown, ill-fitting suitedness, emerging at me still too close in a puddle of jerks and spasms as far across the room from me as I could get him. I wished with all my might that Jeffrey did not exist.

"I had become the Other. In a split second that night, I had moved from the world of the 'normal' to the world of the abnormal, the invalid. I ached in an embarrassment at myself."

What could this tell me now, I wondered, searching out the clues to my existence? Who was Jeffrey? For now, I knew that I must learn the answer. Jeffrey, you see, was no longer only part of a myth thankfully forgotten. Jeffrey was "crippled." And that was me, too, now.

The thought both sickened and fascinated me as I returned to it over and over. What had Jeffrey thought during those visits? My God, did he think, even now? What was his existence like today? For I knew he still lived with Mrs. Stone, a middle-aged woman by now. I pictured him still in the brown suit, still sitting in a pile of small rumples, trapped forever in the never-never land of enforced childhood.

As curious as I was about Jeffrey, I could not bring myself to ask. No information Mrs. Stone or my mother

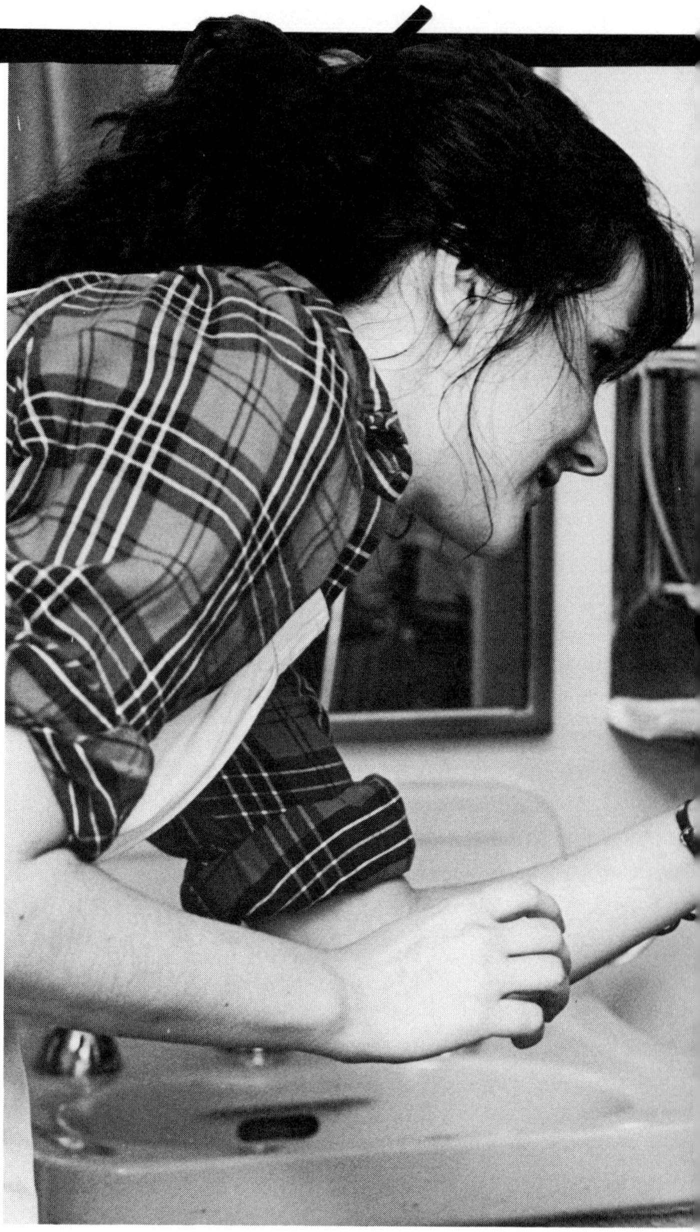

A nurse's aide gives this man a shave.

could give would be the kind I would need. Should I talk to Jeffrey himself, then? I wanted that even less.

Jeffrey's image would dissolve. In his place in my mind arose the childhood visits to the home for incurables. Children all, or so it seemed then. Now as I looked more carefully at the images flowing before me, I saw older people—in their 20's at least. Perhaps older. Why were they there in a children's home? I began to see that all "cripples" were children in the myths. But, in truth, nothing seemed one way or the other in these images. The children didn't exactly seem like children, either. I thought they had no minds. That their bodies must have existed—even worked, after a fashion, somehow—had never occurred to me before. That they were at home in their bodies—intimate with their bodies, as I was becoming now with the motionless part of my body, which belonged to me still and must be taken care of, perhaps as a pet—was a new realization for me.

I turned it over and over, examining it. It was not that they had accepted their bodies but that this was their dwelling where they were to live and could do nothing about it;

"Now I brought out these children of the homes as so many broken, wooden toys from my past and arranged them before me, examining them for the first time with new eyes. I would need to know them now; know them as I had never known them before. They were my precursors. They had been made in my future image and likeness, for we all shared that image: We were the 'crippled,' those who survived."

it was as inevitable as my paralysis was for me. I had never considered this before; never mulled over it. That is, the reality of it had never before been present to me in the way it was now. Now I brought out these children of the homes as so many broken, wooden toys from my past and arranged them before me, examining them for the first time with new eyes. I would need to know them now; know them as I had never known them before. They were my precursors. They had been made in my future image and likeness, for we all shared that image: We were the "crippled," those who survived.

What did I see now as I looked? I looked into souls, now, irrevocably beyond bodies. What infused their souls? What had they thought of my visit to them so long ago? What were their minds doing? How did the minds feel about the bodies?

That it could not be changed, their bodily state? I think that is what they must have felt. That it was their body, morbid as it was said by others to be; it was their body. Not an external condition clapped on but them. Part and parcel.

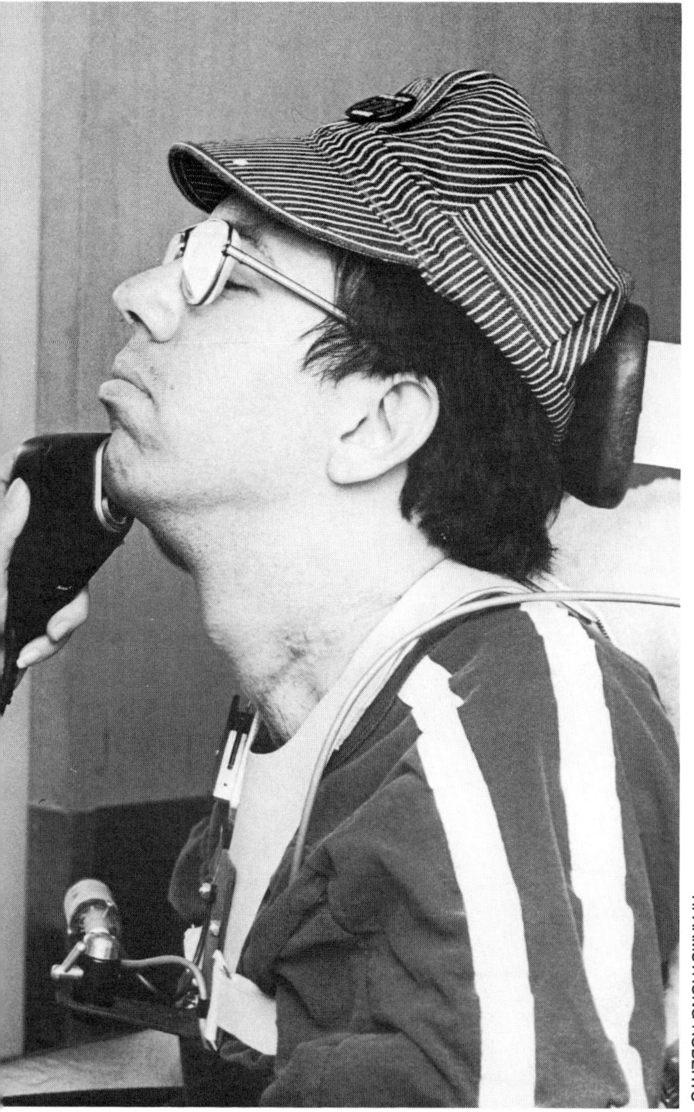

H. ARMSTRONG ROBERTS

Or else they prayed, schemed, and worked, hoping to find a way out. Cures were floated about in the air; a cure was to be prayed for daily. They appeared to have had little else to do with their lives, at any rate. I remember seeing them mostly in beds. Now that I think of it, I know that they could not have needed to stay in bed; they were not sick. But they were in beds, nonetheless. What did they think about this situation? Did they, I wondered, want to be in bed?

Try as I might, I could not really get beyond the images to the reality that must, I felt, be there. The best I could do—and I would have to settle for this, I realized, at least for the time—was to watch the images and study my feelings and reactions. It was all I had. Someday, perhaps, I, a "cripple" would talk to these "long crippled" and see.

For the truth was, I simply did not know. About them. They had long populated a country I was just now entering. I would have to wait and see.

This excerpt from *A Survivor's Manual* begins with S. L. Rosen's days in the hospital right after his accident. He finds himself unable to avoid overhearing his mother and her friends discussing his condition. Their discussion led his thoughts to his own experience with "cripples" (the word he then called us) in his past. What can this teach him, now a "cripple" himself, he wonders.

Permission was given by *Disability Rag*, where this first appeared in July 1982.

PATIENT'S BILL OF RIGHTS

The Patient has the right to:

1. *Receive considerate and respectful care.*
2. *Obtain from his or her physican complete and current information concerning his or her diagnosis, treatment, and prognosis in terms the patient can be reasonably expected to understand.*
3. *Receive from his or her physician information necessary to give informed consent prior to the start of any procedure and/or treatment.*
4. *Refuse treatment to the extent permitted by law and to be informed of the medical consequences of his action.*
5. *Receive every consideration of his or her privacy concerning his or her own medical care program.*
6. *Expect that all communications and records pertaining to his or her care should be treated as confidential.*
7. *Expect that within its capacity, a hospital must make reasonable response to the request of a patient for services.*
8. *Obtain information as to any relationship of his or her hospital to other health care and educational institutions insofar as his or her care is concerned.*
9. *Be advised if the hospital proposes to engage in or perform human experimentation affecting his care or treatment.*
10. *Expect reasonable continuity of care.*
11. *Examine and receive an explanation of his or her bill regardless of source(s) of payment.*
12. *Know what hospital rules and regulations apply to his or her conduct as a patient.*

American Hospital Association, Committee on Health Care

Jean Longwill

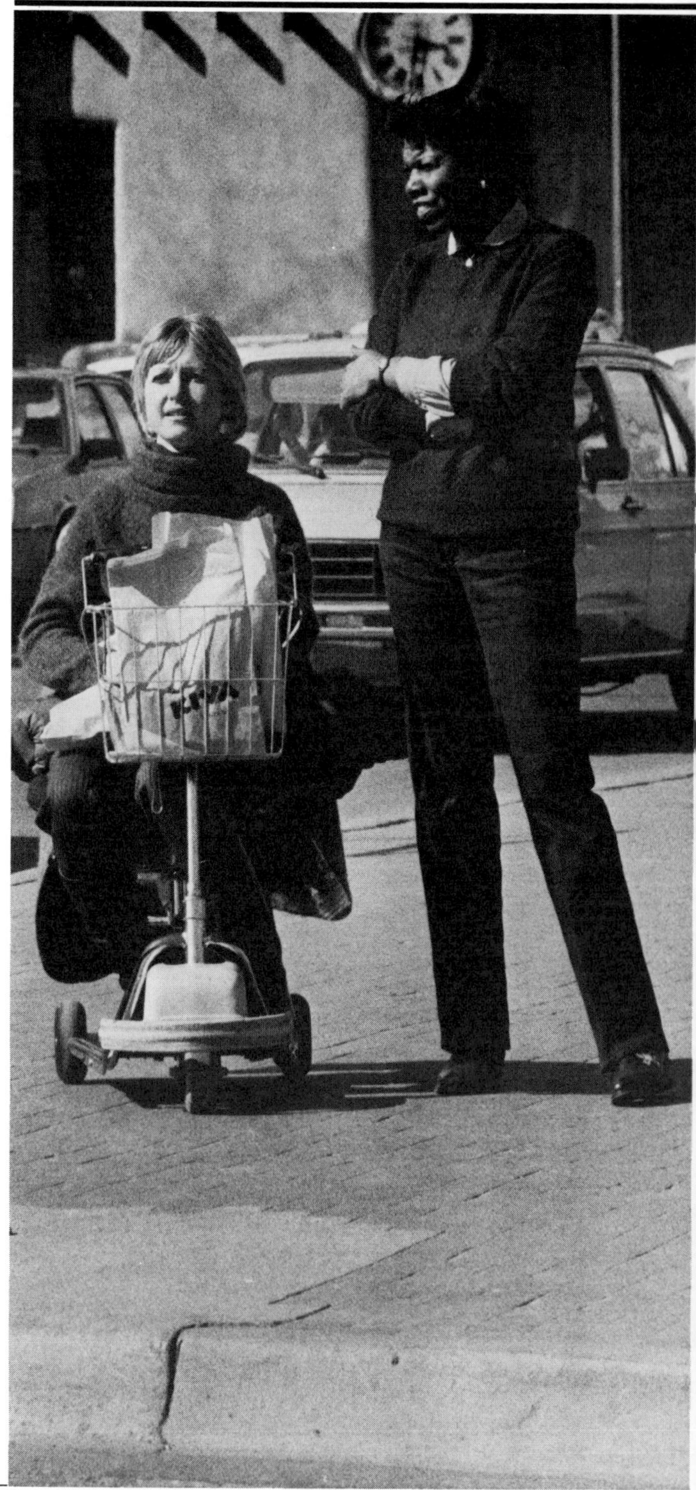

Now, we all go the bathroom, but we don't advertise the fact. One time, I didn't have my regular attendant and one of the young women who was home from nursing school was helping me. I expected her to have a certain amount of professionalism.

The phone rang and she answered it for me. I heard her say—actually I couldn't believe I was hearing her correctly—"Oh, Jean can't come to the phone right now. She's having a BM, okay?" I was astonished. She didn't have to answer the phone that way. Well, she came in for a while and checked me out and the phone rang again. She went out and answered it: "Jean is on the bedpan."

Here she was, a beautiful-looking woman; I loved her appearance. I thought, well, she came out on this cold winter evening to help me, so I am going to keep my mouth shut.

Then the doorbell rang, and when somebody asked for me, she said I was on the bedpan having a problem. Well, I thought, it was about time to stop this; and I did. I said, "I prefer not to have my private bodily functions discussed with anyone who visits or calls." And I asked, "Would you answer the door for your mother and say, 'My mother is in the bathroom sitting on the toilet'?" And she said, "Oh, well, I never thought of it that way."

Shopping in Santa Fe, a woman uses a motorized cart.

ATTENDANT CARE/HOME HEALTH CARE

Attendant care is one of the services most closely associated with the movement for independent living. If they are to live outside a hospital environment, this care is essential for severely disabled individuals:

- ***What is an attendant and what services does he or she perform?***
- ***What are the qualifications required of an attendant?***
- ***What are some factors to be considered in selecting an attendant?***
- ***What benefits can be derived from working as an attendant?***

An attendant is a person who assists a disabled individual, for pay, in personal needs of daily living. Individual needs may vary greatly, and no two clients require the same schedule and services. Typical services required include assistance in dressing, bathing, toileting, grooming, transferring to and from a wheelchair, food preparation, and cleaning.

Tina Grico, an occupational therapist, says she looks for certain qualifications in her attendants. "I feel an attendant should have the ability to accept responsibility and the willingness to take direction," she states. "In addition, the attendant must be willing to learn my needs and be able to relate well to me and to any guests who come into my home." Grico has found that, in order to be dependable, her attendant must live nearby and have access to reliable transportation. "I have to be at my job on time, so my attendant must be here to get me out," she said.

Elma Gilehrist, a home health care attendant, talked of the benefits she gets from her work: "I do my work in a professional way, and even though I work for a salary, the friendship that forms between us is equally important. To me, it is not just a job."

Many Centers of Independent Living have established attendant care placement services. Factors considered in matching attendant and client include the following:

- ***Will transportation or travel time be a problem?***
- ***Are work periods compatible?***
- ***Is there agreement on the tasks that need to be done?***
- ***Are the personalities compatible?***

Each question is indicative of the balancing act necessary on the part of both client and attendant to make a successful relationship work.

Colleges, churches, synagogues, and community bulletin boards are additional resources for attendants. Word of mouth is usually a good way to learn about experienced attendants.

Attendant care services cut across at least three major sectors of the human services system—health care, income assistance, and social services.

Financial assistance for home health aides may be obtained through various government bureaus. Benefits differ widely throughout the country and may depend on whether the state in which you live has Medicaid and allows for home health aides. If you feel an unjust decision has been made, you may request a fair hearing—a trial, set at a specific time, to state your case and to try to bring about a change in the decision.

Community organizations serving people with disabilities can provide information about legal services within the community. Independent living centers either offer legal counseling or make referrals.

Clothes: Their Role in Liberty, Equality, and Fraternity

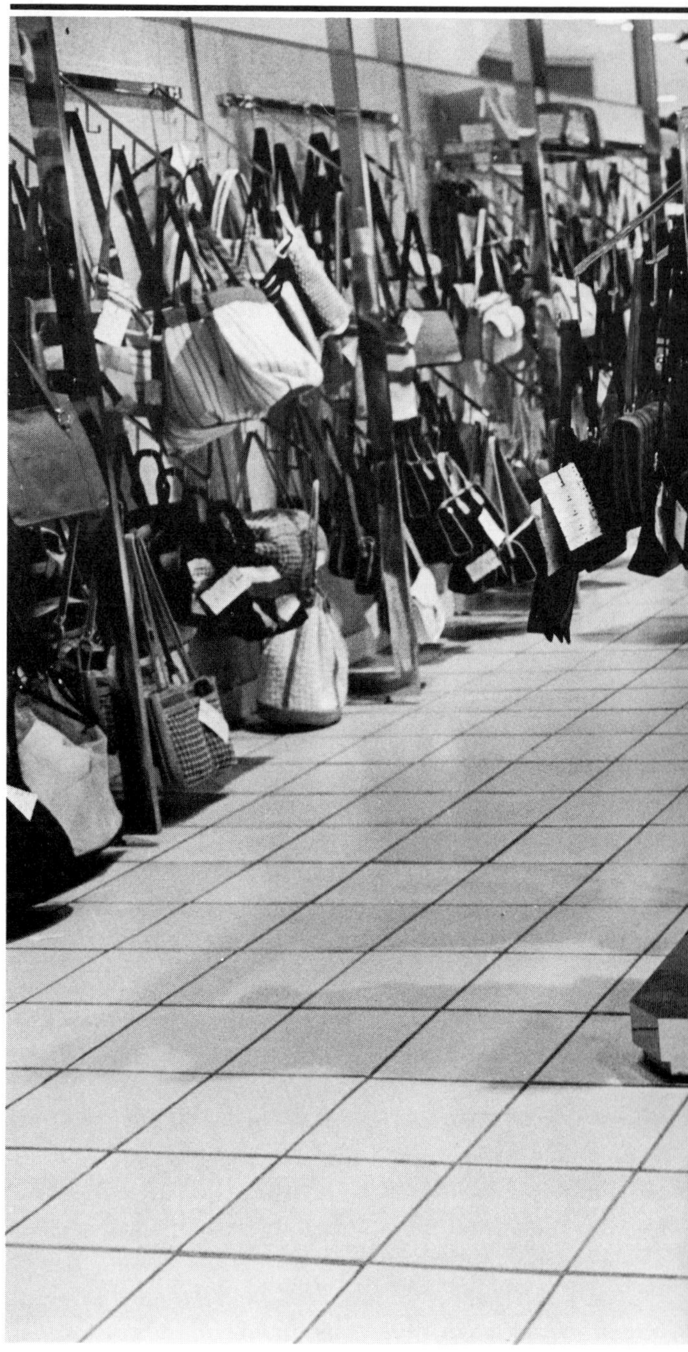

Shopping at the Riverside Square Shopping Mall, Hackensack, New Jersey. The pocketbooks on this rack can easily be reached.

Joan Schute remembers that more and more people with disabilities began leaving home for the first time to enter colleges across the country. "It was not surprising that we began to feel differently," she says, "and this was reflected in how we looked and dressed. We were making personal statements—coming out of the closet.

"One thing that changed within the week I got to the University of Illinois was I started wearing eye shadow and mascara. My body image was not very good," she laughingly admits, "and that's an understatement!"

Dan Morales, a Vietnam veteran and pro basketball player with a New Jersey team of paralyzed veterans, feels "the times they are a-changin'," as the song goes. "I've always been a people watcher, particularly women. The clothes a woman with a disability wears these days says a lot about how she and others see her; it's definitely a combination of the two—the woman and the times in which she is living. Less than seven years ago, a woman in a wheelchair, no matter her age, had on 'sensible shoes,' flat-heeled brown oxfords. A woman I know, who became paraplegic from a skiing accident, wears spike heels and matching panty hose. When I see her, I know we have come into our own."

Tom Clancy has a style all his own. A story about him, which appeared in the Russian language magazine *Amerika*, referred to him as "The Electric Cowboy"—combining his profession in the world of computers and his distinct fashion tastes. Tom's seven-gallon hat can be seen a block away. He chooses a Western string tie for convenience and appearance.

Clancy describes, with his inimitable Irish wit, the shoes he wore when he called Goldwater Memorial Hospital on Roosevelt Island his home after he got polio in the early 1950s. "All men wore these high boots that weighed a ton, fit no one, and were the only thing in the hospital that never got ripped off. They were that awful. Made from the stiffest leather. Parratroopers' boots are soft in comparison. So, if a guy was hemiplegic, he had this one-ton boot that he had to drag along. The women's shoes were not much better, but they did at least have a little more style. Someone probably had a lifetime contract with the city to supply shoes, and we got stuck with them.

"In the basement of one of the hospital buildings was a shoe room with thousands of pairs of shoes in every size—but only one style. That was clothing with a certain mind-

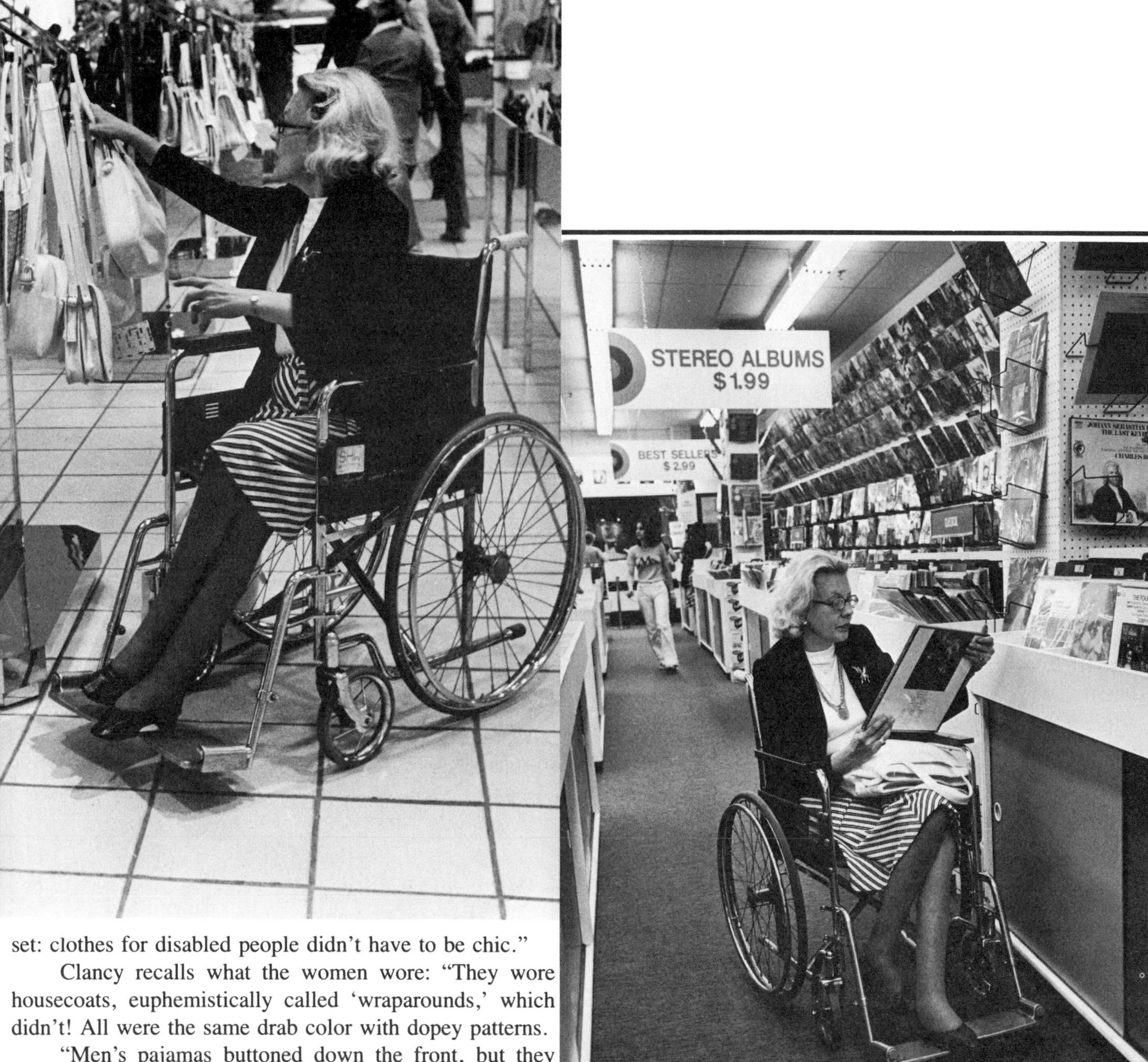

set: clothes for disabled people didn't have to be chic."

Clancy recalls what the women wore: "They wore housecoats, euphemistically called 'wraparounds,' which didn't! All were the same drab color with dopey patterns.

"Men's pajamas buttoned down the front, but they never closed altogether. At all times, a part of you was exposed, so we would turn our head if someone was being transferred from the bed to a chair so as not to embarrass one another."

SYBIL SHELTON/MONKMEYER

Harriet Bell, who was in Goldwater Hospital at the same time as Clancy, puts it this way: "When I was in the hospital, I always wore my own clothes. Before polio, I designed and made my own clothing. Afterward, my husband shopped for me for a while, and as soon as I could get into a store, I did—I headed for Lord & Taylor's separates department. I knew just what would look good on me. It took me two years before I could get there."

Bell recalls: "When I was in an iron lung—where I was many, many times, I wore a pajama top or, if I was very sick, a hospital gown."

Bell, who uses a motorized chair and is quadriplegic, prefers suits with soft, lace-trimmed blouses, two-piece dresses, skirts, and blazers. "I wear regular clothes," she says. "I don't wear anything made for the disabled population because I think they are ugly. I like taffeta half-slips because if I need to change my position in my chair, the material is substantial enough to give the person adjusting me something to hold onto."

Anita Lawson, an occupational therapist, uses regular stockings rather than panty hose because they are easy to get on and off. Her panties are one or two sizes larger and modified by snaps similar to those found on body suits and sold by the yard in notion's departments or fabric stores. Lawson prefers wool blends for winter and cotton knits for summer rather than slippery materials, such as gabardine, which cause one to lose position in a chair. "I would not choose a material that rips easily, but someone can still be practical and gorgeous."

For men's clothing, the consensus is low-slung pants—not too low but below the waist are best. A trick with pants is using concealed snaps or velcro, making it easier for dressing.

"In the past, people with a disability were hidden away, and when you are hidden away, nobody really cares how you look," Lawson says. "I knew a lady who was kept in the attic for forty years because she had seizures. People in nursing homes and hospitals did not object to wearing pajamas and housecoats," she continues. "They were not happy about wearing them, but they had no choice, so it was a negative happiness—apathy."

Disabled veterans returning from World War II in the early 1950s were part of the rehabilitation philosophy initiated by Dr. Howard Rusk: Wearing your own clothing adds to a feeling of personal pride. Those veterans changed long-held societal beliefs: Disabled people could and should take their place in the world of work and in the community, and wearing the same clothing as everyone else helped the transition back into the community.

Home economics departments of universities have taken

Resources: CLOTHING

Attends
Proctor and Gamble
Cincinnati, OH 45202
Aids for incontinence.

Cleo Living Aids
3957 Mayfield Road
Cleveland, OH 44121
Exercise, diagnostic, and testing equipment. Braces, eating, dressing, bathroom aids.

Dri-Pride
Division of Weyerhauser Co.
Fremont, MI 49412
Aids for incontinence.

Geri Specials
Kinderhook
368 Dragon Lake Road
Coldwater, MI 49036
Comfort garments, men, women, children. Designer clothes.

Hill Bros.
39 Ninth Street
Lynchburg, VA 24504
Shoes for women, sizes 2½ to 14, AAAA-EEE.

Independent Living Aids
11 Commercial Court
Plainview, NY 11803
Can-do products for writing, household, and medical self-care.

Montgomery Ward
2825 East 14th Street
Oakland, CA 94616
General catalog.

National Odd Shoe Exchange
R.R. #4
Indianola, IA 50125
Shoes, odd sizes, left, right

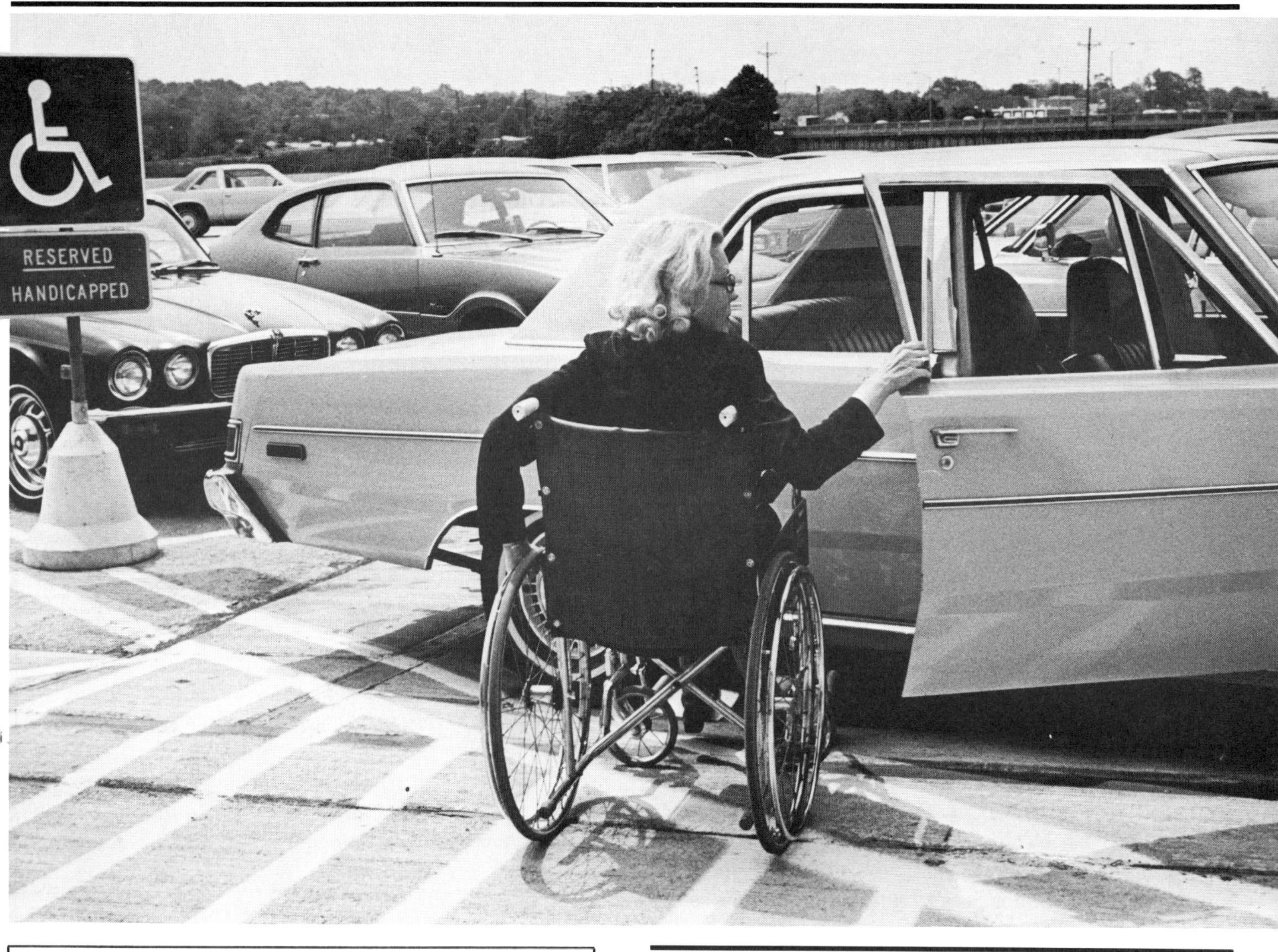

Pirca Fashions
301 Third Avenue
Sacramento, CA 95818
Custom-made design clothing

Sears Home Health Care Catalog
Sears, Roebuck and Co.
Chicago, IL 60607
Mail order catalog for home health needs; surgical hose, mastectomy garments, incontinence supplies.

Techni-Flair
Box 40
Cotter, AR 72626
Interesting, cheerful clothing; men, women, boys. Designer fashions

"I like taffeta half-slips because if I need to change my position in my chair, the material is substantial enough to give the person adjusting me something to hold onto."

on projects to determine the needs of a growing population of people who have difficulty in dressing. Flattering clothing has been designed for people who are arthritic and cannot button clothing or use zippers and for individuals who cannot raise their arms or who prefer clothing to conceal braces or prostheses. More recently, disabled consumers have been asked to advise from their experience on which adaptations and designs would be best.

Equipment

By the time we reach the fourth grade, every schoolchild in America knows about George Washington's assistive aid. That George Washington's teeth were made of wood brings about a variety of reactions and questions, such as: "Did his gums get splinters?" and "When he drank, did his teeth get waterlogged?"

But that is usually the end of our education pertaining to the different assistive aids and equipment that people with a disability might need in order to live their lives.

Mary Lilla Browne,* in 1962, was working as a librarian with the U.S. Army in Korea when she took a vacation in Japan. "During a Japanese tea ceremony, I discovered I could not kneel." The problem turned out to be a malignant bone tumor in her right leg, which ultimately necessitated an above-the-knee amputation.

At the time of the operation, her concern was that no one would want to look at her until she was fitted with an artificial limb. "I had faith, however, that the replacement limb would be indiscernably lifelike," she says, "that my walk would be like anyone else's and that I would have no more problems." As Browne puts it: "The prosthesis industry was not up to the challenge. Ever since 1962, wearing a prosthetic leg has been more exasperating than the amputation itself or the limitations it placed on my mobility and life-style.

"Wearing heels was one of my primary concerns from the beginning," she continued. "Even in the recovery room immediately following the amputation, as I went in and out of the anesthesia fog, I am told I kept talking about high heels."

*__Ms. Browne__ is an attorney who wrote of her personal experience in *High Heels*, published by *Disabled U.S.A.*, upon which this article is based.

Usually, a prosthesis is made to fit into only one of the shoes in a person's wardrobe. For a woman, it is important to wear shoes with varying heel heights. So along with her first artificial limb, she had to have several shanks of different heel heights that attached to the mechanical knee joint. Browne says, "Since I am not very mechanically talented, and to change shanks requires only a certain screwdriver, many times I have called a friend to say I would be late because I was trying to change shanks to match the height of my heels."

This is just the tip of the iceberg of annoyance, most likely. It is necessary to get a precise fitting, and there is great variance in workmanship and attitude. Maintaining a good fit also requires that one's weight not vary by more than five pounds; only with precise alignment will the leg be comfortable and not cause irritation that could lead to infection.

"Ever since 1962, wearing a prosthetic leg has been more exasperating than the amputation itself or the limitations it placed on my mobility and life-style."

Repairs (as with all equipment) are undoubtedly the most frustrating problem for everyone. The need to replace a knee joint on a prosthesis reaches awesome proportions.

Using a mouth stick to dial a number.

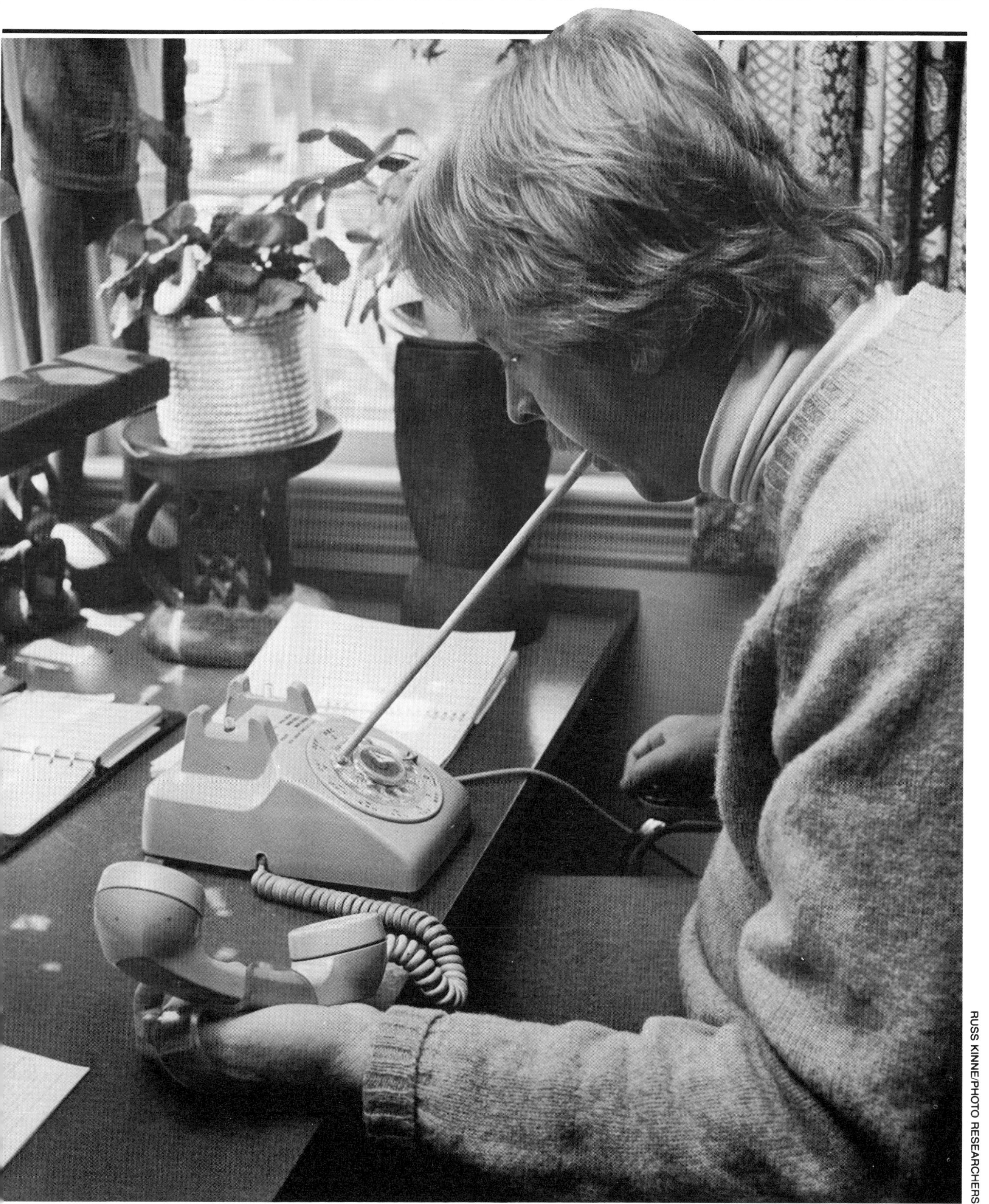

RUSS KINNE/PHOTO RESEARCHERS

"Most artificial limbs are manufactured on the West Coast, and only the manufacturers are allowed to make repairs," Browne says. "So for the time they are being repaired, a person is left with no visible means of support!"

Browne has done some clear thinking and has some answers: "A simple solution would be for every amputee to have a spare leg; but legs are expensive for the individual, and insurance companies won't pay for a duplicate." She continues: "The medical profession bears a share of the blame for what amputees go through. Although insurance practices require a prescription from an orthopedic surgeon, the average surgeon is unfamiliar with the fitting and the design features of prostheses."

Obviously, there needs to be more information exchanged between surgeons and the prosthetists, who replace what is amputated. It is no longer acceptable for a surgeon to convey the attitude: "We saved your life. What more do you want?"

Medical school training needs to include more study about amputation procedures, limb replacement, and an understanding of prosthetic devices. Perhaps someday research will discover how to permanently attach a prosthesis or even how to facilitate limb regrowth.

As for Mary Lilla Browne, she says: "Until these advances are made, I would like to have a leg that allows me to try on shoes of different styles on the same shopping trip, to swim, to climb most any grade, and to wear miniskirts if they come back in style."

A universality of experience exists, whether one is in need of a prosthesis, a watch with Braille numbers, or a smoke alarm that lights—rather than sounding an alarm—for an individual with a hearing impairment.

A person needs to (1) find appropriate equipment, (2) have resources to maintain it, (3) enjoy the partnership of a physician and supplier working together, and (4) encounter an attitude that those who need these supplies are, first and foremost, customers.

Resources: EQUIPMENT

Abledata
National Rehabilitation Information Center (NARIC)
4407 Eighth Street, N.E.
Washington, D.C. 20017
(202) 635-5826 (Voice/TDD)
Toll free: 1-800-34-NARIC

Abledata *is a computerized listing of commercially available products for rehabilitation and independent living; $10 for up to 100 listings; $5 for each additional set of 100 listings.*

Accent Buyers' Guide, 1984–1985
P.O. Box 700
Bloomington, IL 61701

Accent on Information (AOI)
P.O. Box 700
Bloomington, IL 61701

AOI is a computerized retrieval system with a data base of aids, assistive devices, and how-to information; $12 per search.

Centers for Independent Living

Council of Organizational Services for the Deaf
P.O. Box 894
Columbia, Md 21044

Lifecare
5505 Central Avenue
Boulder, CO 80301

Respiratory aids, respirators.

Rehabilitation Centers, Clinics, Hospitals
Telephone

Special telephones, special adaptations made by the telephone company. See your local directory for number and address.

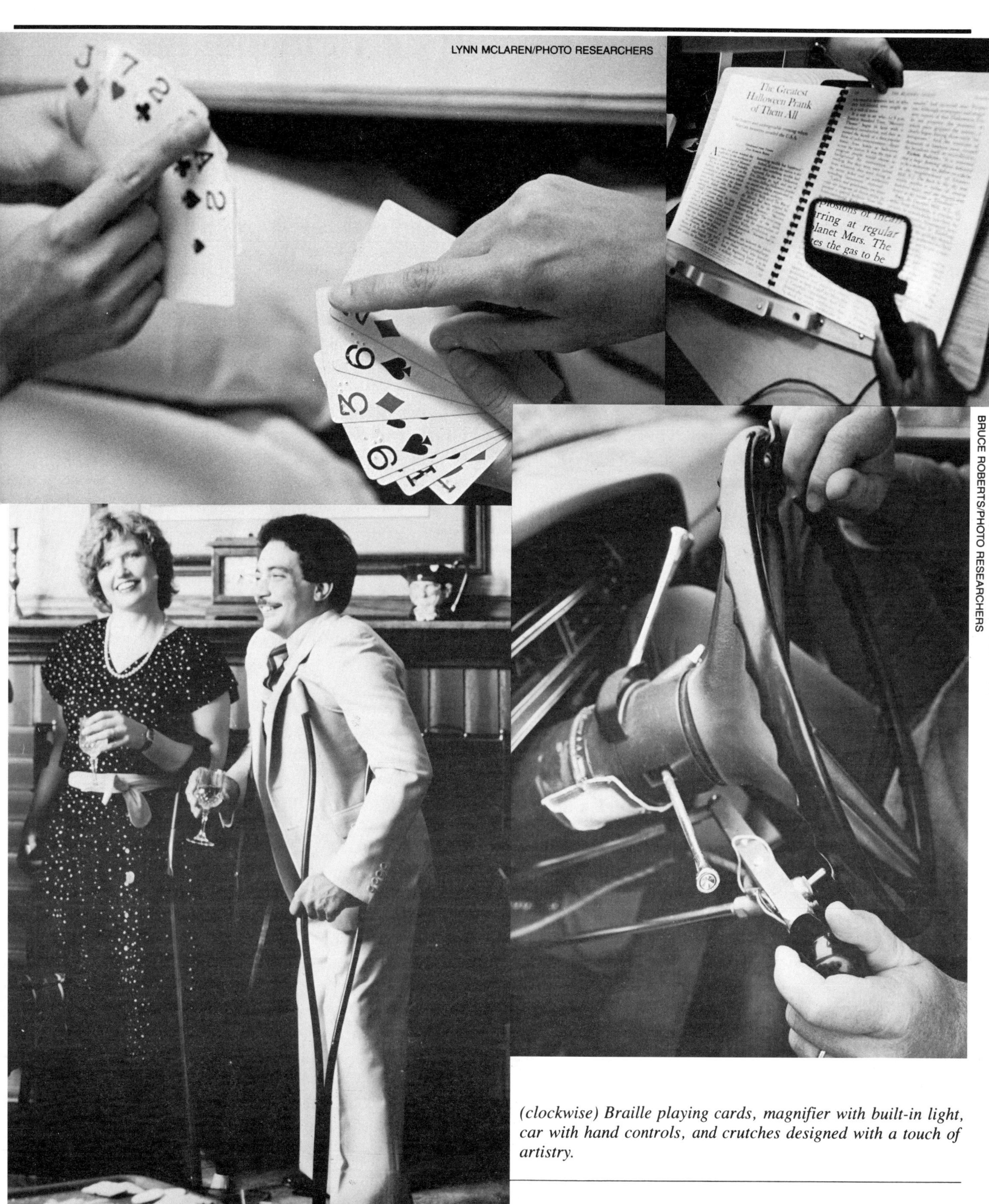

(clockwise) Braille playing cards, magnifier with built-in light, car with hand controls, and crutches designed with a touch of artistry.

Rights of Critically Ill Individuals

- May a competent adult refuse medical care necessary to keep him or her alive?
- Can the family of a critically ill individual stop the medical treatment of that individual if he/she wants it continued?
- Is there a legally binding directive an individual can write authorizing that medical care be stopped if he/she becomes terminally ill?

When an individual is diagnosed by one or more physicians as having no chance for recovery and elects to die without further medical treatment, many people, often with differing viewpoints, play a part in the decision.

The family may disagree. The physician may be caught in the dilemma of the individual's wishes, the differing viewpoint of the family, the concerns of a malpractice suit, and possible intervention by public officials who feel that to stop treatment is tantamount to the individual committing suicide.

In answering the question of whether an individual has the right to refuse treatment, John A. Robertson, in *The Rights of the Critically Ill*, has this to say:

> In general, yes. The right of self-determination and autonomy central to American law is now recognized and includes the right of a competent adult to reject lifesaving medical care. This right is an application of the rule of informed consent to medical treatment. Under this rule, no doctor may treat a competent individual without his free, knowing consent. While the United States Supreme Court has not yet addressed the question, influential state courts have found the right to reject lifesaving medical care to be part of the fundamental constitutional right of privacy.

Many people would like to ensure that they do not have to submit to treatments that prolong life but do not consider its quality. This is now possible by making a "living will," a legally binding directive to one's family and physicians to stop life-prolonging medical treatments when one is critically ill and no longer able to state preferences.

The "living will" is so named because it controls events when the individual is still alive but not competent, in contrast to wills that control events upon death. A legally binding document, the "living will" gives the doctor immunity from civil and criminal liability for withholding care and requires that the doctor leave the case if the instructions are not followed. It also relieves the family of the responsibility of making painful decisions on behalf of a loved one.

Not all states have passed legislation for this type of will, but it is honored in many states. Living will laws have different names, such as natural death, death with dignity, or right-to-die laws. An attorney or legal services office can be helpful in drafting a personal living will. A patient advocate in a hospital or the social service department of an organization serving a disability category would be good resources. The local librarian may have reference material of examples of living wills. Perhaps it would be best of all to create one based on your own wishes.

The "living will" is so named because it controls events when the individual is still alive but not competent, in contrast to wills that control events upon death.

Most people in this country are not allowed to die with dignity. We die in impersonal hospitals, surrounded by aggressive medical treatment, often long after a diagnosis of terminal illness has been made.

Our hospitals impose visiting rules, out of necessity, which keep family and friends away, and often physicians and nurses maintain a distance that doesn't allow us to deal with our dying.

An alternative, humane way was necessary, and the growing hospice care programs have been one answer. There are more than a thousand hospice care programs in the United States. Hospice programs are based in a variety of settings—special hospital units, nursing homes, independent hospice facilities, or in one's own home with round-the-clock telephone access to medical assistance. The hospice movement encourages individuals to remain at home if their needs can be met.

Special units in hospitals or hospice facilities are home-like, often with kitchen facilities, dining room, and places for visiting, and individuals are encouraged to bring mementos from home to add a personal touch. Visiting hours are unrestricted—any and all may visit, including children and family pets—and in some hospices, relatives can sleep overnight.

Most major insurance carriers pay hospice benefits, depending upon an individual's policy. Specific coverage may include nursing care, home health aides, inpatient hospice care, respite time aides for the family, and bereavement support.

Individuals in hospices receive relief from pain and other debilitating symptoms (when possible), but treatment is no longer directed at curing the illness. The quality of life is stressed in hospices.

To find out what local hospice care programs are available, call the social service departments of local hospitals, home health agencies, and visiting nurse associations. The National Hospice Organization, 1901 North Fort Meyer Drive, Arlington, Virginia 22209, maintains an up-to-date, nationwide directory of hospice programs.

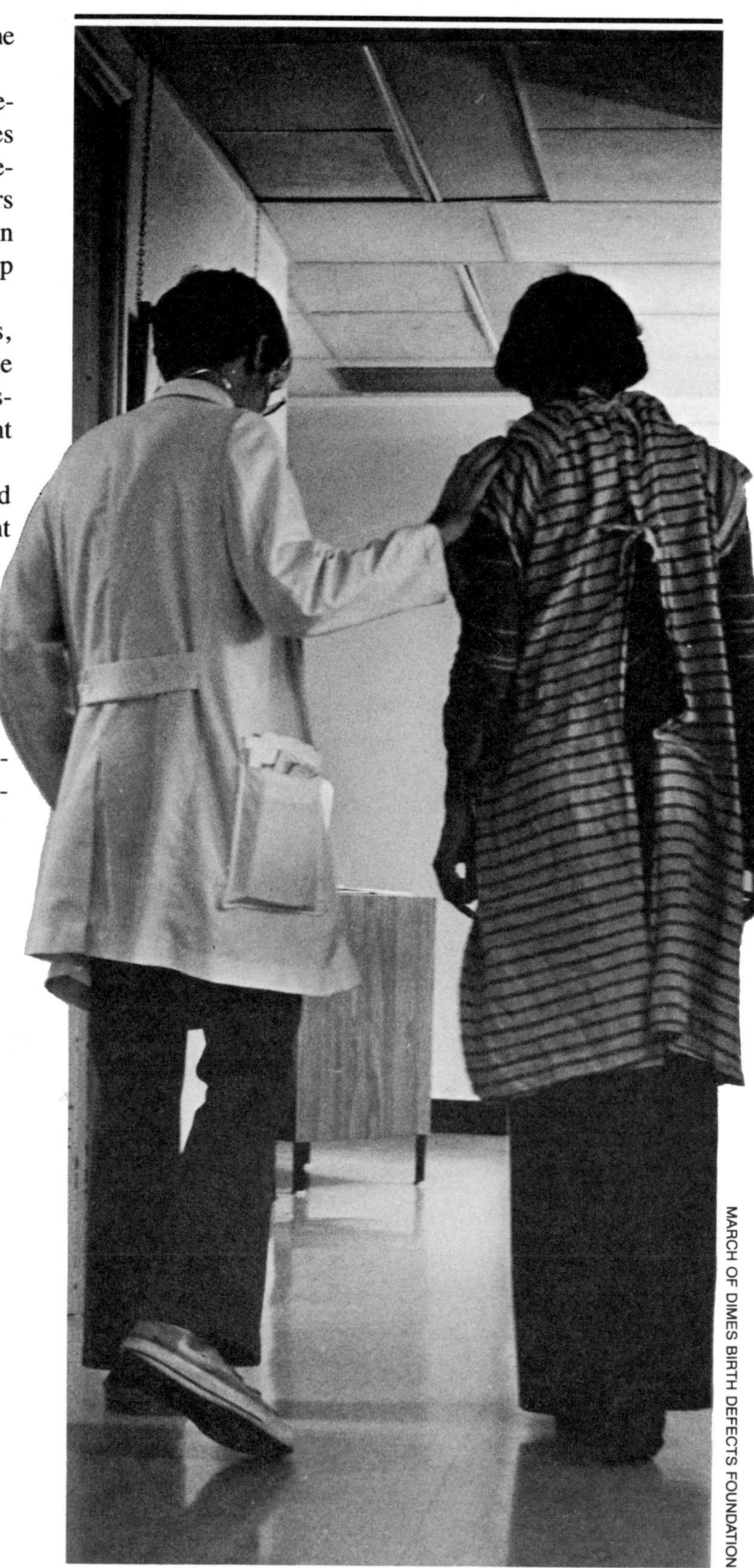

MARCH OF DIMES BIRTH DEFECTS FOUNDATION

A doctor talks to the mother of a new born baby who is in critical condition.

Hermina Jackson

Hermina Jackson watches me drink a cup of tea offered to me by her attendant. Together, we watch the heavy snow outside. The apartment, neatly kept with one bedroom, is in a twenty-story city project.

She remembers, "I used to drink hot water at night when I lived in the hospital, with nothing in it, just to get filled up. We would eat dinner at five, and by ten o'clock, I was starving, and there wasn't anything to eat. I was a teenager, hungry all the time."

On the coffee table are photograph albums. Many pictures, carefully arranged under plastic, mark christenings, birthdays, other happy times.

It is when we begin to speak of writing that permission is given to tape, but not before she asks her attendant to lower the television she has been listening to in the bedroom so it is not recorded.

I'm really interested in writing. I want to tell about myself, what I experienced, how I became the person that I am. I just want to put it down on paper. I think of so many things that I went through . . . that I'm still going through, have to go through . . . just to get to where I am now and be the person I am; to be sure about myself; to know how much I'm capable of. So I just want to share it.

I'm disabled. I'm a disabled woman. I'm also a black woman. All these things have to come out of me. This is what I want to give to people so they can understand. They'll get just a little knowledge of who I am and maybe they can understand themselves, too. It's all balled up inside of me.

Of course, when it happened, I was young . . . about thirteen years old. I had a gunshot wound in my neck. From that day to this, I can't move my arms or legs, or hardly any other part, without someone helping me. I move my wheelchair by putting a stick in my mouth and pressing the stick down on a lever, which starts the motor that moves the chair.

I can remember a time when I could run and skip and do what other kids do. When I was younger, I dreamed about me doing all those things. Even now, I'm not in my wheelchair in my dreams; I'm walking.

I've never been bitter about the fact that I was disabled. But I just couldn't understand it because, when it happened, I just thought I would get better.

Sometimes I would lay there and the nurse would say, "We have to turn the Stryker frame bed around now." I was used to looking to my left side, and when she turned the frame around, I would have to look to my right. I would get annoyed at her because she wanted me to look the other

"I can remember a time when I could run and skip and do what other kids do. When I was younger, I dreamed about me doing all those things. Even now, I'm not in my wheelchair in my dreams; I'm walking."

way. I couldn't understand why she wanted that. She explained to me and my folks that if I didn't turn, it wouldn't heal right. But I was thirteen years old then; how could she expect I would understand? My mother didn't really understand. Your child is walking around outside and then all of a sudden something happens . . . it's very hard. She would ask the doctors a question; sometimes she didn't understand.

My family, we were close. My mother was very strong and she really kept us together, strong. By me being young when this happened . . . and they didn't expect me to live . . . everyone spoiled me. If that hadn't changed, I would never have grown up. That is where my mother played a big part.

After I was in the hospital for a year and a half, I went to a rehabilitation center. My mother came every day, brought me food from home that she cooked, and stayed with me. If I said I wanted a TV or a radio or new pants, someone in my family brought it. My little sister spent so much time there she practically grew up in that place.

One day, my mother was going to a funeral, and she came and brought me some ravioli from a can. (I was about eighteen going on nineteen then.) She warmed it and put a little seasoning in it. She said, "I can't stay too long today." I resented the fact that she was leaving, and I asked, "Why did you make ravioli?" First, she started to explain, and then she looked at me and said, "You know, I just realized there's something I have to do to straighten you out. I have no time now, but I see you are going in the wrong direction and I have to stop you because no one else is going to put up with this. If something should happen to me, no one is going to deal with this." I heard her.

It was the best thing in the world because she was really right. My mother made me strong to the point that she depended on me. Now I'm stronger than anyone else in that family.

After that, if I wanted something I saw in the newspaper, my mother would say to me, "All right, how do you want to go about getting it? How much can you put toward getting it?" If I said, "Mom, could I have such and such?" she would say, "Can you *have*, or do you want to borrow it? If you ask me, can I have something, and I have it, I'll give it to you, but if you want to borrow it, I expect it back." And she meant what she said. If I said I wanted a dress, she would say, "Your size is twelve. Ask one of the nurses or find a way to get it. Do it." I got to the point where I started shopping for her! And this is one of the ways I got to be strong. In this sense, she made me independent.

In another sense, to be strong in a hospital, to stand up against so many crises, now that's another thing! In order to stand up against that, you have to get so fed up and love yourself so much to just say, "The hell with it!" You're not going to worry about how many people like you.

"By me being young when this happened . . . and they didn't expect me to live . . . everyone spoiled me. If that hadn't changed, I would never have grown up. That is where my mother played a big part."

There were always a lot of people around me, and they liked me. It's so nice to be a good patient. That's the best. "She's a good patient." So you try to keep being a good patient. I almost died trying to be a good patient!

I had to have a laxative; at the time, we were given enemas. I just didn't want to hear the nurses complaining so much, so one time I just didn't say anything. Maybe I went three weeks; nobody noticed it. Then I got very sick, running a high temperature and everything. The doctors were all around me. Then they called doctors from another building, and they didn't know what to do. It was one of these big things . . . one said I needed an operation. So my doctor came, he examined me, and he said, "Wait a minute—okay, everybody, leave her alone."

They had already sent my mother a telegram to come, but she was on her way to the hospital and she missed it. The next day, the doctor came in and he sat down and talked to me. "You do this again, you're not hurting anyone but yourself." He looked at me in a special way. Nice.

"There were always a lot of people around me, and they liked me. It's so nice to be a good patient. That's the best. 'She's a good patient.' So you try to keep being a good patient. I almost died trying to be a good patient!"

I had another couple of really good, good people who loved me and cared about me. They were nurses and nurses' aides. Once one of them came over to me; she was on the twilight shift . . . from 3:30 to around midnight . . . and she said, "Let me tell you something. Everyone is not going to like you, so you better start caring about yourself now. If I'm giving you medication, ask me what it is; find out what you're taking and why; look at it; ask me, what's in here? And I'm going to tell you another thing . . . because I wash your ass, don't kiss mine!"

They try to break you. To get over that is like climbing a mountain; you get to the top of it, and you see clear; coming down, it's easy. Because you know who respects you, you know who cares about you; and you feel the same way about them. They undersand and accept you as a human being.

It's very hard because you always want people to like you. And, if you are in this condition, you always feel you're dependent. You feel like you shouldn't say things, talk back. On the other hand, you're killing yourself inside. You know where the respect comes from—inside. All those phony people, they don't mean anything, I've been called a rebel, a bitch; I've been called a lot of things.

When you're in the hospital, you know there are certain rules. You have certain rules, period, in life. You can't just say, "I'm going to rebel." There are certain things that you are supposed to be doing. You have certain responsibilities. Those are not the things you're rebelling against. Being treated like an animal, that's what you're against. If someone does treat you like that, you say something. And if that doesn't get you anyplace, you go further, and you keep going. You don't just let it stop there. I have a godmother, a strong woman and person, who has inspired me a lot. She always told me, "No matter who they are, there is always someone over them." This becomes something very important to remember if you're not being treated right.

One time I had the whole twilight shift against me. I still got what was coming to me. You have to get over the fact that someone is not going to talk to you, too. They try to "freeze you out." Now, one shift is not going to be there all the time; it's going to change; there will be other people coming on . . . maybe some good people who are secure enough so they don't have to try to push someone around.

My mother made a statement one time: "I'm happy that you've changed and are standing up for yourself because certain things I didn't know how to deal with." Even though I was her child, there were things she couldn't control because she wasn't with me all the time. If my mother or another person in my family said too much, they were afraid after they left that the staff would take things out on me somehow.

Your family means a whole lot, but if *you* don't say anything, it's nothing.

I decided to leave the hospital when I was all grown up and had outgrown it. All together, I was in there for seventeen years.

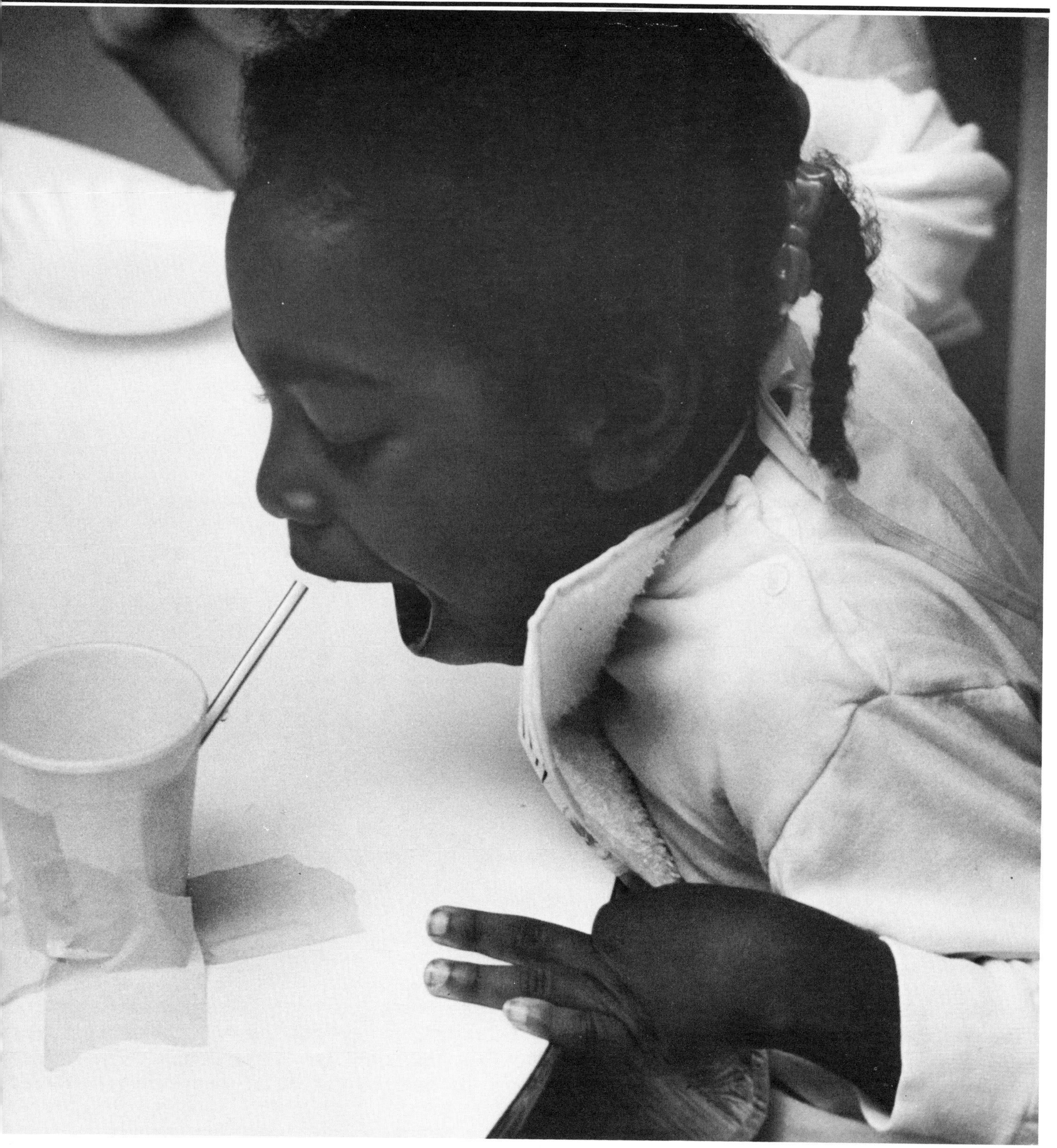

HANNA SCHREIBER/PHOTO RESEARCHERS

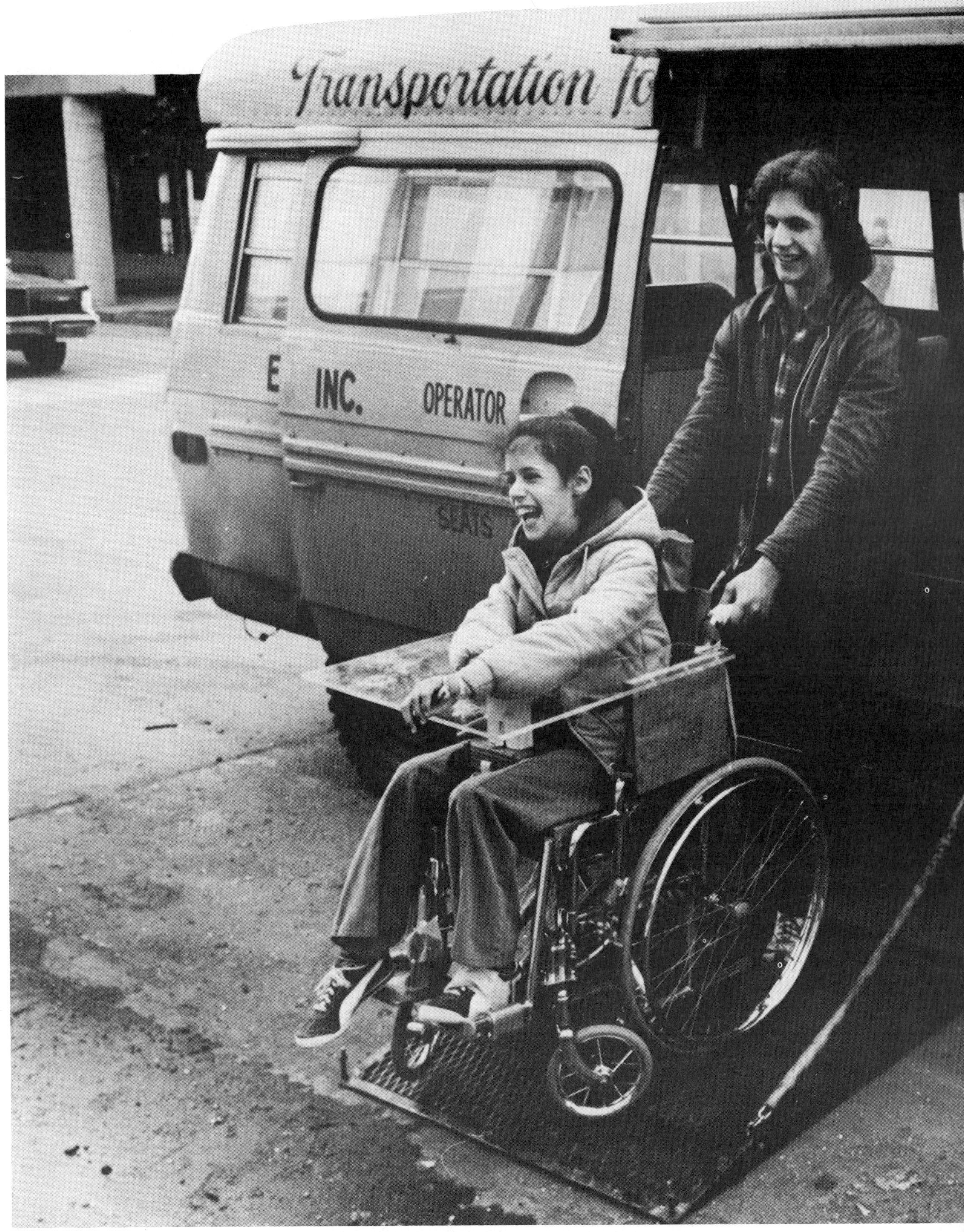
Transportation fo
E
INC.
OPERATOR
SEATS

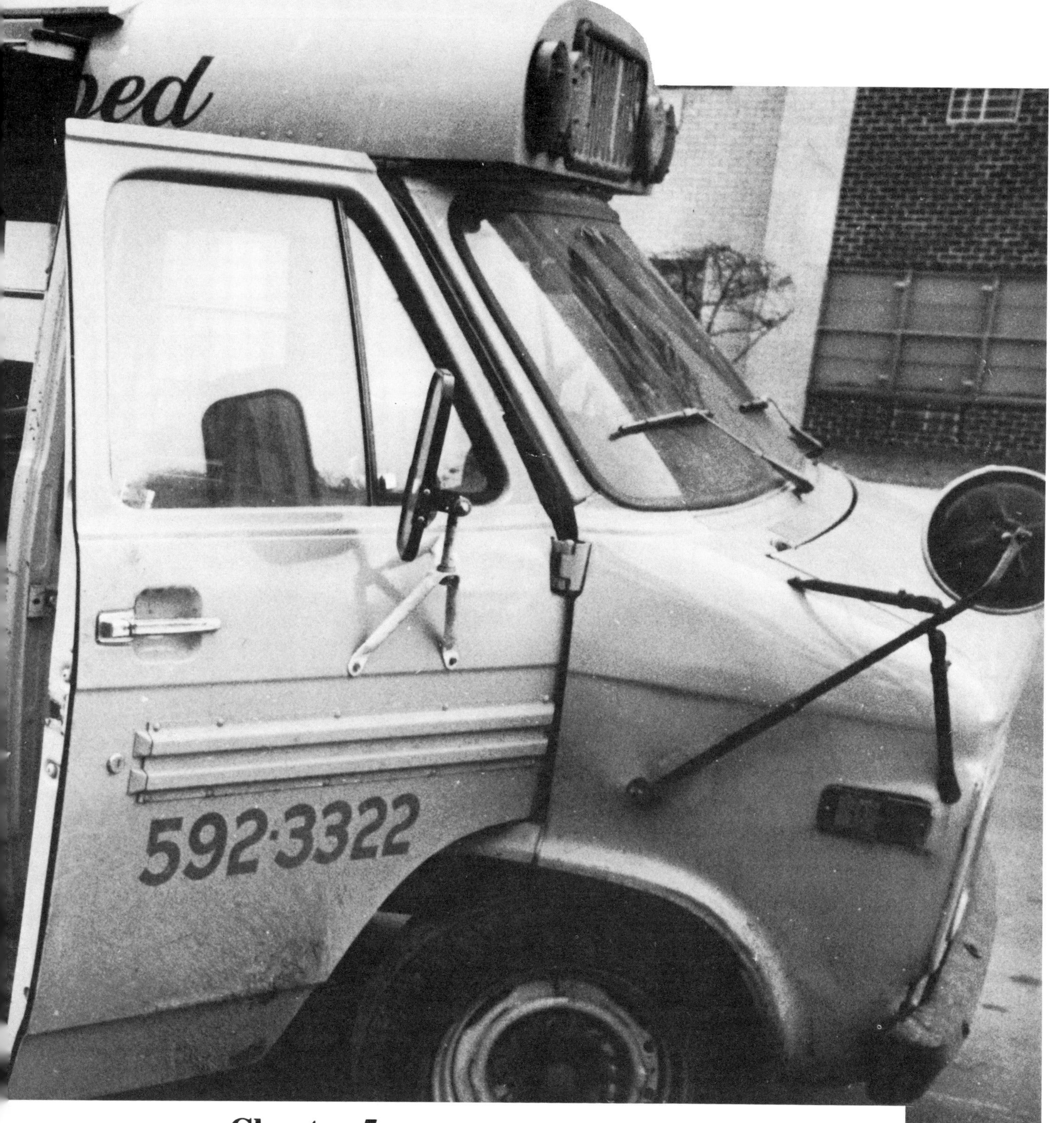

IRENE BAYER/MONKMEYER

Chapter 5

Education Is a Right

Disabled children must be given the opportunity to experience everything that all children do.

Getting Your Rights

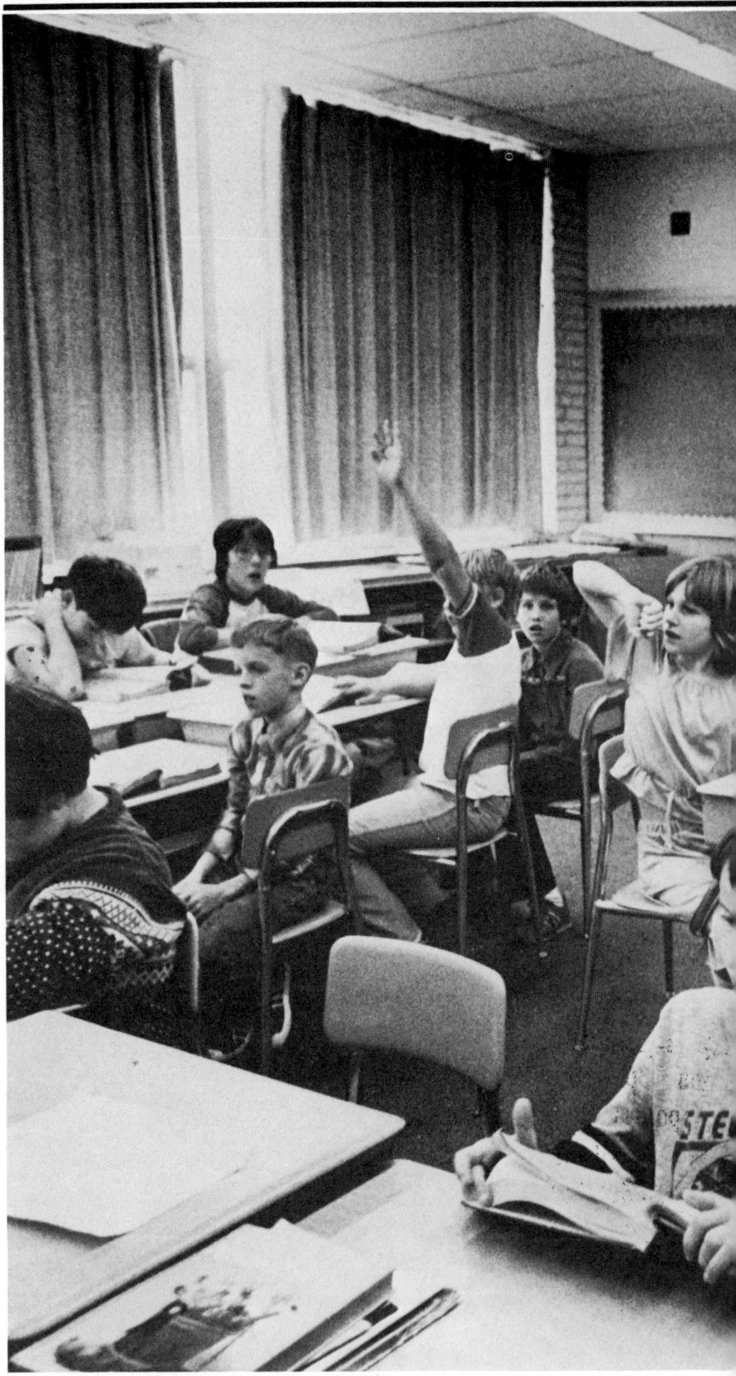

A fifth grade class at the Green Park Elementary School, Green Park, Pennsylvania.

"When you try to get the special help your child may need in school, you begin to feel bureaucracies have been created to break you," says Terry Schmele, whose son, Josh, has a learning disability. "And unless you get good advice about how to fight for your rights, you can come darn close to giving up. But where are you going to go? The public school is the only game in town; it isn't as though you can take your business elsewhere," she adds.

Terry Schmele counts herself very lucky for a number of reasons: Her family lives in a school district whose employees are well trained and sensitive to the special needs of children; and a friend—a teacher's aide—helped the family get appropriate help and provided information about learning disabilities, finding other parents with similar concerns whose children could be friends for Josh.

"Unless you get good advice about how to fight for your rights, you can come darn close to giving up. But where are you going to go? The public school is the only game in town."

First, Schmele joined the PTA and got involved in a committee on special needs education. Meeting other parents gave her some reassurance that she was not alone. Her husband wrote the department of education for a copy of the state special education law. He knew that states vary in what they mandate in education for disabled children, but he was interested to learn that the ages of children eligible for public education vary in different states. Some state provide appropriate services for disabled children at birth—with infant education programs—and help for parents. Oth ers extend the age of eligibility past twenty-one.

When Terry Schmele learned from a parent that ther was an association for children with learning disabilities she wrote for a list of their publications. As she put it, "

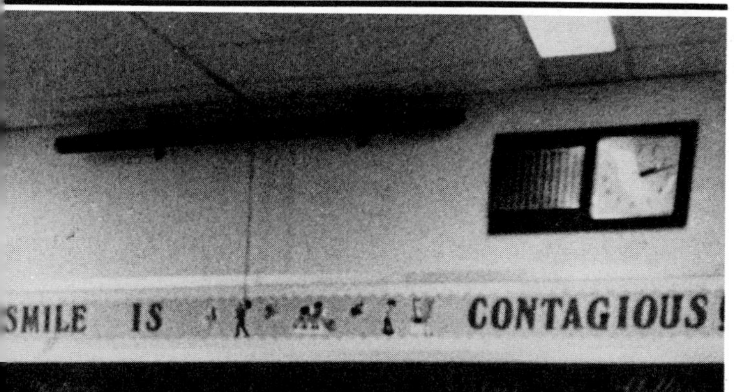

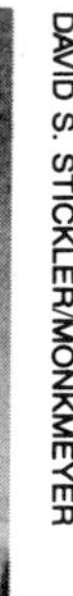
DAVID S. STICKLER/MONKMEYER
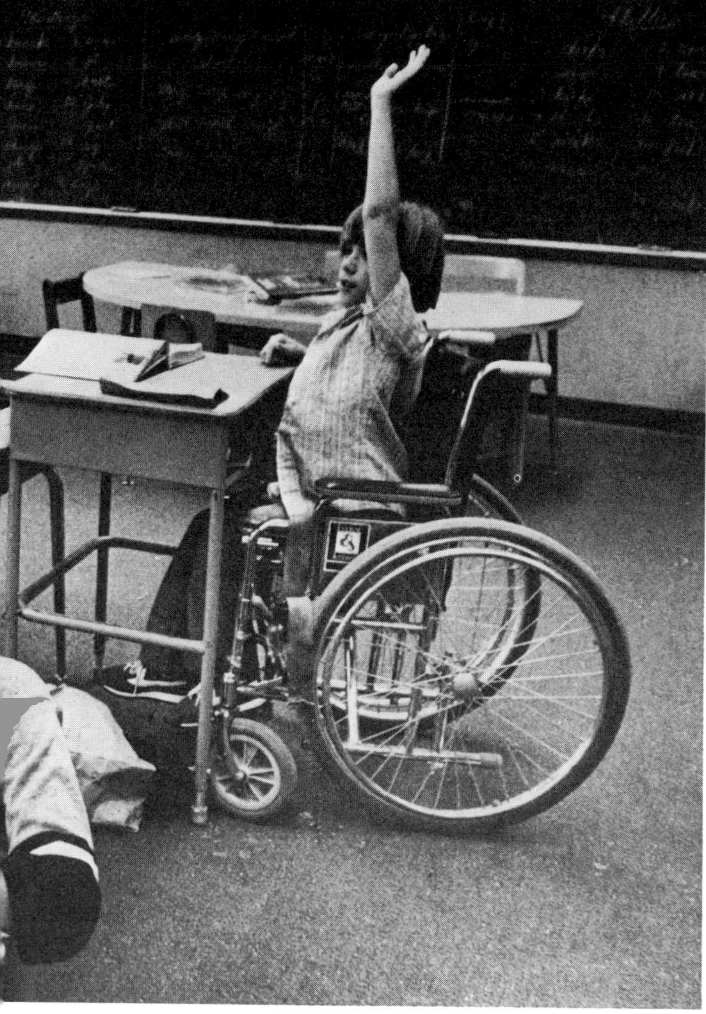

ever knew anyone who had a learning disability, and I was nterested. What I find now is that there are lots of experts vho do not have the answers either."

Terry Schmele's role of parent advocate has had a ositive effect. She remembers her early days when Josh egan to experience problems learning to read words. "I am ne kind of person who is a fixer—I fix things—and this vas something I could not fix," she smiled wryly, "so workng to get Josh the best assistance was a way of making nings better for him, for me, for the whole family. And I was also not someone who could handle authority, and to me, school administrators, teachers, principals, and school psychologists are authorities. Before long, I got over that," she says, "but I cried a lot after meetings at schools. It is amazing how people respond to you when you are prepared, committed to listening, not attacking them, and determined to get what you feel your child needs."

Ten Steps To Take When You Are in Conflict with Your School System

The right of parents to question actions or decisions of schools is clearly written into the Education for All Handicapped Children Act and the regulations for Section 504 of the Rehabilitation Act. Both laws provide legal options for exercising your right to protest. But before you take legal steps, you want to use every available channel of communication with school representatives to try to settle disputes through understanding and persuasion.

Remember: A child with a disability has the right to a free, appropriate education. That right is guaranteed by law.

It is important to be aware of the people you can turn to for advice—and the key officials with whom you should discuss your problems. Here is a checklist you can use to help you take constructive action when things seem to be going wrong. Remember: A child with a disability has the right to a free, appropriate education. That right is guaranteed by law.

1. Talk to your child's classroom teacher and to other school people who are aware of your child's needs, such as the counselor, nurse, school psychologist, or social worker. Naturally, not all of these people are involved in every situation. Discuss the problem you see with any and all of the staff members who do know your child to see if adjustments or changes can be made through new understanding and effort.

2. If these first steps don't work, do be sure to find out who among these school people will be willing to help you go further. Is the teacher sympathetic to your needs? Will she or he stand by your request? Does the counselor have information that will help? Ask them if they will be willing to come to meetings with you or to supply letters or statements in support of your position.

3. Discuss your concerns with other professionals outside of school who know your child, such as your family doctor, pediatrician, psychologist, audiologist, neurologist, or other specialists. Will they support your efforts to get new services for your child? Will they write letters or come with you to important conferences to answer questions? Will they express their views on a tape recorder—for you to bring to the school?

4. Remember to keep notes of your conversations and a file of up-to-date records. This is invaluable.

5. Discuss your complaints with the school principal. Have a clear idea of your reasons for requesting a change in your child's program, and present your documentation. Be straightforward and self-assured. You are an equal in this and other school conferences. It's neither necessary nor productive to be aggressive or apologetic. Approach it as a situation in which both of you are seeking a solution to a problem.

6. Go directly to your district director of special education or director of pupil personnel services if the school is unable (or unwilling) to change its decisions. If no such staff positions exist in your district, contact the superintendent of schools. The superintendent is responsible for all school programs in the district and must be involved if other officials are unresponsive. Again, your notes, records, and other files should be in order. Use them. In all of these conferences, it is important to know what part of the federal and/or state law protects your child's rights.

   It probably will be necessary to have more than one meeting to settle things. When meetings are held, make clear that you would like to have other people present who know your child and are familiar with the problem. Ask to have them included so that the discussion will be as productive as possible. Many problems can be settled just this way.

7. Bring your complaint before the local school board if none of these approaches work. Increasingly, there are members of school boards who are deeply concerned about special education, and they may be able to take action on your behalf. Even if their actions do not bring about immediate results that help your child, school board members can, in the long run, see to it that education programs are developed, that teachers are trained for new responsibilities, and that schools are accessible and capable of meeting the special needs of disabled children.

8. Get in touch with your state director of special education. He or she should have information and advice you can use. State departments of education are responsible for carrying out the provisions of Public Law 94-142. Explain fully what you see as a violation of your child's right to free, appropriate education under the law. Find out what action they can take to help the situation.

9. States are required by PL 94-142 to appoint complaint officers to investigate problems and monitor the implementation of the law. Find out if your state department of education has appointed someone to fill this position. Contact this officer for further advice, clarification of your rights under law, and suggestions for action.

10. Find your allies. In addition to reaching and conferring with these key people, it is important to get support from other well-informed and skilled allies. They include:

    - Members of state and local chapters of parent and advocacy organizations, such as the Association for Children with Learning Disabilities, Association for Retarded Citizens, National Association of the Deaf, United Cerebral Palsy—and groups representing other disabilities. More and more, other parents are now trained and ready to go with you to school meetings, help you decide what to do next, and help you decide how to present your case.

    - Advocates with special knowledge about the rights of disabled children and youth. The number of centers

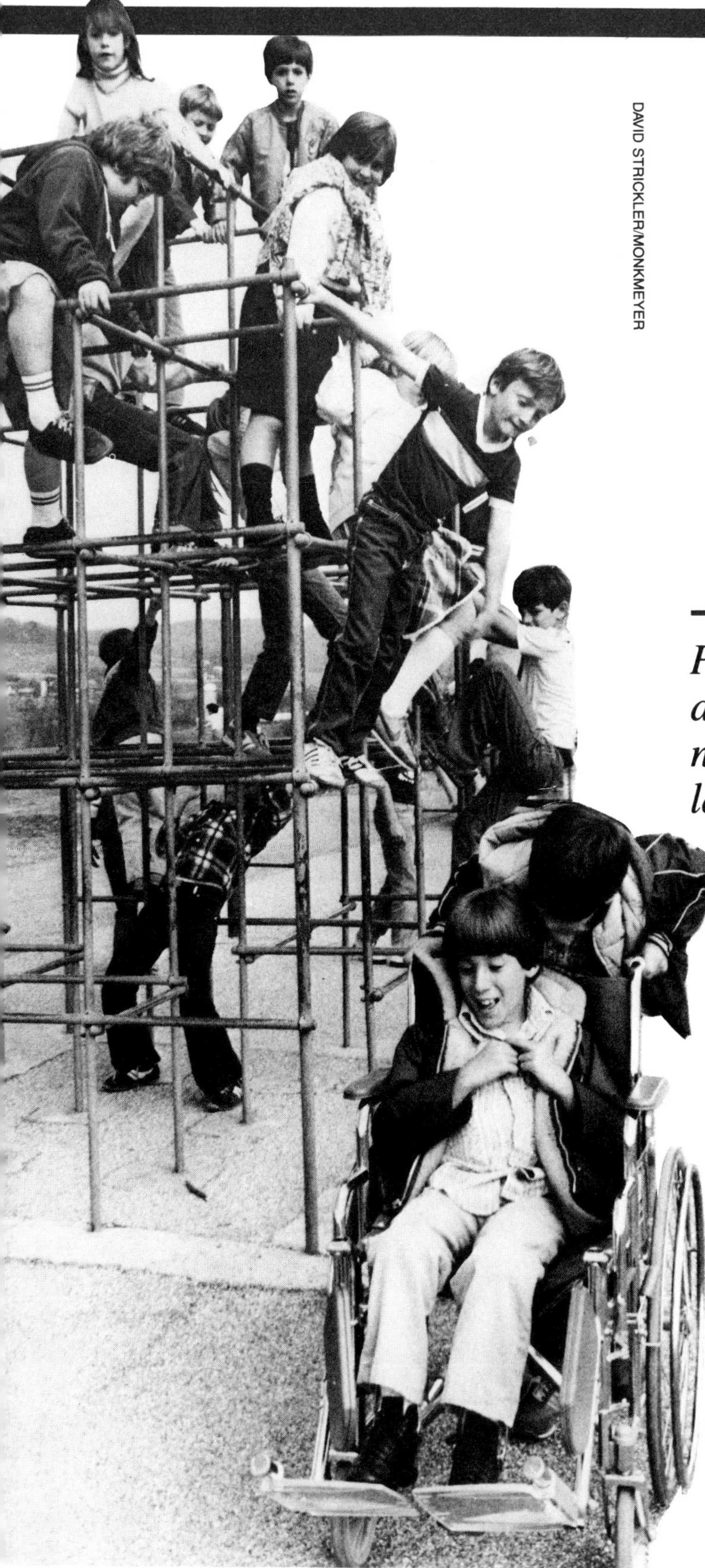

Mainstreaming on the school playground at the Green Park Elementary School, Green Park, Pennsylvania.

providing advice and assistance in obtaining appropriate school programs is growing. Parents don't necessarily need the aid of a lawyer but they often do need someone who understands the law of the school bureaucracy thoroughly. Protection and advocacy centers are set up in every state for children with developmental disabilities. Check also with area college and university departments of special education, as well as independent living centers and organizations for disabled citizens, for other possible leads to local advocates.

- The people you have gathered as your own advisers can help counsel you about next steps if all your efforts to come to an agreement break down. That's when you need to decide whether to call for a due process hearing before an impartial hearing officer, as provided by PL 94-142, or to take other legal action. This is your right, and it may turn out to be necessary; but before you move into legal action, be sure that you have done what you can to solve problems through the methods already outlined.

Parents don't necessarily need the aid of a lawyer, but they often do need someone who understands the law and the school bureaucracy thoroughly.

Each state has specific steps for due process hearings and appeals. Write to your state department of education for information about state rules and regulations. Find out if a manual describing educational rights has been written for your state—and get a copy. Take the time to study your alternatives and get all the help you can from other parents, teachers, and advocates so that you can be as effective as possible in defending your child's rights.

Portions of this material appeared in the newsletter of *Closer Look* and is reprinted with permission.

PEOPLE TAKING CHARGE

- *See that all disabled students can and do participate in after-school activities, in assembly, the cafeteria, and gym. If this is not taking place in your child's school, find out why. Start with the teacher, work your way up to the school board.*
- *If physical therapy, speech therapy, occupational therapy, catheterization, or other special needs are prescribed for your child, it is essential that these services be delivered.*
- *Check to see that the PTA includes special needs of disabled children in their meetings, and let them know your concerns.*
- *If there is no parent advocacy group or you are not satisfied with the one in existence, start a new one.*
- *Invite teachers, school counselors, principals, and teacher assistants to meetings.*
- *The bulletin boards of day care centers, libraries, supermarkets, housing developments, churches, and synagogues are good places to post notices of meetings. Try a direct calling campaign and invite parents and others to meetings.*
- *Know your rights. Keep up to date with any changes in order to become an effective advocate for your child and others.*
- *Coalitions can fight more effectively than individuals. Join together with other organizations. Learn about the work taking place in the state office of organizations, such as United Cerebral Palsy, Muscular Dystrophy, Epilepsy Foundation, etc., which include advocacy for special education for all disabilities.*
- *Learn the organizations in your community involved in disability rights educational efforts and join them. A number of these organizations have educational legislative representatives on local, state, and federal levels. Find out who they are and about the work they are doing.*
- *Community newspapers usually assign a reporter to cover educational subjects. Call the newspaper and find out the reporter's name. Send press releases concerning special education and notices of all meetings.*
- *Organizations should send press releases to the media, newscasters, and TV and radio stations for coverage of their work and events. Follow-up calls can be made to determine if additional information is needed to create further interest.*
- *If there is a special education department in a local college, contact the chairperson of the department and invite the individual to attend your meetings. Perhaps the chairperson or other professors could be guest speakers. Similarly, parents may be willing to share their experiences with students attending the college.*
- *As a citizen and constituent, visit your representative to Congress at his or her local office and introduce yourself. Let your representative know your position on special education.*
- *If there is a particular issue that is to be voted on, start a letter-writing campaign to the Washington office. Get the address and zip code from the local office. It has been said that as few as ten letters from constituents can influence a vote.*
- *Write all political representatives and share your stand on special education. Find out when state assemblymen and state senators will be in your community. Arrange a meeting to discuss your viewpoints on special education. A well-organized and well-informed group may be the best bet.*

Phyllis Rubenfeld

Phyllis Rubenfeld has done almost the impossible in education—she has gone from home instruction to a doctorate of education Ed.D. The president of the American Coalition of Citizens with Disabilities (ACCD), she has worked her way up through the ranks. We have organized and marched together, and we enjoy a warm friendship.

Late one afternoon, we sit drinking coffee in the student hangout at Columbia. The wood-paneled room with its high ceiling is almost empty of students. Outside, snow is falling for the fourth consecutive day. Occasionally, a student comes in and, recognizing Phyllis, waves and points in the direction of the snow with a smile of resignation.

"A few of us who are disabled were in here last week talking about what this weather means to us," she says earnestly, expressing the feelings of dependency that come up at this time of the year.

My special education class for orthopedically disabled children was self-contained in a public school classroom and had several grades (I believe it was fourth through eighth grade) in one class. Each grade sat in a different row.

Every day, we were given sheets of questions and little blue books. I am convinced that's why, to this day, I have an aversion to test books—they're blue, also. But those were not test books; they were answer books. We had a lot of question sheets, and we were taught how to copy the answers from the blue book onto the exam sheets we were given. Whoever could *copy* the answer best was the one who got the highest grade. You were even cheating on cheating because a cheat can figure out how to cheat to get an answer.

That's how we were taught. It was a very interesting way to learn!

We were taught all subjects, except in either the morning or the afternoon, I forget which, when we washed the chalkboard. The 7th and 8th grades were very cooperative. Those of us who could raise our arms would wash the top part of the board; those who couldn't would wash the bottom. After washing the boards, we would bang the erasers out the window, clean our desks, clean the teacher's closet. We did this every day. That was going to school; that was our "education."

As inadequate as it was, it was school. But I didn't get to stay in school long. I only went for one year, and then I was stopped from going and put on home instruction.

The reason was, in those days, you had to be able to do everything by yourself; you had to take care of all your bodily needs unassisted. They wouldn't allow other students to help you. My problem was I could not get off the toilet alone; it was too low and there were no such things as grab bars.

There were kids in another classroom—that was the class with the cardiac and tuberculosis conditions—who were really tough; I'm not sure why. Some of the girls lived in my neighborhood and knew me. They would come into the bathroom and help me off the "john," with the teacher not noticing. For several months, we got away with this, but then they caught us and saw I was being assisted. A letter was sent to the board of education, and I was immediately stopped from going to regular school.

"Some of the girls lived in my neighborhood and knew me. They would come into the bathroom and help me off the 'john,' with the teacher not noticing. For several months, we got away with this, but then they caught us and saw I was being assisted. A letter was sent to the board of education, and I was immediately stopped from going to regular school."

Home instruction was a unique experience because of the teacher assigned to me. She had a very positive effect on me; if it hadn't been for her and for my family, I don't know what I would have done academically. She was a little weird in the sense that she was completely committed to her work, my education—quite unusual for home instruction. From about a third grade reading level, I was raised in all subject areas; I was in the seventh grade at the time. Not only did I achieve grade level, but every morning when she came in, we saluted the flag—in my bedroom. I mean, I was going to school! I was doing what other kids in regular school were doing. I could talk about saluting the flag, singing whatever other kids sang, "God Bless America" or "The Star-spangled Banner."

She took me to see my first operetta, *The Love of Three Oranges*. A whole system was figured out where all the kids going to the operetta had to meet at the subway station. She also taught me how to travel alone. She had to do a lot of persuading to convince my mother it was okay, but she did it.

In the summer, she went to Europe and took reams of film. When she came back, we met in her home on a Sunday and, through the pictures, I saw Europe.

The only extremely upsetting thing that she ever did—without, of course, knowing it—was take pictures of me walking into an auditorium. I had never seen myself walk other than in the mirror in physical therapy when I worked at the parallel bars, and there you are walking very slowly—you try to walk very straight and not limp. So you don't really know how you look when you walk; when you limp, you don't feel you're limping. I guess people think you do, but you don't. I looked at myself, and I was so upset; I said, "God, do I walk like that?"

But she had such confidence in me, in all her students. I can't imagine that she could have believed I would have gotten out of high school. When I had her as a teacher, I had to learn. I would be given cards with division on one side, multiplication on the other. My father didn't know math, but every night he would do those flash cards with me.

"Most kids on home instruction didn't take exams because you were not going to engage a disabled child in competition. Blind, paralyzed, deaf, mentally retarded—it didn't matter because everyone was looked upon as being the same."

Most kids on home instruction didn't take exams because you were not going to engage a disabled child in competition. Blind, paralyzed, deaf, mentally retarded—it didn't matter because everyone was looked upon as being the same. There was no reason that I, or any other disabled kid, regardless of the disability, could not compete. But she gave exams! She gave spelling tests; we had to do compositions. I had to do so much for her; I was constantly working.

Then, when I got to high school, things changed; I went to regular school one year. It was really hard, although I liked it. I had a lot of trouble socially. When guys would make advances, I was very suspicious because why would they be interested in me? I'm disabled. First, I thought they were crazy, really strange people. It was interesting because attention usually came from the guys who were the most popular; they were the "jocks." The girls were nice, but it was difficult. Academically, it was horrible. I wasn't used to a classroom; there's a lot of competition. If I didn't understand something, I couldn't keep raising my hand and asking. The pace was much quicker.

I'll never forget one French teacher who said, "I am going to give you a hint for the exam." This was a long time ago, and I still have not forgotten it because it was so meaningless to me. "Remember," she said, "when I am correcting your grammar, the pants always fit the jacket." To this day, I don't know what the hell she meant! Everyone sort of nodded. "They know," I said to myself, "and I don't know what this lady is talking about."

I liked school; I liked the idea of going to school. I worked in the dean's office, the library, everywhere. It was so new, so different; it was terrific. I even read the Bible in assembly. It was a big honor. I don't remember how I got up the three steps to the stage. I think I may have crawled. That never, ever stopped me.

"That there were steps, that the campus was so large, didn't faze me. It was a fact. The place was large; it had steps; so what? I asked people to help me."

That was the reason I was physically able to go to Brooklyn College. That there were steps, that the campus was so large, didn't faze me. It was a fact. The place was large; it had steps, so what? I asked people to help me. The campus being large meant to me that if I had German at 9:00 o'clock in the morning in Boylin Hall, I would next schedule art in Gershwin Hall at 11:00 o'clock. I never programmed myself, as most students do, with classes back to back. I had to give myself an hour in between each class. I did this as a freshman and sophomore. But as a junior, I became a little brazen; I scheduled classes back to back and arrived at the second class a little late.

For the first two years, I was in that school day and night. I planned six courses, which covered the entire day, so I would never be a minute late to class. No one could say I was late because I was disabled. I never discussed this with anyone; it was just something I had to do. The wanting was always there. I couldn't get into Gershwin Hall because there were no rails. There were three steps inside two halls where classes were held, in addition to all the steps on the outside. If I sat down on a step, I couldn't get up by myself. I was dreadfully embarrassed. I always prayed that no one would ever see me shimmy up those steps. And if they saw me, I'd act as though I didn't know they saw me.

The steps inside were nearly impossible. The only way I could get up them was to lean against the wall, sort of crawl up the steps, and then shift my way over to the door. The door opened out, and it was, pardon the expression, a

"During the snow, it was a big problem. I needed help wherever I was going. I couldn't go anywhere alone."

"blind" corner. Miraculously, I never got knocked down. How I did that I don't know because all of a sudden I would appear there, just praying no one was coming out the door from the other side. If I had been hit, I would have been thrown down all the steps.

I guess one of the reasons I didn't ask for help was that I traveled from one class to the next on my hour break. I would travel when I knew most of the other students were in class. It wasn't during change of class, so the traffic wasn't as great. I would stand in the hall for hours; there were no chairs anywhere. But that didn't matter.

During the snow, it was a big problem. I needed help wherever I was going. I couldn't go anywhere alone. I'd usually ask people in my class to help me to another building.

If I had an hour break, I would want to go to the library and do some work. I couldn't do that if it was snowing. I spent a lot of time just staying put, standing around. If it was raining, I'd get drenched because I couldn't go from building to building fast enough to stay dry. Sometimes when there was a change of classes, I would ask just anyone if they would let me hold their arm, help me get up the steps, carry my books.

"After being on home instruction, you are totally not socialized. You don't have the experience or know-how to take an exam."

I was a lousy student my first two years in college—very, very lousy. I was not good academically. Pure and simple. That was a reality.

First of all, I think those of us who have been on home instruction have certain deficits. I have talked to many people who were on home instruction, and I think they feel as I do. There are certain deficiencies that will, perhaps, be with us forever. To this day, I have them, even though, for the most part, I've done well in graduate school and in my doctoral work.

After being on home instruction, you are totally not socialized. You don't have the experience or know-how to take an exam. When you go to school, you learn how to take exams—not because you are taught but because you do it every day. You know how to take an exam; you know how to read, what to read, what to skim. Where did I have a chance to learn this? How do you know how to write a paper if you've never been taught or have never done it before?

When I was at Brooklyn College, taking notes, what did that mean? Taking notes meant to me (you won't believe this) recopying the book! My parents certainly could not help me. They were European and not that well educated. My mother just kept wanting to know why I was writing so much. I said, "I have to take notes." I was sitting there rewriting a book.

Some of my teachers in college were interested in me but not in the first two years because the courses were all liberal arts and you took anything and everything before you chose your major. I think a lot of the teachers were shocked. Remember, in the late '50s and early '60s, very few disabled people went to school, let alone college! In a way, I was a novelty.

My sociology professors especially tried to understand me. They would pull me into their offices and say, "You have such good ideas and speak so well in class, but when you write a paper, we're not sure what you're talking about." The teachers had no idea why I could talk in class and not be able to take exams or write papers. They wondered who this person was, as though I came out of the forest. Really, it was peculiar, even though they were kind.

They wanted to know what kind of problems I had. I told them that, except for two years, I never went to school; the rest of my education was at home. They would just look at me. It was so strange to them. Some of them tried to help.

So my first two years were very, very difficult; I got a lot of Ds. I think the reason I got Ds is because I studied so hard. That sounds ironic, but the only reason I passed with Ds was that I studied so hard. I didn't know which end was up. I also thought when you studied you had to memorize pages. If you've never learned, you don't know any better. It seems so inconceivable at times.

I took chemistry one semester. As one of my required courses, there was very little choice. You have to raise your arms when you reach for the materials and to do the experiments. And I can't. So I went up to the professor, a relatively nice woman, and told her, "I can't raise my arms." No one could help me because the lab period was timed for each experiment, so by the time someone was finished, the class was over. I said to her, "Maybe if you could put the test tubes on a lower table, I could do it. I don't have to stand with everyone else." (What's the big deal?!)

The chemistry professor said, "I'll have to check it out with the chairperson." It seemed a little weird just for a lower table. She did and the okay was given. They brought in a lower table with all these test tubes and whatever. One day, the chairperson came into class and said, "You can't do it." I don't have any idea why I didn't get hysterical, since I always cry about everything. The reason I wasn't allowed to do it was because I might break something. So I told him I knew what the rules and regulations were. If you broke it, you had to pay for it. He probably thought I was crazy because what did that have to do with the fact that that was "normal." I said, "If other people break it, they pay; if I break it, I'll pay." That also wasn't his concern. His concern was that I might "hurt myself" or that I might blow something up in my face. Well, so could everyone else. Anyway, I couldn't take chemistry. Then what could I do? I had to fulfill that requirement, so I went to see the dean, whom I'll never forget.

When I told him what had happened and that I needed an equivalent course, he said to me, "People like you who can't raise your arms shouldn't go to college." At that point I got totally hysterical. I called him every name my Brownsville upbringing had taught me. I was cursing and at the same time I was crying hysterically.

One of the professors, Professor Erickson, heard someone screaming and came into the office. He was surprised to see me there, crying; that was not my usual stance. He took me out of the office. I was sobbing uncontrollably. He asked me what was wrong, and I told him. He said, "I don't see why we can't work something else out." He said the purpose of taking a science is X, Y, and Z, and you can take physical anthropology and satisfy the same X, Y, and Z. "You can hold a skull in your hand, can't you?" I said "Yuch!!" He said, "It's dead!" I said, "Isn't there skin on it?" "No," he said. Then I started to feel better. I guess he didn't know what my disability was. Did I have polio or cerebral palsy?; did my hands have spasms? I said, "No, I can hold it." That was it; it was worked out, and I took physical anthropology rather than chemistry.

Those first two years were so difficult; they were horrible. If you saw my transcript, you would die. The third year, when I started to get into my major, things got better. I wanted to major in education, but they wouldn't let me because disabled people couldn't be certified as teachers. So I majored in sociology so I could go into social work.

In looking back on that period, I realize I always tried to accommodate myself to the situation by not asking for anything unless it was absolutely impossible, therefore necessary.

I first wanted to be a teacher. Since I lived in a very poor neighborhood, I then decided to be a welfare worker. My idea of a social worker was to give money to all the people who needed it. I was going to be a "nice" social worker because I used to curse my welfare workers.

My parents always supported anything I wanted to be. My disability played a very small part in their minds. My mother always had this thing that I should be a lawyer. Something about that was scary to me. But I always thought there was something about helping people I really liked. So I just always felt I could be what I wanted to be. I was scared, though. Periodically, at night, I used to start crying and say, "I'm going to fail the test."

I had contacted the Office for Vocational Rehabilitation (OVR) while I was still in undergraduate school in Brooklyn College. I was told they paid for your books, transportation, whatever. I didn't get special transportation; I could take the school bus. I never told my parents that I called the OVR. Brooklyn College, a city school, cost $5 a semester, so it was not a prohibitive expense for my family. I told the OVR, when I called, that I was disabled and wanted to go into social work—I heard they provided these services. Over the phone, they asked me what my disability was and to describe it. I did, and they said, "No, you can't go into social work; you're too disabled; you can go into speech therapy." I said I didn't want to go into speech therapy. "Well, we won't support you." I never told my parents I called because I thought they would say (though they never did), "For the money, you should go into speech therapy."

Then I graduated, and I worked for a year and a half before I went to graduate school. I went back to OVR and again they said I couldn't go into social work because of my disability. "Why am I too disabled?" Their answer was, "because you can't jump!" Apparently, *all* social workers jump! "What does jumping have to do with being a social worker?" "Well," they said, "when you do recreation, you need to jump." "I want to go into case work and then the therapy aspects of social work," I said. "No," they said, "you can't jump." And they were serious; you had to jump.

I made another appointment with them, told them that I knew a guy who had muscular dystrophy and wanted to go to law school. That, they said, was a bad risk, and they would not sponsor him. He sued, had a fair trial hearing, won his case, and went to law school. I told them I knew the situation and I was going to do the same thing, sue them, if they would not sponsor me. And, of course, I started getting very angry; I was yelling. I also told them I didn't think they had any right to decide whether I could go to school or not. I thought the school itself should decide that. The profession should decide if I could go into it or not, not the Office of Vocational Rehabilitation. With my carrying on, they decided to sponsor me.

I am convinced that OVR continues to function that same way today. The students that scream the loudest and engage in threats are the ones who get what they deserve. OVR also has professions that they sponsor in cycles. I have two friends from "the year of the speech therapist." I am not "the year of the social worker" because they didn't want me to go into it. My year, too, was probably the beginning of the speech therapy cycle because they thought that in speech therapy, you just sit at a desk, which is also not true.

"A constant in society is that there is prejudice against the person with a disability, no matter his or her credentials."

But the Office of Vocational Rehabilitation continues to think in categories—this year is the "year of the lawyer or rehabilitation counselor." By doing this, they flood the field, and people can't get jobs.

A constant in society is that there is prejudice against the person with a disability, no matter his or her credentials. However, the OVR also trains people based upon society's prejudices. It is more acceptable for the person with a disability to become a rehabilitation counselor than to get a master's in business administration. Institutions of higher learning and rehab centers discriminate . . . how often do you find people with a disability in the business world with a title? You can probably count them on one hand. So OVR follows that pattern, and they are reinforcing these discriminations. They don't see it that way, however. They claim they are being realistic; they are not going to train someone in a field in which they cannot be employed after completing their training.

My father wanted me to be a doctor, though not necessarily a medical doctor. Then he could go to the shop every day and say, "My daughter is a doctor." I was in graduate school in social work, but I may have started to think of postgraduate work when he kept telling me his dream. I would tell him, "You have to be smart to get a Ph.D.; I'm not." He would say, "You cried in high school, you cried in college, you cried in graduate school. You always say you can't, and yet you're doing it."

"I went back to OVR and again they said I couldn't go into social work because of my disability. 'Why am I too disabled?' Their answer was, 'Because you can't jump!' Apparently, all *social workers jump!"*

I also think a great deal of influence in thinking of doing postgraduate work had to do with the fact that I was working in an academic situation. Other situations don't lend themselves that much to working on a doctorate.

A woman I worked with was extremely bright. She made it sound so simple. She would say, "It is just an extension of your undergraduate work." One summer, I decided to try it. What could happen if I took one course and failed?

In my mind, I thought, "If I fail, I'll throw myself out of the window." But I was trying not to be too neurotic about it. One hot summer day, I went to register with the woman I worked with. The place was dangerously inaccessible, down in the basement of a brownstone; the steps were broken and steep. She practically carried me down and dragged me up afterward. She stayed with me the whole time.

I had a choice of two courses that were being given: economics or political science. I had been working 14 years full-time, along with going to school, and I was not new to decision-making, but, for the life of me, I couldn't decide between the two courses. I was panicking! "My God, I'm entering a doctoral program!" After the two courses were described to me, political science sounded more interesting. When I filled out all the cards then had to check "doctoral program," I became extremely anxious. I thought, "What am I undertaking?" (I felt I was undertaking guaranteed failure.) From the time I went down those broken steps, I got a master's, completed all the course work for my doctorate, and transferred into special education, which is where I wanted to be in the first place.

It's sad; my father died. He missed seeing his dream come true. His daughter is a doctor.

I feel I made it in spite of the educational system foisted upon me. That's it in a nutshell. Now, in classes with people going into special education, I see them, I hear them, and I find most of them highly offensive. Then I say to myself, "Why should I get so upset? They are like everyone else. They are like the people who came before them." Then there are people who remind me of that teacher I had in home instruction. That one wonderful teacher! Usually, I feel I made it in spite of the others. Their programs actively discouraged me. I had to fight them to move ahead. Because I have a disability, they did nothing in terms of academic preparation.

You would have to have an enormously strong ego to go from home instruction to college, practically fail the first two years, and still keep on. I don't know where that comes from in me. There is that incredible, striving, enormous drive. It still goes on; it hasn't stopped.

I suspect if a psychological test was ever done, and I'm sure they probably were done on me, it said, "This person is an obsessive-compulsive." Everything negative that they could possibly think of would be found. "I'm going to do it, come hell or high water"; that has absolutely always been my attitude. There are so many forces working against people with disabilities that if they don't have that kind of positive, obsessive drive and incredible motivation, they are not going to succeed.

Susan Lo Tempio

I went to a Catholic high school. Nobody was in a wheelchair. I was the only one. There were no other students (or teachers) with disabilities. In my last year, there was a freshman who had cerebral palsy, that's all. I had total mainstreaming before they knew what the term meant!

Then I went to the University of Illinois. I had to take many tests before I was allowed to attend the school: IQ tests, vocational aptitude tests. In addition to the tests, disabled students had to see whether you were physically able to be in school. It was a humiliating experience for me.

At that time—it was 1968—there were about 150 people with disabilities in our program. I understand that now there are a lot less because since then many other campuses have made accommodations for disabled students. In those days, I had only two choices: Illinois or Hofstra.

They had never heard of "the movement" in Illinois, and it was a very paternalistic program. The man who ran the program was our "Father" and pretty much told us what to do. We were supposed to be loyal to him and to his rehab center before we were loyal to the university or to ourselves. He said, "I am here to help you grow up and be independent adults." But, in essence, in your junior or senior year, you realized what was going on and you rebelled. Some kids never caught on and were always grateful to "Father."

There was a kind of separatism that took place on the campus, fostered by "Father" more than by us. He wanted us to remain a clique, 150 "friends." You play the clique game for a while and then realize that it is a false society; that is not the way the world is. As soon as you got involved in your curriculum, declared a major, and hung around with the same people all the time, they became your friends. I made lifelong friends whom I still see from time to time and correspond with.

Just because people are in wheelchairs doesn't mean they have to be your best friends. Yes, you have a lot in common, but, no, you don't have a lot in common, too.

Why not choose? Everybody else does. Most of my friends from college days are disabled, but if they weren't, they'd still be my friends because I love them for who they are—they are good people.

We grew up fast. For a lot of us, it was the very first time we had ever been away from our parents. A lot of disabled kids are very dependent on their parents for everything. Away at college, you couldn't be dependent on them anymore. You had to take care of yourself—financially, physically, and emotionally. In fact, a lot of people who leave home don't make it on their own if they aren't in a college or group home situation first.

When I went to the university, there was a whole new identification issue. It was a time when you had to identify yourself as a disabled person. Before then, I was the only disabled person that I knew in a society where I was the minority. At Illinois, there was this whole "Gee, wow, everybody is in the same boat as I am" feeling. That is why I became involved in the wheelchair sports program. I traveled from one end of the country to another in the athletic program. I participated for two and a half to three years. I was a cheerleader, basketball player, and anything else they wanted me to be—and I did it all from my chair. It was a real freeing because you shared with people things you never could share with anybody else. And that is a good part of your growing, I think.

Sports proved to yourself, as well as to others, that you could do it. Up until then, you had watched basketball on television but never dreamed you could do it yourself. But now you could play, too. So, yes, it was to prove to people that you had skills like them and also to prove to yourself that you could do anything you set your mind to.

In high school, I was completely integrated in terms of the curriculum: school activities like the honor society, the Latin club, and all that. But when it came to social things, I was not integrated. I would go to dances with girls, but I never dated in high school. I went crazy in college! I found out I was a woman, and I had sexuality connected to me. As a student, I was in college, but on a social level, I was still in high school. There wasn't much rhyme or reason, and there were numerous crushes and countless broken hearts. Sometimes, I was involved with disabled men; most of the time, I wasn't. College was very painful in terms of men and dating. I had a lot of catching up to do. But I learned very quickly; I am still learning, and I feel like I am still trying to catch up, even now.

The Smiths

All of our children are adopted. Danny and Teddy are twins we adopted who became a part of our family when they were twenty months old. Those first months of their lives were not the best, needless to say, and contributed to their disabilities. There was a lack of environmental stimulation—they only had each other. The first year of their lives together was spent in one crib in a rather neglectful situation, and their foster home was not the best. So there was a lot of making up to do.

It wasn't until the twins were in kindergarten that it became apparent that they had some auditory memory problems, and a speech problem. They didn't have a chance to do the babbling and other mother-child responses that normally occur during the first two years. That's where we are now. We're doing speech therapy, going back to the babbling sounds, producing sounds over and over again so the boys know how to form these syllables with their teeth and tongues. They also have an eyesight problem that has contributed to the lag in their learning to read. These problems really weren't evident until they were in kindergarten and began trying to learn basic skills.

Even before kindergarten, we thought Danny and Teddy might have a learning problem. We had the boys in nursery school and thought it would be good for them, being with other children, making friends—not in the neighborhood. I requested preliminary testing with the learning disabilities workers who visit all the different schools—but they really didn't find anything definite. The only thing they would tell me is that the twins were average but on the low-average side for four-year olds. That concerned me a little bit because their birthday is January 19th, so they were chronologically at the oldest end of their age group. I would do little tests at home; I would ask Teddy to go to the refrigerator and get me the bread. He'd stand there staring at the refrigerator, and he didn't know what I meant by "bread." Or he'd try to ask me something simple like, "Where is the ball?" but he couldn't think of what the word for ball was.

Those little things bothered me, but I couldn't find any proof. In the middle of their kindergarten year things began to show up, and I requested very extensive testing through the district special education department. When the results were in, the teacher at first suggested that we keep them in kindergarten a second year, but I thought that would be a waste of time since they were already six years old. I felt sure of my convictions, so we went ahead and enrolled them in a special education class. When the program was presented to us, I had another moment of insecurity, wondering if I had done the right thing.

I had all these myths in my mind. Danny and Teddy are very sweet little boys—outgoing—and I feel they're really quite well adjusted. They have no behavioral problems. My greatest fear was having them in a class with children who did have behavioral problems. I didn't want them to learn any bad habits. I'd really worked very hard to help them be as sweet and nice as they are. It was several months after talking to people at every level of the special education staff, from the district superintendent right down to the teachers and social workers, before we knew the special ed class was the right place for them. I'm very pleased with the makeup of the class.

"It wasn't until the twins were in kindergarten that it became apparent they had some auditory memory problems, and a speech problem. They didn't have a chance to do the babbling and other mother-child responses that normally occur during the first two years. That's where we are now."

By sorting out our own feelings, we separated problems into categories of legal problems and social concerns. Since they're not in class with the neighborhood kids, we worried about reintegration and wondered how to keep up those social contacts. We've overcome any problem they might have had through participation in Indian guides and through going to other kids' houses after school to play, so that really hasn't been a problem. They've maintained all their friendships in the local school district; we anticipate that when they're reintegrated in a couple of years, it'll be just as if they had been in the class with their neighborhood friends.

In addition, they have some advantages as perceived by their peer group; for example, Danny and Teddy have an ice rink they can skate on at their school. And there are all the real educational advantages they're getting, which don't mean anything to the peer group but do to the parents. Some of the advantages are: small class size, special training of the teachers, very close supervision, rapid progress, and some of the innovative programs, like the Chisenbop math they're doing. It's just amazing; Ted has grasped that like crazy. He's just a whiz at math.

All of this has occurred within a short time—a little while ago, they couldn't even recognize a dozen letters of the alphabet. It takes a lot of intensive training, and we work together at home, too—under the teacher's direction. We have flash cards, sight word cards, and, when they were doing their alphabet, we had A, B, C flash cards.

We've had a lot of success, but it depends a great deal on the particular special ed district and even more on the particular teacher. There's certainly no guarantee that just because the institution's taking special ed money from the federal government that they're doing the job. Many people move after researching the different special ed districts and choose the one they think is best for their child.

We picked our house where it was for two reasons: first, because when I joined the bank, I thought we should live in the community; and, second, that district (and particularly that school) is one of the best in the country. We live one block from a high school that is renowned for its scholastic achievements and has a remarkable curriculum.

The progress the boys made was visible from the first day. The change in attitude was the first indication—very immediate and very real. They came home and they had assignments; they had to watch the news. They thought of what they were doing as work for school; they had goals to accomplish. Maybe that's partly the transition from kindergarten to first grade, but it's also a very special attitude of their teacher that they went from a kind of goofing around, playing games experience to something with goals and with assignments. Once they had that frame of mind, which was almost immediately, the progress started.

They've maintained their good self-image, which was really important to me, too. I didn't want them to be in a regular class and be the last and not feel good about themselves. This has not been a problem at all. Their achievements in this special class have been just amazing. They've progressed very nicely, and when they've had trouble in certain areas, we've worked on them without lowering their self-image. If there's a problem with something, we find another approach. Sometimes, you run into a little snag when you reach a new plateau in reading that's particularly difficult—a certain sound for instance. The school will call me and tell me about it, and we'll talk together and find out whether we're pushing too hard. Their teacher will call me on her lunch hour if she's had a problem in the morning, and we'll talk about it.

"There's certainly no guarantee that just because the institution's taking special ed money from the federal government that they're doing the job."

The class size really facilitates her giving clear thinking to each child because she can work with each one as an individual. There are eleven children in the class now; they started with seven. There are two certified teachers. The children get a lot of verbal encouragement and can see their progress. They're only dealing with a learning disability. They get less frustrated than our third-grader, who's in a regular class. Again, regarding peer pressure, especially with their brother, they have that ice rink and they take special trips, so they have things to talk about that he doesn't do and vice versa. And, of course, in the family, there's no discussion about any limitations—none at all.

In a sense, I guess that's really part of our philosophy. You can do whatever you want as long as you don't think you can't.

I think one of the things that's important about our particular school district is the parents. The people in the community are very child-oriented. They're very concerned about the scholastic offerings of the schools. The PTAs are active; we have caucus meetings that the school is involved in—general town meetings for all citizens—and if there's a particular concern, then people have the opportunity to speak out.

Only when there is parent concern, intervention, and responsibility has there been this kind of push, even with an effective school superintendent. He needs the parents' support; he needs their voices. I think parents we know feel that they have something to say; they have the opportunity for input, and most of them have taken that opportunity and found the time to get involved.

There may be many people who have a child who would benefit from special ed who wouldn't get involved; they would put the child into a regular school situation. I think if those parents choose not to, it's part of their own ego problem. In effect, they're saying, "My child isn't learning disabled; he just has a bad teacher" or "He's had bad luck." Parents think of excuses why their child isn't doing too well in school instead of trying to dig in and gain a perspective and find out why and try not to blame themselves. I think that's another problem; a lot of parents blame themselves.

Even in the best cases, there's probably a year or two delay beyond what should be the optimum time for getting a child into special ed. Very few parents recognize the learning disability and take action immediately. Most parents wait and see what will happen next year. I think that's the school's approach, also. The teachers, even the principals, are aware of that kind of emotional feeling on the parents' part, and it's almost as if they're afraid to come right out and tell you that your child needs special ed; "Let's wait another year, keep him back another year, and see how he does. If that's no good, then we'll talk to the parents." I think it's because of the strong reactions they get from parents who say, "No, that's not my child you're talking about."

Parents have to become more accepting of special ed and its goals, and they need to gain the realization that their child doesn't fit into the mainstream immediately. What's needed is parent education. You just can't take parents by the scruff of the neck and say, "Hey, look! You gotta do something for this kid!" You've got to bring them around slowly. It took the better part of a year for us to bring ourselves around. We went through it in stages. Danny and Teddy had been in junior kindergartens, Montessori programs, and before that, nursery programs. We had a lot of indications; there was a lot of testing. They went to a special ed, district-operated summer camp the year before. It was a sort of trial run for us to see how that would turn out. So it was a slow decision, even for us.

We had made a point of asking questions and talking to different professional people—asking off-the-record opinions of the children's teachers, at the university, and of parents whose children were already in the special ed program. My experience has been that there are very few people who aren't interested in pursuing it a little further. For some, it's due to personal curiosity; in many cases, it's out of a situation that somehow touches them personally—a child or a grandchild who is having difficulty in school or who is exhibiting behavioral problems directly related to school activities. Many people want to compare the local school system with one somewhere else or they want to see if it would benefit their child to stay where they are or move to a different district or state.

Whatever the reason, parents have the responsibility to exhaust every avenue in their search for the best educational environment for their child.

ASSERTIVENESS IS/IS NOT

ASSERTIVENESS IS:

- ***Expressing your needs clearly and directly***
- ***Expressing your ideas without feeling guilty or intimidated***
- ***Sticking up for what you believe your child needs—even though professionals may not agree***
- ***Knowing your rights and how to get them***
- ***Documenting what your child needs and all facts pertaining to his or her case***
- ***Treating professionals like partners***
- ***Effective communication***
- ***Conveying your feelings of self-confidence when you communicate with others***
- ***Advocating effectively on your own and your child's behalf***
- ***Self-reliance and independence***
- ***Persisting until you get all the services your child needs***
- ***Analyzing a problem and pinpointing areas of responsibility before you act***
- ***Agitating to get necessary legislation passed and get it implemented***
- ***Organizing for change***
- ***Having a positive attitude at all times***

ASSERTIVENESS IS NOT:

- ***Beating around the bush before stating your needs***
- ***Feeling too guilty or afraid to express your needs***
- ***Agreeing with professionals—no matter how you feel—because "professionals know what's best"***

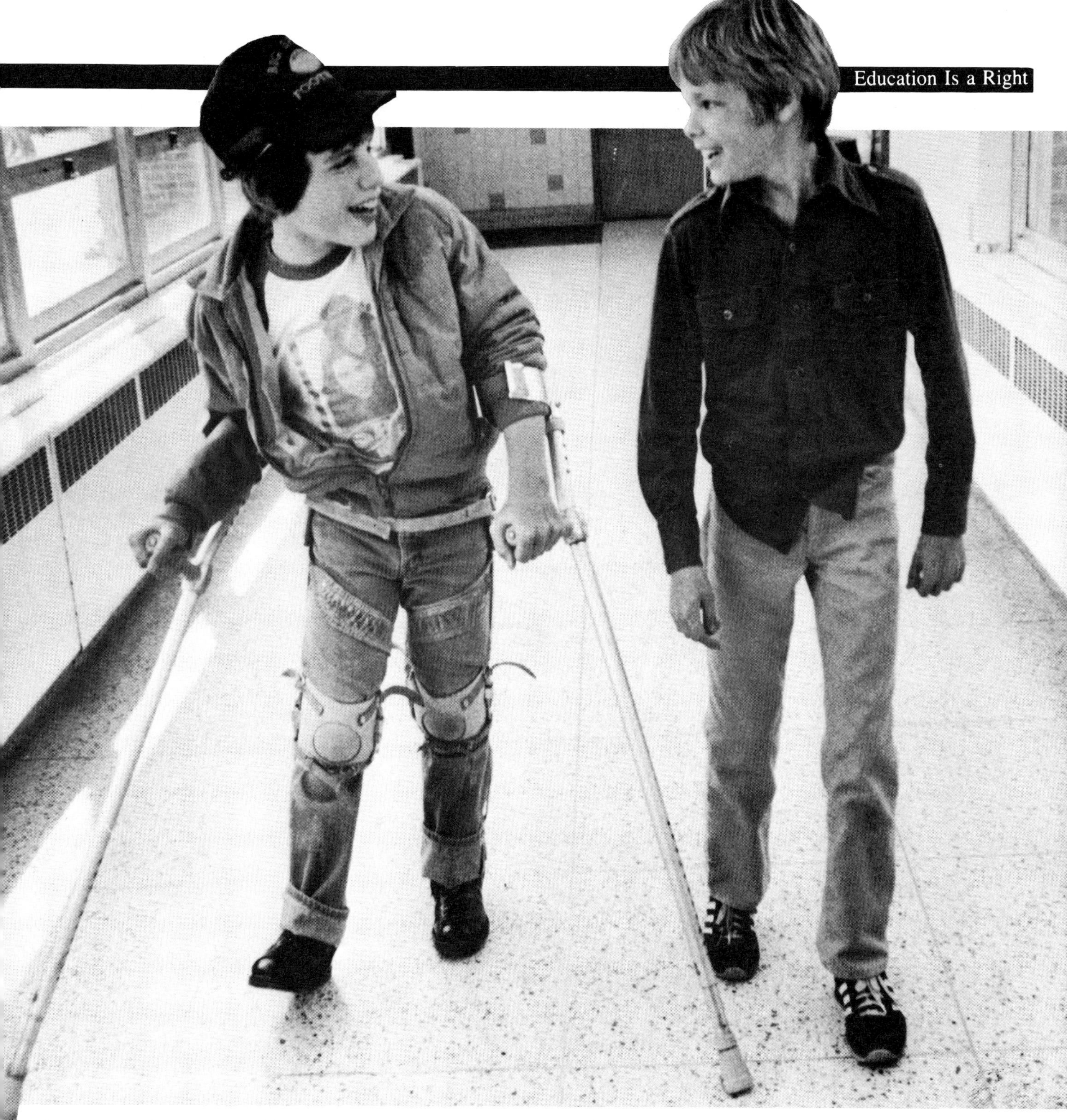

- *Ignorance about your rights*
- *Leaving everything to others because "they know how to do these things"*
- *Apologizing when asking for what is rightfully yours*
- *Ineffective communication*
- *Begging for what is legitimately yours by law*
- *Abdicating to others your right to advocate on behalf of your own child*
- *Reliance and dependence on others*
- *Giving up when you run into red tape*
- *Acting precipitously before you get all the facts*
- *Letting the politicians "take care of laws and all that political stuff"*
- *Acting "only" on your own behalf*
- *Giving in to defeat*

—Charlotte Des Jardins

What We Did When We Found Our Child Was Deaf

Judith Raskin

Joy was born in 1967 and, like most parents, we assumed that our life would proceed as we had planned. That was not to be. At six months, we noticed something was wrong with Joy. We did some crude tests of our own and deduced that Joy had a severe hearing loss. We made the usual round of pediatricians and specialists only to be told, "Wait a while, and bring her back in a year." Of course, we were being "overanxious because she's your first child." Finally, I went to a prominent specialist and said, "I want to take Joy to Boston for some tests. Please arrange it." The doctor did some preliminary tests and felt there was reason for concern.

We arranged for some tests at Massachusetts Eye & Ear Infirmary, where it was confirmed that Joy had a severe hearing loss. Here my story differs from many others. I had a very understanding and supportive doctor, who said, "This is a terrible shock, I know, but it will be all right. I know of an excellent program in Boston for hearing impaired children and their families."

We visited Emerson College and enrolled in their "family centered program." Joy was tested again and fitted for hearing aids. At Emerson, we were taught about hearing impairment. Most importantly, working with our child and working with professionals, we were taught that *we* were the experts and that we knew more about our child than anyone else. Dr. Luterman's program at Emerson was responsible for directing our actions and our lives.

I gained a great deal of confidence in myself and my child at Emerson and put it to good use. I visited various state and regional programs. I questioned state and local officials about their plans. I complained, constructively, about the lack of services. My daughter was doing very well, but I felt a powerful urge to join with other parents—to share my joys and frustrations, to plan for our children, and to impact the system. I became a "political animal." Some people say I was born with leadership qualities; I feel they were acquired out of need. Whatever the case, I emerged as a leader of a parent group I became involved in. I would say I am typical of the leaders of the "parent movement." We see challenges and rise to meet them, with strength and skills we were unaware we possessed.

As my skills grew, I realized that changes must occur, not only for my child but for *all* children. I was moving into the "noncategorical" realm. Sensing that major change must occur legislatively, I became active in lobbying local, state, and national legislators. I learned how to present testimony effectively, how to reach legislators, and I learned the power of written material. I joined with representatives of various disability groups to form a coalition.

"I became a 'political animal.' Some people say I was born with leadership qualities; I feel they were acquired out of need."

This was the first statewide group in New Hampshire representing *all* disabilities (noncategorical). The first year, I was elected chairperson of the legislative committee and then became president of the coalition.

I have been told that I am a "model" for other parents. Perhaps it seems that way to some. However, I believe that many parents are able to reach the heights I have; all they need to do is try. I am not unusual; I know many other parents who have done what I have done. I want to see more.

Our coalition grew in numbers, strength, and expertise. We started working with other parents who were having difficulty finding services for their children (this was before Public Law 94–142, when disabled children could be, and were, denied appropriate services). We worked for or against legislation. We got the different disability groups talking to one another. But in order to accomplish the necessary tasks, we needed not only personnel but money. In 1976, one of our members noticed an R.F.P. (request for proposal) in the *Federal Register* for an information center for parents of disabled children. Although none of us had written proposals before, several of our members spent a few days writing and revising, and we submitted a proposal to establish a center in New Hampshire. To our delight, we were chosen for funding!

After much discussion with my family and a great deal of support from my husband, I stepped down as president and applied for the position of executive director of the new center. While my professional background was heavily business, I did have a great deal of experience in working with parents, organizing, writing newsletters, working on legislation, etc. I was eventually chosen to lead the new organization.

We received very little money to set up the Parent Information Center (PIC). The first year $38,000 was allocated to serve the entire state! We were able to supplement this and, in three years, have tripled our budget. We have accomplished a great deal in the three years of our existence. We have been able to do so because of the tremendous energy and commitment of the staff. They work long hours (many evenings and weekends without extra pay) in primitive conditions (no fancy offices and equipment here). However, we are all aware of how we are hampered by inadequate funding.

Millions of dollars are spent each year training teachers and support personnel for their new roles under PL 94–142 but little or no attention is paid to training parents for *their* new role. Parents are the least prepared of any group for this critical participation.

We have worked very hard to give parents these skills. We do this through:

1. *One-to-one contact*. Parents are able to call us and discuss their problem in depth with one of our parent counselors, who will listen to the problem and help the parent plan a course of action. Ongoing contact is maintained until the problem is alleviated.
2. *Training*. The center provides training sessions throughout the state on various subjects. The standard training session is in two parts, the first dealing with the process and procedures involved in obtaining special education and related services and the second dealing with the writing of the I.E.P. (Individualized Education Program) and parent/professional communication techniques. We also offer tailored training sessions to parent groups, school groups, etc., who call and request training.
3. *Training of professionals*. While the bulk of our training is for parents, we recognize that educators must also be trained. We find that good training programs for professionals are sorely lacking. Therefore, we provide training to specific groups of educators—teachers, principals, superintendents, school boards. We have found that where both parents and professionals have been trained and have knowledge of their responsibilities, very few major conflicts arise.
4. *Printed materials*. We have developed a variety of materials for both parents and professionals that is available to anyone who requests it. We also have compiled information on specific disabilities, parent groups, educational programs, services, etc., that is available.
5. *Assistance in due process procedures*. While the due process procedures have been established so that parents can complete the process by themselves, without having to hire a lawyer, we find that many parents are overwhelmed by the steps involved in preparing and presenting their cases. One of our staff will assist parents in gathering information, deciding what needs to be introduced at the hearing, and understanding the process. We will also attend the hearing with the parents, giving them some much needed "moral support." Our staff will assist the parent from initial call through the due process review, if necessary, stepping out only if the case must go to court. Unfortunately, we find very few lawyers at the present time who are experienced in special education law. At the present, PIC is usually the best source of information and assistance for parents going through due process, and the services are free!

> *"The philosophy of the Parent Information Center is simple: parents working with parents."*

The philosophy of the Parent Information Center is simple: parents working with parents. Our staff is well aware of the problems parents of handicapped children face; they have "been there." This gives us a great deal of credibility with other parents.

One of my fears is that programs like the PICs, which have gained a great deal of expertise and credibility in dealing with the parents of disabled children, will fall by the wayside because of foolish economy measures, such as cutting money from the wrong programs. Parents helping parents is a successful model, one that cannot be duplicated by a bureaucracy. Only through well-trained, vigilant parents will PL 94–142 be able to remain intact.

It is hard to believe, at times, that my life has taken such direction from my daughter. What some think is a tragedy—the birth of a disabled child—has strengthened me and given me a full and rich life, both personally and professionally.

Joy is now a healthy, happy thirteen-year-old. She attends public school—she has always been integrated into public school with hearing children—and does very well. Contrary to the norm for deaf persons, her reading level is very high, three years beyond grade level. She is the model deaf child; she also happens to be very well adjusted. I have no fear that she will be anything but successful in whatever she chooses to do with her life. We have been very lucky; we had a very bright, talented child, who happened to have parents who were willing to work and fight for what was best for her. But she should not be thought of as "atypical." What has worked for us can and does work for other children and other families. But parents need to know what is right for them and follow their instincts. Then go out and make waves!

"Parents need to know what is right for them and follow their instincts. Then go out and make waves!"

Judith Raskin began the Parent Information Center in Concord, New Hampshire. At one time, a network of parent information centers reached from Boston to Chicago, Cincinnati, Concord, and South Bend. Other parent information centers have been established, some have consolidated, and some have closed because of lack of funding. Contact an independent living center, your local school board, service organizations, such as United Cerebral Palsy or Easter Seal Society, for the nearest Parent Information Center.

WEE PALS by MORRIE TURNER

DO WE CALL YOU HANDI-CAPPED OR DIS-ABLED?
8-3

CALL ME CHARLOTTE
MORRIE
©Field Enterprises, Inc., 1981

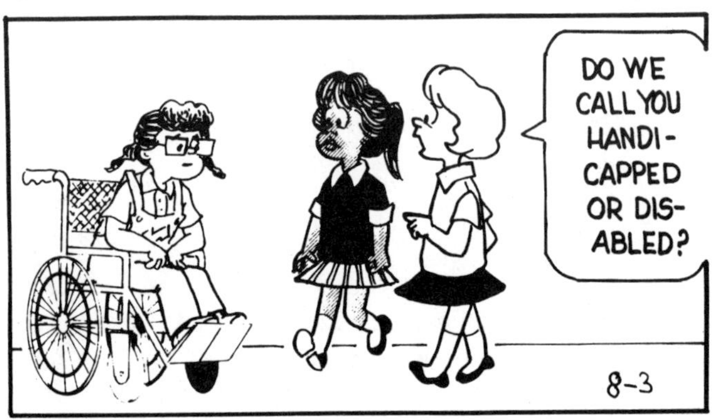

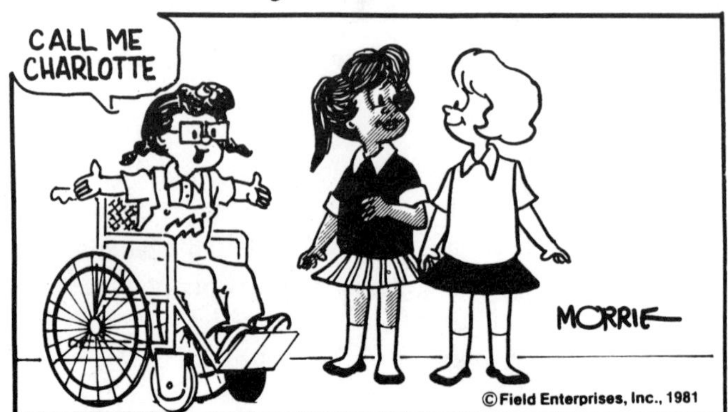

Judy Rogers

Judy is interested in the personal experiences women with disabilities have giving birth. This is prompted by the birth of her son, whom she nurses in an antique rocker in her living room. We have come together for an evening of work, but the California air makes us giddy, and we sit drinking coffee and talking about all the Easterners who have made the trek to Berkeley.

My parents pulled me out of the school for handicapped children when I was in the third grade because they saw me identifying with the children with worse disabilities. But the problem was that I hit a different prejudice in the regular schools. They were afraid of me!

What does it say to a child when there's an air raid drill and he or she doesn't get to go and find that air raid shelter? It's sort of, "You know, when it [disaster] comes, you ain't going to be one of them [the ones who are able to save themselves]." That's what I felt. They stood there saying they were trying to protect me so I wouldn't get hurt, but the underlying message is, "She'll never understand or be able to do what we tell her."

"What does it say to a child when there's an air raid drill and he or she doesn't get to go and find the air raid shelter? It's sort of, 'You know, when it [disaster] comes, you ain't going to be one of them [the ones who are able to save themselves].' That's what I felt."

I sat with the assistant principal watching all the kids going to the air raid shelter. I was allowed to participate when we had a fire drill and went outside but not when we had an air raid drill—it was very strange.

And when my friends would stay to eat at school, I couldn't eat with them because I couldn't carry the lunch tray. God forbid if the tray fell and hit another kid and I got another kid disabled; then where would we all be? So I had to eat with the special A and special B kids, like I was a real menace to society, me and my tray! Eating with the A and B kids was real scary to me because it was so controlled.

My father came to school—he was an advocate—and screamed, so I got to go and eat with my friends. The best thing the OT (occupational therapists) ever did in my life—it's why I became an OT—was to teach me how to carry a tray.

You were forced to play in gym if you were mainstreamed. I couldn't really do half the gym games well, and when it came time to choose teams, I was the last one picked—the competition was so stupid. Why did the kids have to choose? That way, it always made me feel bad.

There are all sorts of other solutions, and you just have to make it known that the alternatives are there.

Rights and Recreation

We believe in the work ethic in this society, and the concept of free or leisure time has been equated with idleness and seen as wasteful.

We continue to place high premiums on work and productive activities that contribute to the economy, but in recent years, our society has invested energy in recreational activities close to the point of a national frenzy.

The word leisure comes from the Latin *licere*, meaning to be permitted. It describes the way of living in ancient times when only a select few were able to have time to reflect without the pressure of other responsibilities.

Before the return of disabled veterans from World War II, few opportunities existed for recreation. It was the introduction of wheelchair basketball in rehabilitation programs for veterans injured during World War II that made us realize that people with disabilities could play.

In England, in 1944, at the Spinal Injuries Centre at Stoke-Mandeville Hospital, Sir Ludwig Guttman introduced a full range of sports activities, including swimming, archery, and table tennis, as part of the total rehabilitation for everyone treated in the spinal cord injury unit.

This project had a profound effect and brought to participants a sense of pride and capability. After leaving the hospital, many people returned to compete in sports. This led eventually to a sports center and a Special Olympics that takes place at the same time and place as the World Olympics.

Sir Ludwig Guttman was eighty when we visited him at the Stoke-Mandeville Hospital. About the sports program, he said, "If I was asked of what I am most proud in looking at my work as a physician, I would have to answer: the introduction of sports into the lives of people who suddenly become disabled."

Starting with wheelchair basketball teams of veterans from World War II, Korea, and Vietnam, a collective consciousness in this country, backed by legislation, has made accessible recreation more prevalent—but still far from universal.

The Rehabilitation Act of 1973 authorized training and research that directly or indirectly had a major impact on recreation services for people with disabilities. Some funding was allocated for projects to determine the ways to make recreational activities available for everyone.

The Architectural and Transportation Compliance Board was also created at that time to "investigate and examine alternative approaches to barriers confronting disabled individuals, particularly with respect to public buildings and monuments, parks and parklands." Their mandate was to study ways of eliminating what had kept people with disabilities out of places that belong to everyone.

The 1978 Rehabilitation Act significantly expanded the scope of these services and included recreation as a component of rehabilitation in certain programs.

In recent years, sports have enabled people with disabilities to develop physical skills, develop relationships, experience challenges and competition, and take advantage of the opportunity to organize and operate national and international programs.

Sports have done more than anything else to give both able-bodied and nonable-bodied individuals a sense of belonging.

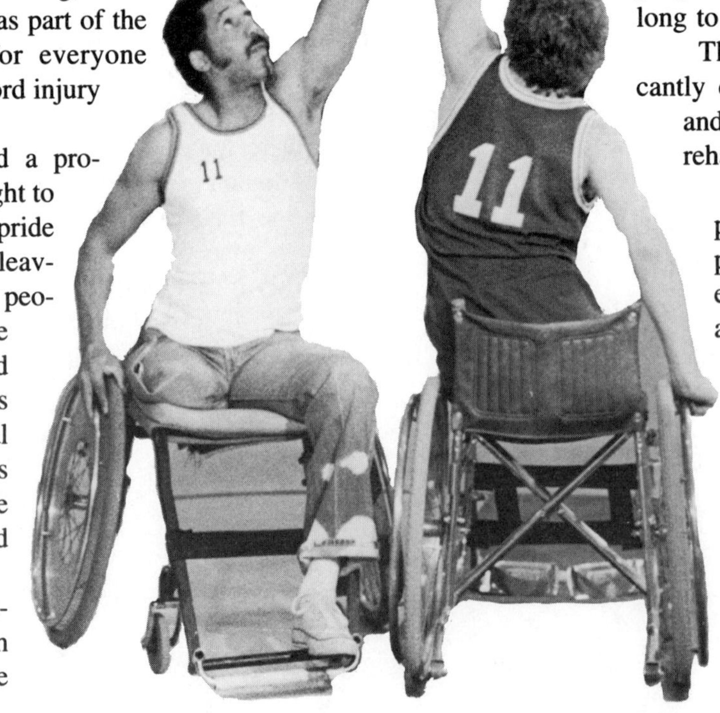

MIMI FORSYTH/MONKMEYER

Resources: SPORTS

American Alliance for Health, Physical Education, Recreation, and Dance
Unit on Programs for the Handicapped
1900 Association Drive
Reston, VA 22070

American Camping Association
5000 State Road, 67 North
Martinsville, IN 46151
Provides information on children's camps, many of which serve children with disabilities.

Boy Scouts of America, Scouting for the Handicapped
1325 Walnut Mill Lane
Irving, TX 75308-3096
Open to boys with all kinds of disabilities, ages 8 to 20. Disabled scouts participate in the same activities but at a slower pace and are included in regular packs and troops.

Disabled Sportsmen of America, Inc.
P.O. Box 5496
Roanoke, VA 24012
Hunting and fishing.

4-H Youth Extension Service
United States Department of Agriculture
Washington, DC 20250.

Girl Scouts of the USA, Scouting for the Handicapped
830 Third Avenue
New York, NY 10022
Girl Scouts does not provide a separate program for disabled girls. The philosophy is to mainstream disabled children into regular troops. There are troops in special school settings that use the same materials as girls in the mainstreamed programs. Open to girls ages 6 to 16 (age 20 for mentally retarded young women).

Handicapped Boaters Association
P.O. Box 1134
Ansonia Station, NY 10023

Handicapped Scuba Association
1104 El Prado
San Clemente, CA 92672

International Committee of the Silent Sports
Gallaudet College
800 Florida Avenue and 7th Street, N.E.
Washington, DC 20002

International Foundation for Wheelchair Tennis
2203 Timberloch Place, Suite 126
The Woodlands, TX 77380

International Wheelchair Road Racers Club, Inc.
165 78th Avenue N.E.
St. Petersburg, FL 33702

Louis Braille Foundation for Blind Musicians
215 Park Avenue South
New York, NY 10003

Minnesota Outward Bound School
1055 E. Wayzata Boulevard
Wayzata, MN 55391
Wilderness recreation.

Mobility International USA
P.O. Box 3551
Eugene, OR 97403

National Archery Association
1750 E. Boulder Street
Colorado Springs, CO 80909

National Arts and the Handicapped Information Service
National Endowment for the Arts
2401 E Street, N.W.
Washington, DC 20506

National Association for Sports for Cerebral Palsy
66 East 34th Street
New York, NY 10016

National Foundation for Wheelchair Tennis
3857 Birch Street, Suite 411
Newport Beach, CA 92660

National Handicapped Sports and Recreation Association
Capitol Hill Station
P.O. Box 18664
Denver, CO 80218

National Spinal Cord Injury Foundation
369 Elliot Street
Newton Upper Falls, MA 02164
Marathon racing.

National Wheelchair Athletic Association
2107 Templeton Gap Road
Suite C
Colorado Springs, CO 80909

National Wheelchair Basketball Association
c/o AARA
815 N. Weber, Suite 203
Colorado Springs, CO 80903

National Wheelchair Basketball Association
110 Seaton Boulevard
University of Kentucky
Lexington, KY 41506

National Wheelchair Softball Association
P.O. Box 737
Sioux Falls, SD 57101

North American Riding for the Handicapped Association
Box 100
Ashburn, VA 22011

The Paralyzed Veterans of America
4350 East West Highway
Suite 900
Washington, DC 20814

Rehabilitation—Education Center
University of Illinois
Oak Street at Stadium Drive
Champaign, IL 61820
Football.

Special Olympics, Inc.
Kennedy Foundation
1701 K Street, N.W.
Suite 215
Washington, DC 20006

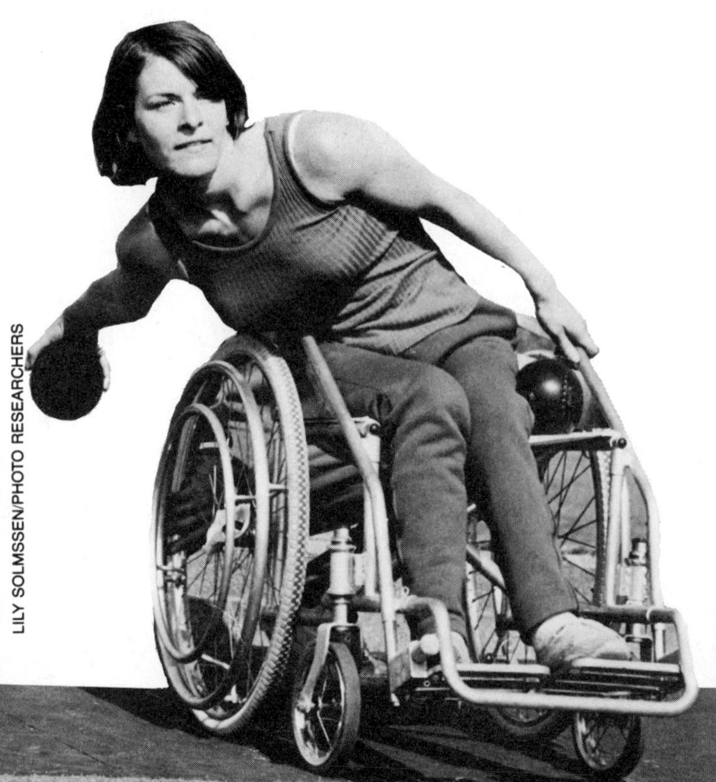

LILY SOLMSSEN/PHOTO RESEARCHERS

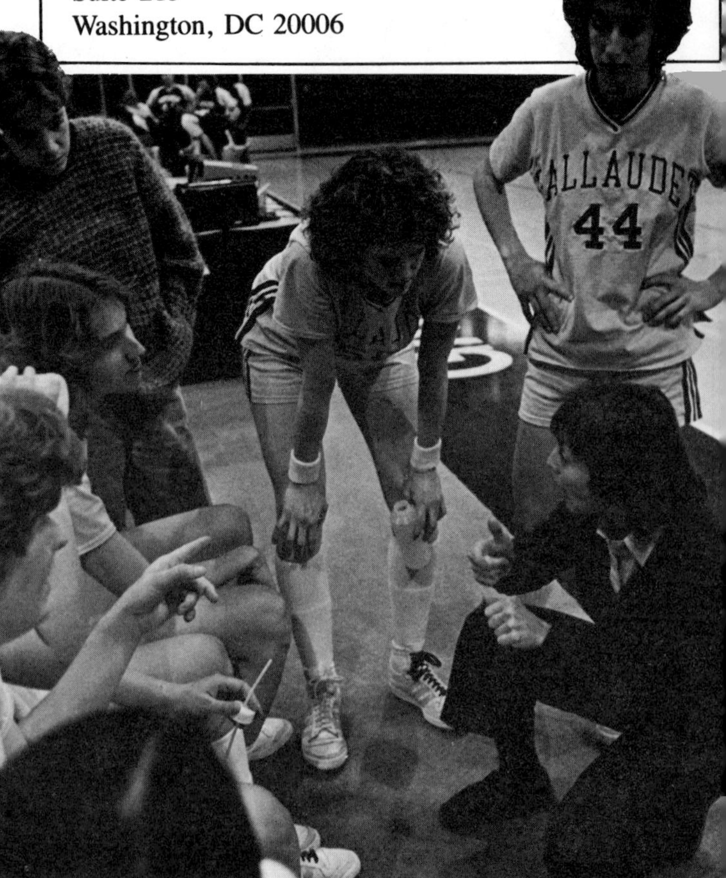

GALLAUDET UNIVERSITY

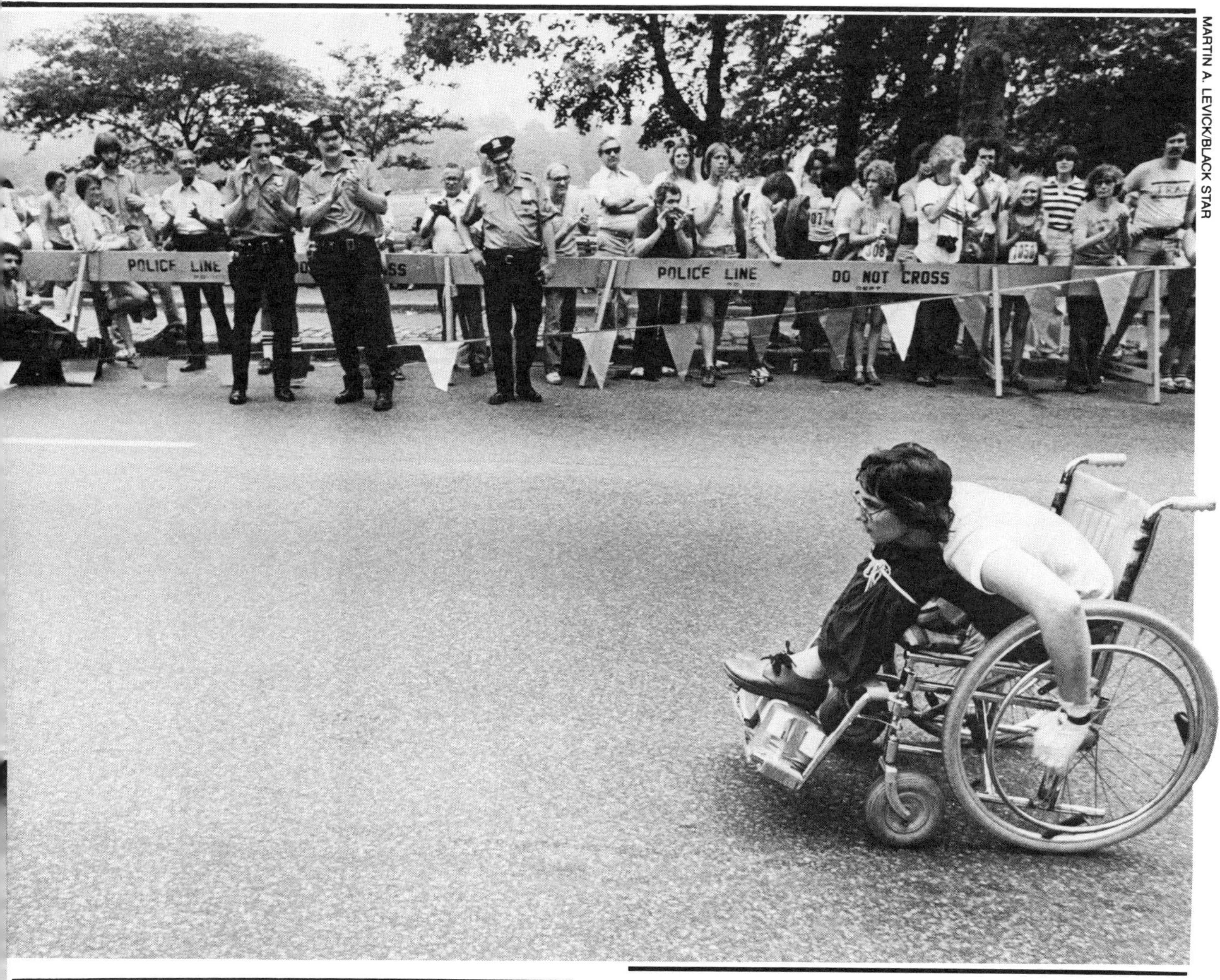

MARTIN A. LEVICK/BLACK STAR

United States Amputee Association
Route 2, County Line
Fairview, TN 37062

United States Quad Rugby Association
811 Northwestern Drive
Grand Forks, ND 58201

Wheelchair Pilots Association
11018 102nd Avenue
Largo, FL 33540

Sir Ludwig Guttman was eighty when we visited him at the Stoke-Mandeville Hospital. About the sports program, he said, "If I was asked of what I am most proud in looking at my work as a physician, I would have to answer: the introduction of sports into the lives of people who suddenly become disabled."

Publications

When people need information and have exhausted all places, they write to "Dear Abby." Abby appears in 750 newspapers; she receives 11,000 letters a week.

Many of these questions are about how to find physicians familiar with the disabilities of the writers or their family members; how to find attendants; or how to find attorneys who will represent individuals in getting their rights. Abby answers these questions in her columns, with straightforward and helpful advice.

Several newspapers carry columns written by a reporter with a disability who is experienced in finding local resources. Up to now, newspapers have underestimated the number of readers seeking such information.

A wide variety of publications are available to individuals with disabilities. Publications of organizations serving specific disabilities have funds to sustain outstanding newsletters that cover federal, state, and local issues. Some consumer newsletters showed promise but stopped publishing because of lack of money.

Ray Cheever, founder of *Accent on Living* and *Buying Guide*, and Gini Laurie of the *Rehabilitation Gazette* have been publishing information for people with disabilities for many years.

Disabled USA, a magazine of the President's Committee on the Employment of the Handicapped (PCEH), addresses a cross-disability readership, and offers profiles of individuals and updates on legislation.

The Exceptional Parent, a magazine for parents and professionals, publishes eight times a year and is informational and supportive. The magazine sells outstanding books of interest to its readers.

The Disability Rag, published by Cass Irvin and Mary Johnson, is a forum for opinions and a literary magazine of merit. "Into the Land of the Myths" by June Price, and portions of "Telethons" by Anne Peters have been reprinted in this book with permission of *Disability Rag*.

LIBRARIES

When you are looking for information on equipment, travel, clothing, or, indeed, any of the subjects covered in this book, try the local library, universities with special education departments, independent living centers, rehabilitation centers, Easter Seal Society, United Way, United Cerebral Palsy, or the Muscular Dystrophy Foundation.

The National Rehabilitation Information Center (NARIC) is a rehabilitation information service and research library that will attempt to answer questions.

NARIC has a listing of many publications and their addresses, including those mentioned here.

To contact NARIC: National Rehabilitation Information Center, The Catholic University of America, 4407 Eighth Street, N.E., Washington, DC 20017; (202) 635-5826 Voice/TDD; 1-800-34-NARIC.

COMPUTERS

William Roth, Ph.D.

Make no mistake. Computers have a special service to perform for people with disabilities. Efforts to develop special equipment for disabled people are under way. Perhaps more significantly, computers, peripherals, and software in general improve all the time. Both sets of technological developments enhance the promise of computing.

Resources: COMPUTERS

Association for Special Education Technology
P.O. Box 152
Allen, TX 75002

Center for Special Education Technology
Council for Exceptional Children
1920 Association Drive
Reston, VA 22091
(800) 345-8324

Committee on Personal Computers and the Handicapped (COPH-2)
2030 Irving Park Road
Chicago, IL 60618
(312) 477-1813

Computer Uses in Speech and Hearing (CUSH)
Department of Speech Pathology and Audiology
University of South Alabama
Mobile, AL 36688
(205) 460-3627

DEAFNET
SRI International
333 Ravenswood Avenue
Menlo Park, CA 94025
(415) 326-6200
(415) 859-4771

National Clearinghouse on Rehabilitation Training Material
Oklahoma State University
115 Old USDA Building
Stillwater, OK 74078
(405) 624-7650

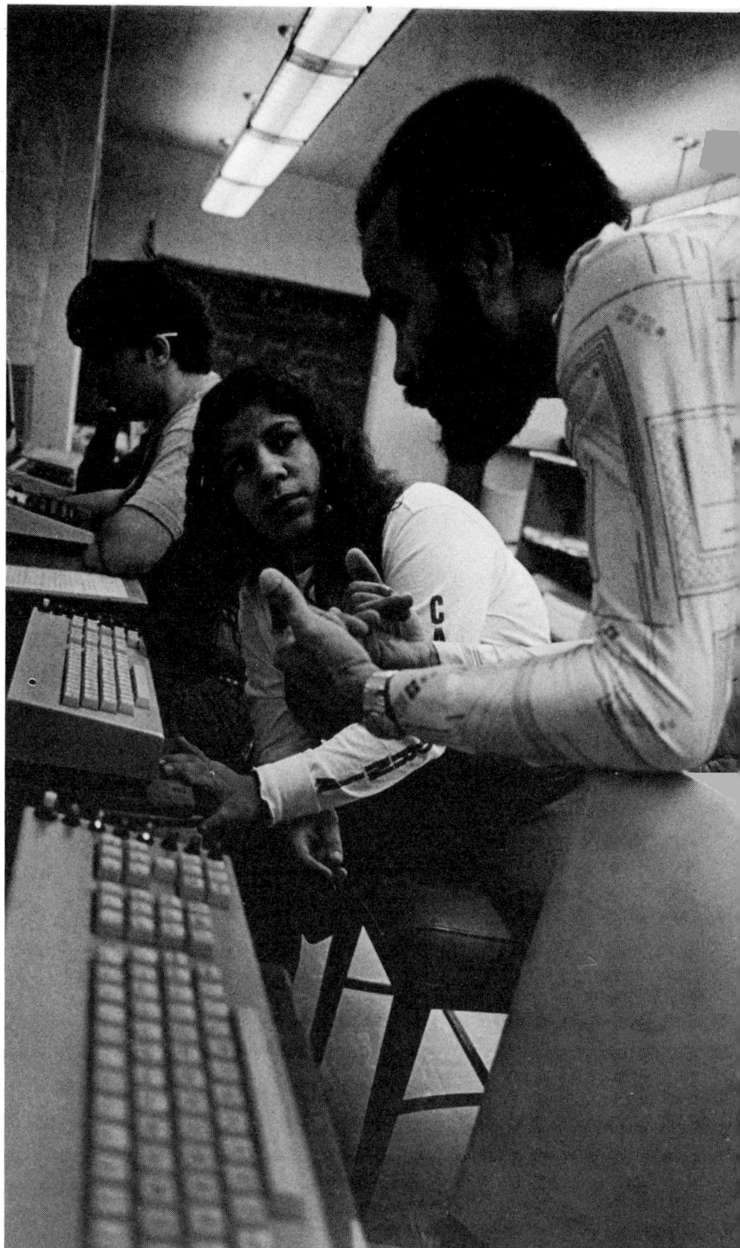

GALLAUDET UNIVERSITY

National Rehabilitation Information Center
The Catholic University of America
4407 Eighth Street N.E.
Washington, DC 20017-2299
(202) 635-5822
(202) 635-5884

Special Education Software Center
LINK Resources, Inc.
3857 N. High Street
Columbus, OH 43214

The Technical Resource Center
1820 Richmond Road S.W.
Calgary ALB T2T 5C7
Canada

Trace Research and Development Center
S. 151, 1500 Highland Avenue
Madison, WI 53706
(608) 262-6966

Publications

The CATALYST
W. Center for Microcomputers in Special Education
1259 El Camino Real
Suite 275
Menlo Park, CA 94025
(612) 248-3294

Closing the Gap
P.O. Box 68
Henderson, MN 56044

Communication Outlook
Artificial Language Laboratory
Michigan State University
East Lansing, MI 48824
(517) 353-0870

Computer Disability News
National Easter Seal Society
2023 W. Ogden Avenue
Chicago, IL 60612
(312) 243-8400

The Computing Teacher
International Council for Computers in Education
University of Oregon
1787 Agate Street.
Eugene, OR 97403

A blind computer programmer reading a Braille print out.

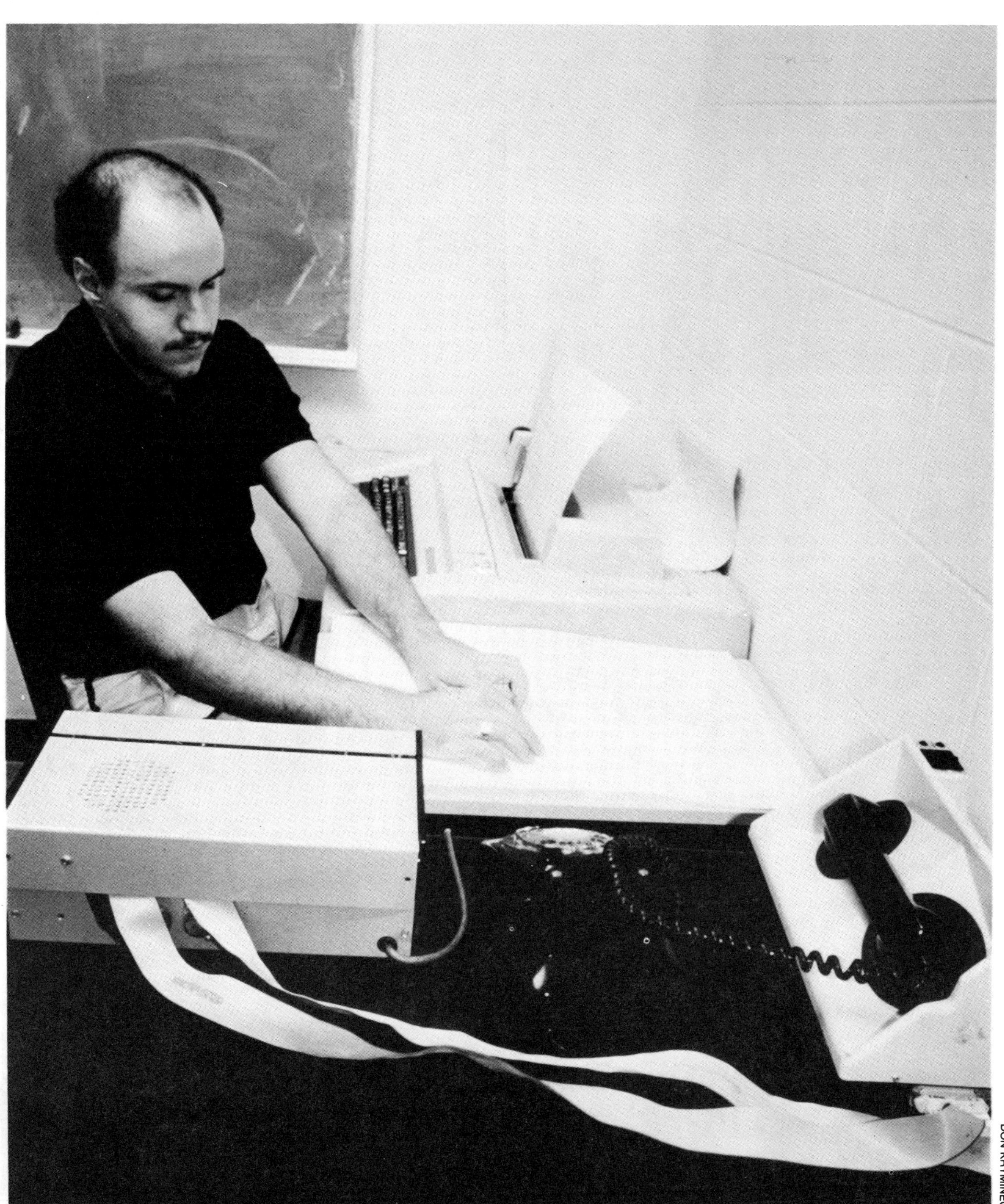

DON KRYMINEC

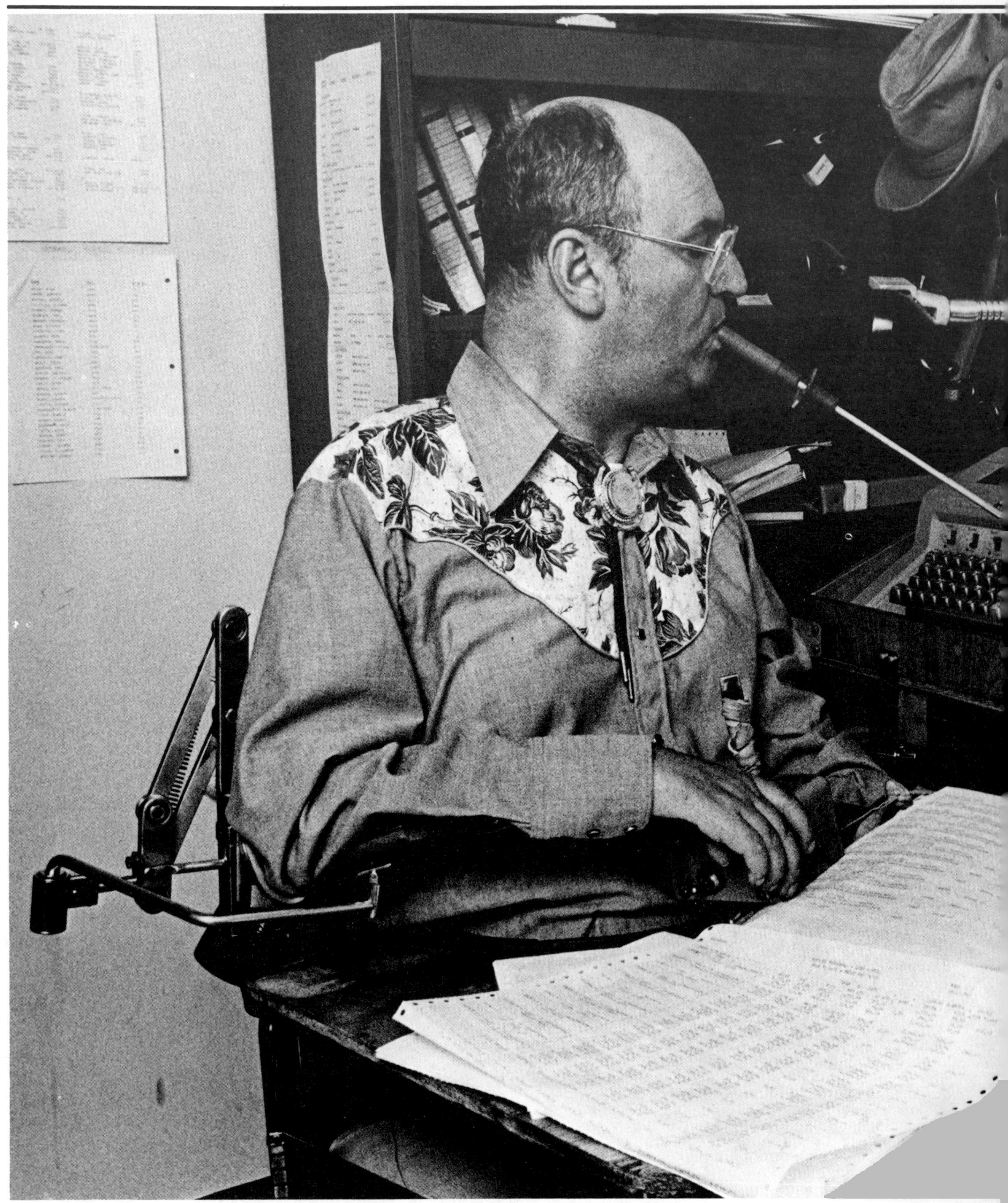

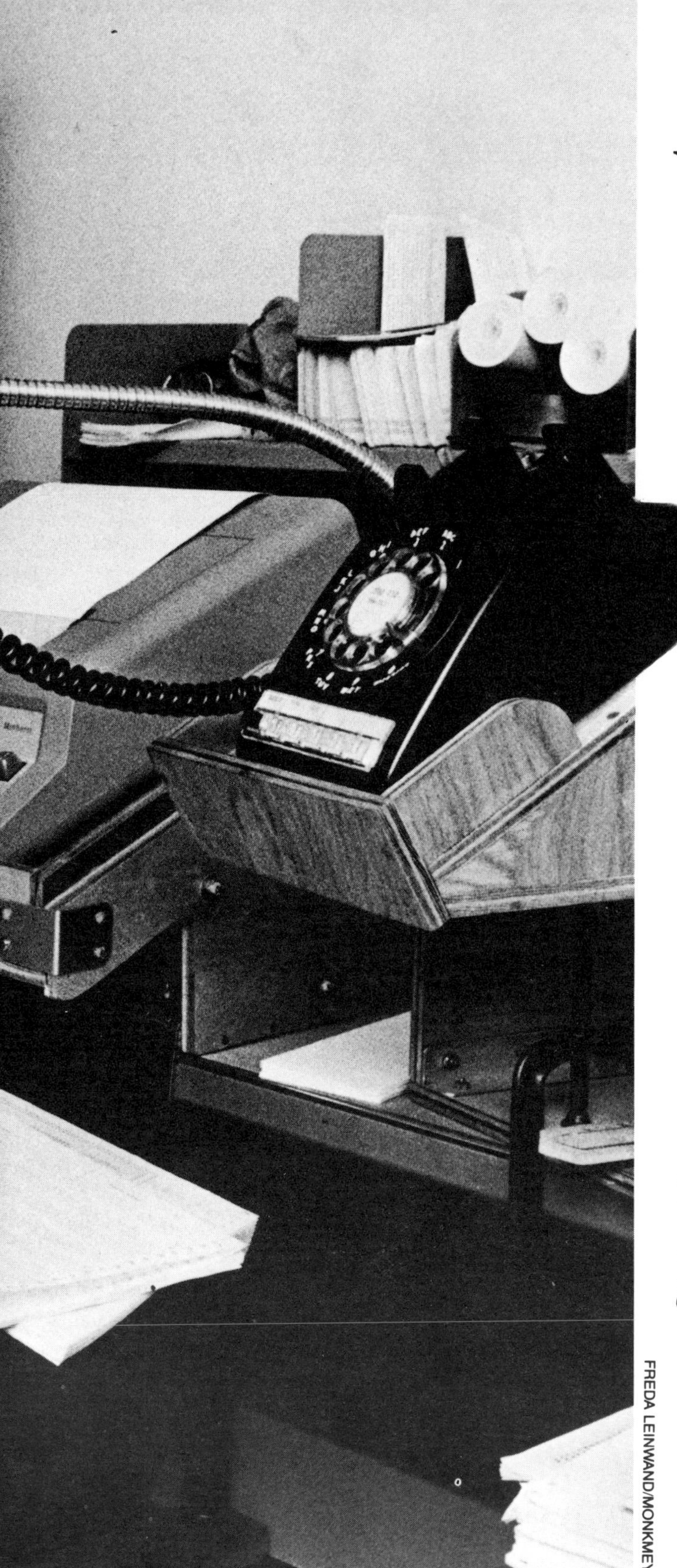

FREDA LEINWAND/MONKMEYER

Chapter 6
Work and Money

Tom Clancy is Manager of Administrative Systems, New York University Computer Center.

Work and Money
Harriet Bell, Ph.D.

Everyone is expected to work in America—except people who have a disability. The message has been clear; disabled people need not apply. So they haven't.

Some disabled people have been allowed to work in sheltered workshops or run newspaper stands, sell pencils or shoelaces or apples. And one became president of the United States.

Many people with hidden disabilities—epilepsy, diabetes, cancer, high blood pressure, pain, kidney disorders, and mental illness—have lied (or managed to slip by the company doctor) and been employed. Then there are disabled people who are willing to work but who pass their days looking at reruns of "I Love Lucy."

"Everyone is expected to work in America—except people who have a disability. The message has been clear: disabled people need not apply. So they haven't."

Once the whole country backed disabled people in getting jobs. After World War II, the G.I. Bill paved the way for disabled veterans to compete with other job applicants. Disabled Korean and Vietnam veterans were not as lucky; the climate in the country had changed. Without a solid job offer, the laws created to protect returning disabled veterans did not mean much.

The job ladder is different for people with a disability. It is not likely that one of us will begin in the mail room, work our way up, marry the boss's daughter, and become a vice president. Harold Krents, a prominent attorney who is visually impaired and the inspiration for the play and movie *Butterflies Are Free*, describes the dilemma this way:

> It was not merely a matter of wanting to go to Harvard University. I *had* to go to Harvard in order to get an opportunity to attend one of our finer law schools.
>
> I graduated from Harvard, cum laude, in June of 1967 only to discover that the doors to most of our nation's outstanding law schools were closed to me because I happened not to see. Eventually, Harvard law school reconsidered its initial rejection of my application, and I was admitted.
>
> For a student with sight, the amount of reading required to do well in one's law studies is overwhelming. For one without sight, it is almost beyond accomplishment. I knew as I toiled through the difficult first two years of law school that it was not enough simply to graduate from Harvard. If I wanted to secure employment with a good law firm, I had to graduate with better grades than most of my colleagues.
>
> So I had people reading continuously to me for 13 hours a day, five days a week, for two years. My day was not over with the departure of the last reader at 10 P.M., for at that point, I would take Braille notes on the class lectures that I had missed; they were supplied to me by friends who were kind enough to tape record them. For two years, I did not go to sleep before 3 A.M.
>
> Why did I put myself through this ordeal? Why did I subject my body to a torture for which I am still

paying a decade later? I did it because it was the only way that I could secure employment that would enable me to develop my potential to the maximum degree. For all of us, of whatever minority, employment is the major goal we seek.

Eventually, I was fortunate enough to find a prominent law firm in Washington D.C., willing to give me the chance to show what I could do.

The vast majority of disabled people now seeking employment wish nothing more than the chance to "make it or break it" on their own. In a society as humane as ours, no citizen should be constantly required to do vastly better than those in the majority in order to achieve maximum employment potential.*

In America, one of the wealthiest countries in the world, most disabled citizens, senior citizens, and the poor—even with assistance—live below the poverty level.

This means my monthly check barely covers my basic needs, and it requires a balancing act to rent a place that doesn't eat up my budget, a place close to transportation and near shopping. I carefully live within my budget—at a great sacrifice. What my neighbors take for granted—having friends over for dinner, going to a movie, visiting their children—are things I can't do.

"I carefully live within my budget—at a great sacrifice. What my neighbors take for granted—having friends over for dinner, going to a movie, visiting their children—are things I can't do."

I have arranged a good life for myself. After living in a hospital for twenty-five years, I now live in my own apartment. Since I am quadriplegic, I have full-time attendant care. At the same time I have a personal and private, independent life. I do not tell you about my life for you to be sympathetic or marvel at my accomplishments. I tell you because for too long there has been an attitude that people who genuinely need assistance are "on the take." For too long a myth has existed that disabled citizens receive too great a portion of the pie. This cannot be true when so many of us are barely getting by.

A myth continues only when there is confusion. What is more to the point:

- There *is* enough money.
- The laws change so fast we can't keep up with them. Our economic survival seems to depend on the whims of whatever administration happens to be in office.
- Money is used as a scare tactic; money polarizes us, turning "us" against "them."
- Even people who are permanently disabled are required to be examined every six months in order to continue receiving assistance.
- Disability is the one minority group anyone can join at a moment's notice.

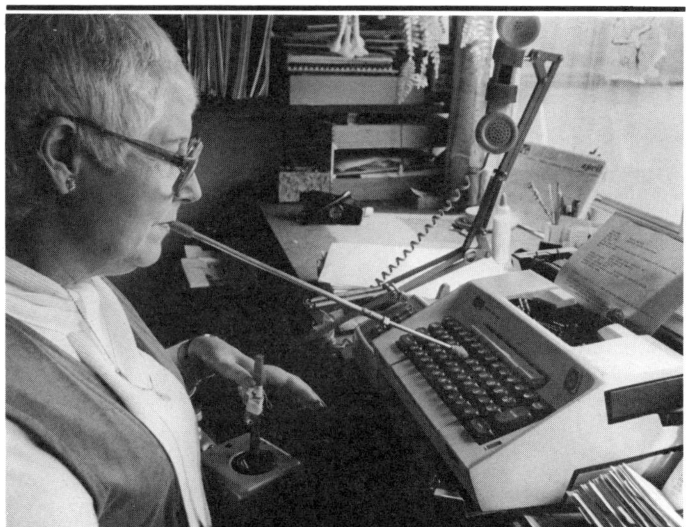

AGNES ZELLIN

Dr. Bell typing. She also uses a computer at the Polio Information Center, Roosevelt Island, New York.

* **Harold Krents**, *The Human Dimension to Affirmative Action for the Handicapped.* U.S. Department of Labor Employment Standards Administration, Office of Federal Contract Compliance, April 1980.

John

I don't think I am prejudiced against people with disabilities who accept a check and genuinely need it. But I feel the system is set up to discourage individuals from taking a risk, giving up that check, and believing in their own worth. If they start a job and it doesn't work out, the waiting period to get reinstated can take a long time. What do you live on in the meantime, I'd like to know, if you can't work?

In 1949, I was making from $18,000 to $20,000 a year. That was a really good living then. In September of that year, I got polio, and from that point on, my total income from the company I had been working for was $38—two weekly disability pay checks of $19. Then they stopped; I don't know that I remember as much as a "thank you" from them.

I had a job I liked and was well qualified for as a wholesale food representative for an institutional house. After I left the hospital, right from the beginning I decided to create my own kind of work. I wouldn't accept the restrictions imposed on me if I accepted a Social Security check. As I recall, no one was coming at me with job offers.

Four times out of five, when you are out looking for a job, carrying a "stick," you have to accept that people feel all you are capable of is "handicapped-type work." Employers think anybody with a "crutch" or disability can only do one thing—take one part of something and put it together with another part—assembling something. The average person has been preconditioned, perhaps by the local fund drive for the sheltered workshop. You get little or no recognition for any ability. This may not be 100 percent true, but it's darn close.

I was out of the hospital, but still in a wheelchair, when a friend of mine came out from Boston to have a picnic barbecue. This was in August 1950, during the Korean War. My friend arrived and told me he had been able to buy the last bag of briquettes the market had; he had gone all over town looking for it. Charcoal was being used in foundries because of the war and was in very limited supply. During the picnic I remembered that a friend of mine in New Hampshire made lump charcoal in kilns. So I said, "Hell, take me into the house." They rolled me in, and I called my New Hampshire friend and told him what I had in mind. He said he would supply me with all the charcoal I could sell.

I figured if I could get someone to drive me, I could go to all the shops and gas stations, get orders, and start making some money—I needed it. My wife drove me around. She was about six or seven months pregnant at the time. We sold a bunch of charcoal, and we got our share of stares, too.

"I tripped over something, bumped into him, and knocked him down on the floor. His catalog fell to the floor and opened up in front of me at the diving equipment section. . . . So I decided to take a chance on diving equipment, gave him $150 to prepay freight, and started what became the skin diving industry in New England."

People are curious about the sex life of people who are physically different—the baby my wife was pregnant with was conceived when we were checking out the "equipment" to make sure it all functioned properly—both of us had polio, so we were more curious than anybody else! That fall, the barbecue season was over, so we didn't have anything to sell, but we went around to thank all the shops for their business. One fellow told me to come back in the spring with more charcoal and to add other picnic items.

That winter, I wrote to several different companies to get other picnic items to add to the line. Five manufacturers' representatives came to my house where I had set up an office.

The fellow who sold picnic coolers came, and as he

was leaving after I had gone through his catalog, I started to get up to walk him to the door. I was somewhat less steady on my feet then than I am now. I tripped over something, bumped into him, and knocked him down on the floor. His catalog fell the the floor and opened up in front of me at the diving equipment section. It turned out that he sold that as well as the picnic items.

I remembered, years before, going to the beach shops when I worked summers in Maine, trying to find a pair of underwater goggles—no one seemed to carry any merchandise of that type.

So I decided to take a chance on diving equipment, gave him $150 to prepay freight, and started what became the skin-diving industry in New England. Five years later, I literally owned it. We used to run beach demonstrations; there would be as many as 25,000 people to see a frogman and what his equipment looked like. So it was a big time show biz!

Then, in 1956, there was a nationwide truck strike, and it became necessary to move my inventory. I figured Florida had a skin-diving boom in the winter that died in the summer. When I got down there, I discovered that diving season was much the same as it was in New England, maybe starting a month earlier and ending a month later. I called my attorney, closed out my business in New England, and stayed on in Florida, where I've lived ever since.

At that time, there was a lot of misinformation about where to go diving in Florida, so I contacted the Chamber of Commerce throughout the state and offered to answer any inquiries they received. I was hit with an avalanche of mail, but I wasn't making any money.

At the same time, I was running a political campaign, but the candidate didn't quite win the election and I wound up with a bunch of his bills. Convinced he would win, I had put all my eggs in one basket. One Thursday afternoon, not knowing which end was up because we had been cleaned out in the campaign, I said to myself, "Where do I go from here?" Because we were a couple of months behind in the rent, the landlord who owned the house in which we lived said we had to pay the rent by Saturday night or get out.

That night, I decided to put together a diving directory. I had one in mind, drew up a few pages, and the next day went out and made some calls on diving shops. Everybody bought advertising space and placed orders for copies. By Saturday afternoon, I had $3,000 to put into the bank! That got me into the writing field, and I have built up a publishing business, producing three major directories. It has been a lot of sweat, but I am an optimist by nature.

There are a lot of people who will cheer for you, but when it comes down to saying, "I am a banker. Come in, and I'll arrange a loan for you," that's when the stumbling blocks come up.

The system has changed somewhat since Congress passed a bill allowing disability benefit checks to be resumed within a short time after a person is no longer able to work. It reduces the fear of being completely cut off with no job and no benefits. Red tape can get in the way.

"There are a lot of people who will cheer for you, but when it comes down to saying, 'I am a banker. Come in, and I'll arrange a loan for you,' that's when the stumbling blocks come up."

It takes less than six months, certainly no more than a year, for that benefit check to become integrated into the family income. The family becomes dependent upon it as a result; it diminishes the effort and desire, on the part of many families, to allow the disabled family member to be in the position of not receiving a guaranteed benefit check. To discontinue it is making a sacrifice, with too many unknowns.

I feel very sorry for people who have the capacity to take advantage of the free enterprise system, to work, who don't.

The Job

Frances Lynn

I don't know what's been happening to me lately. Maybe it's because I am not doing anything much—just reading, watching TV, talking to friends on the phone, and thinking. I've been doing a lot of thinking lately. I wonder how many disabled people are like me?

Mom says it's a phase I'm going through. Mom's usually right. Mom says it's because I have finished college and have not decided what to do next; she said that if I had gotten a job right away, I would be fine. "Work is good for what ails you." She also said that I must accept the fact that, since I am "handicapped," it will be hard to find someone to hire me.

I keep looking for a job and reading and watching TV and thinking.

Maybe if I lived in the city . . . I can't go anywhere by myself out here because we don't have any sidewalks. We don't have any buses either, so, accessible or not, I can't use them.

On Martin Luther King's birthday, the TV stations showed films of him when he came to Louisville to march for "open housing." Good or bad, right or wrong, King and the others marching had to be courageous. They must have wanted something very badly to go through all that.

What they wanted was to live anywhere they chose in the city. That's not such a big deal. Black people live just about anywhere they want today—there is a law that says they have the right. But the day King came to Louisville to march, there was no law. He marched and demanded equality in housing, and he did not even have a law to back him up!

I asked my mom if she thought I had such courage. She said of course I did; all "handicapped" people have courage. How else could we cope with our lives?

She says I think too much; she says once I get a job, I will not have time to think about such things. I wonder . . .

I don't know anyone who is disabled (except for Barbie, who's fifteen). One semester when I was going to community college, a girl named Sherry was in my orientation class. She appeared older than me and disabled in a different way—although she used a wheelchair, too. She didn't talk too well and she pushed herself around in the chair by using her feet and by going everywhere backward; sometimes she would bump into people who were not watching where she was going.

"I realize now that the reason I had such a strong urge to stare was because I wanted to know what she looked like—and what I looked like to other people. I don't really know how I look!"

I noticed I wanted to stare as much as anyone else. But Mom always said that it's not polite to stare, so I would look away, too. (I wonder if she thought I was avoiding looking at her?) I realize now that the reason I had such a strong urge to stare was because I wanted to know what she looked like—and what I looked like to other people. I don't really know how I look!

Mom said that I was better off not getting to know Sherry because "you two are not alike at all!" And anyway, most people were not disabled, so I should learn how to get along with "most people."

The only people I know who are disabled are old. A lady who sings in the choir with Mom has a son who is disabled, but he never goes out. She asked me to call him sometime and talk to him. "You could really cheer him up; you seem so happy all the time, and you two have so much in common; he doesn't know anyone else confined to a wheelchair." I called him. Mom made me. He talked to me for two hours! About baseball, football, World War II, and model airplanes. He's thirteen, and we have nothing in common but the fact that we use wheelchairs, and now—because I talked to him—he is in love with me! I really needed that!

"Segregation is a bad thing when you do not choose to live that way. But I cannot help wondering if disabled people would be different if we spent time together, if we knew each other, if we shared experiences, if we talked to each other."

I want to know people like me! I need to be with people who have the same experiences.

Segregation is a bad thing when you do not choose to live that way. But I cannot help wondering if disabled people would be different if we spent time together, if we knew each other, if we shared experiences, if we talked to each other.

I have noticed that black people have a pride in being black. They say, "Black is beautiful," and they believe it. And women are starting to write plays about themselves saying, "I Am Woman," as though that is important. On public TV, I saw a show on the women's suffrage movement, and one woman walked onto a racetrack and was run down by horses and killed to draw attention to the fact that she would do anything to secure rights for women—even die for those rights.

I don't know if I could die for another disabled person, but maybe that's because I feel no pride. I'm not beautiful. I'm not capable. I'm not important. I am weak. I am helpless. I will never be able to take care of myself. At least, that's what my mom says.

I don't have a job yet. I called the state employment office, but they said I would have to go down there, and Mom says that we should wait until it is not so cold. And besides, Uncle Jake's car is on the fritz and Pop can't stay home from work to take us.

Mom says, "Don't worry if no one hires you; you're 'handicapped.' It's going to take time." And then I read about a woman who types with a mouth stick and earns $11,000 a year—and wonder why I should not be upset!

About two months ago, Mom came home from her ladies' church meeting all excited and told me about a job at our church.

"What does it pay?" I asked.

"What difference does that make? A job is a job. You know, after looking for almost a year, you can't afford to be picky, young lady. And besides, it's right here in the neighborhood so we don't need to worry about a car—we can walk to work!"

Mom sat down and talked seriously about the job. I had never been this close to a job before and I began to get scared. A job, that's a big deal! Just thinking about it made me tired. But Mom and I talked more and she seemed to think it would work out fine for me. So I screwed up my courage and she called the pastor's wife (she's in charge of the office) and made an appointment for an interview.

I was very nervous that day. My interview was for 11:00. (Mom told the pastor's wife how hard it was for us to get ready before that hour. I told Mom I thought that was a bad thing to tell a future employer. But Mom said we had special circumstances and people needed to know that.)

Sometimes I can't decide if I like or want to be special. Being special is nice when you can go to the front of the line at a movie theater. But it isn't so nice when your dad says, "I have a crippled daughter. Can I bring her in early so we can avoid the crowd?"

"Being special is nice when you can go to the front of the line at a movie theater. But it isn't so nice when your dad says, 'I have a crippled daughter. Can I bring her in early so we can avoid the crowd?'"

Well, I went for my interview, but Mom did most of the talking. I would have rejected the job right away if it had been up to me.

But nothing the woman said discouraged Mom. "If it

gets to be too much for her, well, I can help." The pastor's wife said we should take our time and think about the job. They did need someone right away, but she thought for us it was important to make the right decision. "It is a lot of work, even for someone who is not 'handicapped.' If you decide to take the job, we will do everything we can to make it easier for you, as long as we get the job done."

I'll be honest with you: I did not want to take the job. I told Mom about my worries. I thought it was too much work for anyone. I know I didn't know much about money, but I thought they were not going to pay enough. Mom said since it was church work, indirectly, I should think of it as "an offering." I could not help wondering if they would pay a "real" secretary that tiny salary or if it was because I was a beginner. I also wondered why the last secretary quit.

I took the job. Mom assured me that she would do everything to make sure I was a success at it. She said she would not fuss about getting me ready every morning—I was supposed to work every other Saturday, too! She said she would do some of the typing here at home if it got to be too much. "Really," Mom said, "those people are getting

"I can't tell [my mom] I am beginning to be afraid that 'someday' is not going to be here soon enough."

two for the price of one." Finally, Mom said she would even persuade Dad to help me buy an electric wheelchair so I could go to work on my own. I thought that would take a lot of persuading since we don't have any sidewalks out here. But Mom seemed to read my mind and said she would promise Dad that she would walk me to work and make sure I did not get run over. Like I said, Mom wanted this job more than I did.

I guess that's why she was not angry with me when I woke up crying in the middle of the night. I was so exhausted, I could barely sleep, and when I finally did, all I could dream about was typing. It is still hard for me to type this now. (But at least this is all me—Mom is not helping me with this.)

Mom is too busy these days to help me now. You see, when I realized I could not do that job, Mom was hired in my place.

I guess I will not get that wheelchair now.

I have never been involved with an organization for disabled people. I was not sure I wanted to be around other disabled people. I am also not familiar with any of those groups, and I don't really know which one I should join. Mom would probably not take me to a meeting even if I wanted to go. Uncle Jake would, but Mom thinks that the world is not made up of handicapped people and that I should "live in the real world."

That expression is really funny—especially coming from my mother! She wants me to live in the real world, yet she is working at my job and I am staying home!

I always thought that when I got a job, everything would change. And it surely has! But it has not changed the way I expected. And it has not changed for the better. Not at all.

I don't like it, and I don't know what to do about it, or if I should do anything—or even if I have a right to feel this way!

I used to dream that someday I would be like those disabled people who have their own job and their own van and a home and someone to live with them. And it would not be my mom—it would be someone who would work for me, and I would not have to stay home while they went out.

"Someday," I used to think. But I don't think that anymore. I guess when it gets right down to it, I am not like the disabled people in those magazines. I am not courageous. I am not strong. I am not very good at being a disabled person. I know I should not have these feelings, but I do, and I don't know what to do about it. I would talk to my mom, but I can't tell her this. I can't tell her I hate my/her job. I can't tell her I am beginning to be afraid that "someday" is not going to be here soon enough.

I hope, I pray there is nobody else out there like me. But if there is, and if you got out of the trap, please, please, tell me how. And tell me soon!

A series of letters written to the *Disability Rag*, Louisville, Kentucky, have appeared since the newsletter began publishing a number of years ago. Frances Lynn is a pen name. The author has this to say:

> Frances is a kind of person I want to be able to pull out of her experiences, to get her on a road where she is accomplishing much more. I am economically more advantaged and have more education than Frances, so being her allows me to express some of the insecurities people would expect I no longer had. The experiences Frances has are real.
>
> People began relating to Frances when she was going to go to college. And readers started writing letters telling her how to overcome the problems she was having.
>
> For people to believe that Frances is feeling their feelings, they have to grow with her. And I don't want her to grow too fast because I don't want her to leave some people behind.

A Way For Frances

June Price

My early postschool memories remind me that it's astounding any of us can get through those years with any sanity at all. But I needn't try and tell you what it's like; you live it, as I once did. I would like to share some of my experiences—they may be of help or consolation.

It took me nine years from the time I finished school to realize it was pure stupidity to do "traditional" work. I, too, had my share of nightmares . . . I could hardly make three "telephone sales" calls without breaking down 'cause I hated it so. I patched holes in tablecloths (with Mom's help, of course) for thirty cents an hour, but it was "something to keep her busy!" I glued thermometer pieces together, using highly toxic glue that stuck to my fingers and infiltrated my weak lungs (but Dad made me a special board to make the job more efficient, which, I guess, was to help me hate it less, which didn't work). Etc., etc.

"Somehow, my parents began to realize they had less control over my life. They even began to respect me more, I think."

I finally decided this "work" business wasn't worth it for me. What I did find, finally, was that I fit one job perfectly—that of a "consumer advocate." I had gotten involved with groups and organizations. Very slowly, but I had. They told me what skills I had. And I found myself enjoying it. They'd find me rides to meetings in people's vans and such. (Call some. You might find the same thing.) I met new people, learned new things, and accomplished something for "the cause."

When I was living at home after high school, I really could see no future for myself. I had tried commuting to college for two years but quit finally due to those commuting traumas. I knew I was totally dependent upon my parents for everything; I couldn't even get into the living room without help getting over the carpeting, much less get anywhere else. I envisioned nothing but a nursing home future. Period.

Somehow, though, things began to evolve in me. Ever so slowly. I think the advocacy work I was doing with the organizations was finally paying off inside me, perhaps. Life just started changing.

I got an attachment to make my manual wheelchair motorized, which meant that two or three times a year, Dad would take me shopping, but I could shop alone for the first time ever. I could use the motor when going to a meeting if I was picked up in a van. And if an agency wanted me at a meeting or to speak at some event on their behalf, I could go—if they'd pay for the transportation. And they did.

Then affordable "special" transportation came to my community. When my motorette unit broke, I got a standard power wheelchair, which I was "allowed" to use more often (and though Dad still complained that it made too much noise in the house, I wasn't letting those objections matter as much to me anymore). I started going more places by myself. Somehow, my parents began to realize they had less control over my life. They even began to respect me more, I think.

I got chosen in a state lottery, of all things, to move into the first housing for the disabled in the state. I was given only a couple of months in which to make my move. The housing units were in another city, and I hadn't the slightest idea how to hire an attendant, where to find one, or how to live on my own. So I turned it down. I just wasn't ready. But even though my parents still thought, certainly, that I'd never be able to survive in that setting, they were beginning to think I had options. Maybe.

I remember so often thinking that even with all that was starting to exist, it was never meant for me. I remember thinking "independent living" was an elusive dream I was foolish to chase. At thirty-one, I found I could no longer bear residing in my parents' home. I knew I needed my own space. I began thinking that maybe even nursing homes weren't all that bad . . .

Then it happened. I went, by myself, to look at a vacancy in some new apartments for the elderly and handicapped, not really knowing what to expect. The manager told me the place was mine if I wanted it—but that I had to sign the lease within three weeks.

"I remember thinking 'independent living' was an elusive dream I was foolish to chase. At 31, I found I could no longer bear residing in my parents' home. I knew I needed my own space. I began thinking that maybe even nursing homes weren't all that bad . . ."

This time, somehow, it felt right; I was ripe for the move at last. I told my parents I was taking the apartment (although I was scared to death at the time—both for myself and for them).

At first, they said nothing. Later, my dad came to me and said, "I don't care what you say, you'll never make it." (Don't you just love the confidence parents have in their disabled children's ability to make it on their own?)

Then he added, "And another thing: You can't even get yourself a glass of water. How do you expect to live alone?"

Independent living, dear Dad, means that you don't store your glasses in the cabinet above the sink and that you see that there's a cutout so that chairs can get under the sink so you can reach the faucet!

I moved. Believe me, Frances, you don't know nightmares until you move!

But again, ever so slowly, just as they had before, things began to improve once I was on my own.

I'm now thirty-five. I've been living in my own apartment for nearly three years. I have my power wheelchair. I hire my come-in aides. I use the subsidized special van service. I cook all my own meals. I even get my own glass of water.

My parents are doing well, too. Mom got a real job.

Life has changed for me. My imagination could never have created the fantasies I now live so smoothly.

I, too, used to read about those people who could manage a chain of department stores from their iron lung. I don't want this to sound like that—or the woman who types with her mouth and makes $11,000 a year. But you don't have to surrender to the Great Crip Fate if you don't want to. Your day will come. Prepare for that day.

Try to determine what you would like from life. Do you want to move? Do you want a power chair? Do you want more disabled people to talk with? Whatever it is, set goals and go for it. But don't expect miracles. Nothing will come easy, and life, for the most part, will always be an uphill struggle. But you will, indeed, get your day. Trust me.

By the way: I have found some work—or it has found me.

I'm still very involved as an advocate. I'm on a slew of committees, and I also get paid well for doing in-service trainings and speaking to groups. (I set a price, and they pay it! That's self-worth!) I've formed my own nonprofit corporation, which sets up camping opportunities for people with muscular dystrophy. My job is volunteer coordinator—the only paid job in the organization, but it's a start.

This letter was received by the *Disability Rag*, Louisville, Kentucky, in answer to "The Job" by Frances Lynn. It is reprinted with permission.

John Flack

John Flack welcomes me into his office and hands me a cup of steaming English tea. I have taken the morning train up from London, and although the sun is shining, a wet snow covers the ground.

A small heater in the corner of the office takes the chill from the air. There is a factory just beyond us where communications devices, designed by John, are assembled.

His work means a great deal to him, especially because his inventions assist people in communicating, and he is sensitive to feelings of isolation.

It's so easy to talk to him and to enjoy his humor.

This building in which I now have my business was, oddly enough, the old Labour Exchange, the place in England where disabled and elderly came for their weekly benefits. I used to have to come here for my dole money.

I was looking for employment, and the exchange had me go to several firms in the area. Well, I could do quite a few things because I had learned radio and television servicing at college. But no one they sent me to was interested in employing me at a decent wage, which wasn't very surprising because this is a small town.

Several firms offered me jobs but at very, very low salaries. I would have taken one of them, but my parents, especially my mother, said, "No, you can't take employment at that sort of level; it just isn't worth it. There is no financial advantage. Employers are going to reap considerable benefit from your training and should pay for it."

I was being offered four pounds a week, which would have been about $8. At that time, a nondisabled person in a similar junior level position would have been earning about $30 a week.

I didn't find employment and continued searching around. Then I decided to start a little firm mending car radios, which was very profitable in the summer. In winter, no one seemed to bother too much because they didn't have to keep the children entertained during the holiday trips. So that business folded; but I hadn't declared it to the authorities, so nothing in benefits was stopped.

One day, the exchange rang me up and said there was a position open for a wireman/technician for a research project at the hospital where I had once been a patient. I remember the day clearly when I went to be interviewed. I was very enthusiastic and eager to get the job. I was offered close to $30 a week, which, by my standards, was a fortune! Never had I dared hope to earn that much in my first job. I said yes and started working the very next day.

Although I was pleased to have the offer of a job, I was appalled, really, to go back to the same hospital where I had once been a patient for two and a half years; I particularly didn't want to go back to some of the memories it held for me.

However, I liked my first job working in a laboratory in the hospital. It lasted for about three years. We developed special equipment for the disabled: a unique electronic system that allowed people who did not have use of their hands to switch on equipment—telephone, television set, tape recorder, electric shaver–unassisted. It is still used today, somewhat modernized.

"I was being offered four pounds a week, which would have been about $8. At that time, a nondisabled person in a similar junior level position would have been earning about $30 a week."

Money became scarce, and as it ran out, people started resigning. The draftsman left. I applied for his job and got it. The design draftsman left. I applied for his job and got it. The design engineer then left. I applied for and got his job as well! That shows the awful state of things, particularly since I never got a raise in salary—only prestige, status, and lots of work!

Soon after, the group I worked with formed a private firm to continue this work, and I continued on with them. Although we moved to a new facility, we had financial worries similar to those we experienced in our small laboratory in the hospital. All the employees, myself included, had contributed a considerable part of our wages for several months. It was time for me to make some decisions about my future should the company ultimately go under—the direction in which it certainly seemed headed.

I'm a person who sees an opportunity "through enlightened self-interest"—I just saw an opportunity, actually. My feeling was that, should the company fold, there would be nobody around to mend the existing equipment that I had helped to develop. In addition, I also wanted to start a business of my own, with my own ideas.

"What we try to do with our equipment is encourage professional people and parents to fully utilize the system by creating a little circle of friends who wouldn't have gotten together with a disabled person otherwise. This gives the disabled person an opportunity to meet people, even if it is only for an hour a day, one day a month."

In order to start a firm, I first had to stop and learn about transistors, which was something I wanted to do. As soon as I'd stopped and learned about that, integrated circuits came in, then the microprocessing system that is now being used. An American invention, it enables computing techniques to be done in quite a small physical setup. This sequence took me two years, and then I was ready to proceed.

I began a company that manufactures an apparatus of my design that, when connected to a typewriter, allows a person who could not otherwise communicate to use a series of switches that are coded to achieve letters and, in some instances, words. Instead of pushing keys, switches activate the typewriter, producing the letters on paper. For those without full use of their hands, but the ability to move a switch, this equipment allows sentences to be typed out.

If I feel good about anything in the system I've developed, it is that it allows people who use the equipment to socialize. The big problem, if you are stuck in a home or a residential group center, is that you might meet somebody while you have your meals, but often that is the only social contact you have. I feel extremely sensitive to isolation, as I am alone.

What we try to do with our equipment is encourage professional people and parents to fully utilize the system by creating a little circle of friends who wouldn't have gotten together with a disabled person otherwise. This gives the disabled person an opportunity to meet people, even if it is only for an hour a day, one day a month.

Tom Clancy

Twelve years ago, when I went to work, I didn't know from nothing. But I was lucky; I had a boss who was interested in me. Most people are very intimidated by someone who is disabled. Some people are terribly intimidated by the fact that I can be so disabled and still think. They can't cope with that. So they resent it, and they fight it. It hurts. Other people find it difficult to compete with me equally because they feel handicapped in their own way—I have this advantage: you can't pick on a "cripple."

I learned somewhere along the line that I had to argue with people purposely so they could feel free to fight back. I had to somehow even it up. By doing that, right now I am politically unacceptable in my working situation. I am the outsider. If they can beat me, then they can have what they want, but I don't agree with what they want to do because they're wrong!

I'm as equal as anyone else, and beyond that, I'm a threat because I'm competent. I know my business. I know how to cope with people. I know how to motivate people, and this is a tremendous threat to the other people who are in charge right now.

I may have gotten away with things in the past because I was disabled, but now I don't get away with them. I'm equal and I'm a competitor. But at the same time, I have this advantage. A year ago, when I got my evaluation for my annual merit increase, they said that some of my attitudes have to do with my disability, and I said, "No. They have to do with my mind."

When I first started working here, I hurt my back getting in and out of the van traveling to and from work. When I started working, I was terrified. I worked with Joe, and Joe reminded me, years later, that I was white as a sheet for three months—I just couldn't believe that I could handle this, that I could cope with it.

In Wonderland, the Red Queen said to Alice, "Here, you see, it takes all the running you can do to keep in the same place. If you want to get somewhere else, you must run at least twice as fast as that."

But those first few months were utterly terrifying. I felt that I had to do twice as much as anyone else—of course, I couldn't ask anyone to help me! I started in the summer, a tremendous advantage because you don't need so much—no coat, no hat, no gloves.

The first year was frightening, and then I began to realize that I could do the things that I had done before I had been in the hospital. If you hear stories about leaders and followers and all that sort of stuff, there is a certain truth to it. I began to assume a sort of leadership-type role, and that fit perfectly. Noting could fit better. I can't do the physical work. I can do the leadership work. The encouragement, development, and teaching—all of that stuff comes naturally, so I fit right in with it.

My title is Manager of Administrative Systems. I have nine people reporting to me. Before I went into the hospital, I had been a shop steward and foreman of a large, industrial bakery, so I was used to having people working for me. And within a couple of years here, it has evolved into a managerial position. People seem to like to work for me. I am able to get along with people, get mileage out of them. It's not so much what I know but that I can convince other people that they believe in themselves. Everything that goes on in this department, people can come and ask me questions, and I supply the answers. That makes me valuable. I also have my own terminal to work through the machine, like everybody else. I press the keyboard with my mouth stick. I can't use my fingers at all.

It takes a long time to get the kind of confidence I've built up. When I first came here, I was afraid to get my coat taken off. I have to be independent. I have to be functional. I have to not be different from other people. It is a psychological thing. It took me a long time to realize people wanted to help me. To realize and accept that people were sitting around waiting for me to ask them, and I didn't ask them.

I was absolutely terrified that if I needed help from others, it would jeopardize my job. "You have to be so much better if you are disabled" is, in part, true; but it is also a psychological manifestation of feelings that because you are disabled, you are less than someone who is not.

If I were not disabled, I would be earning a lot more money and have a lot more responsibility.

There are some feelings that you just have to learn to let go of. You don't quit, you prioritize; and you can let up on some of the negative drive and put that energy where it will benefit you. That's what I'm trying to do.

Anita Lawson

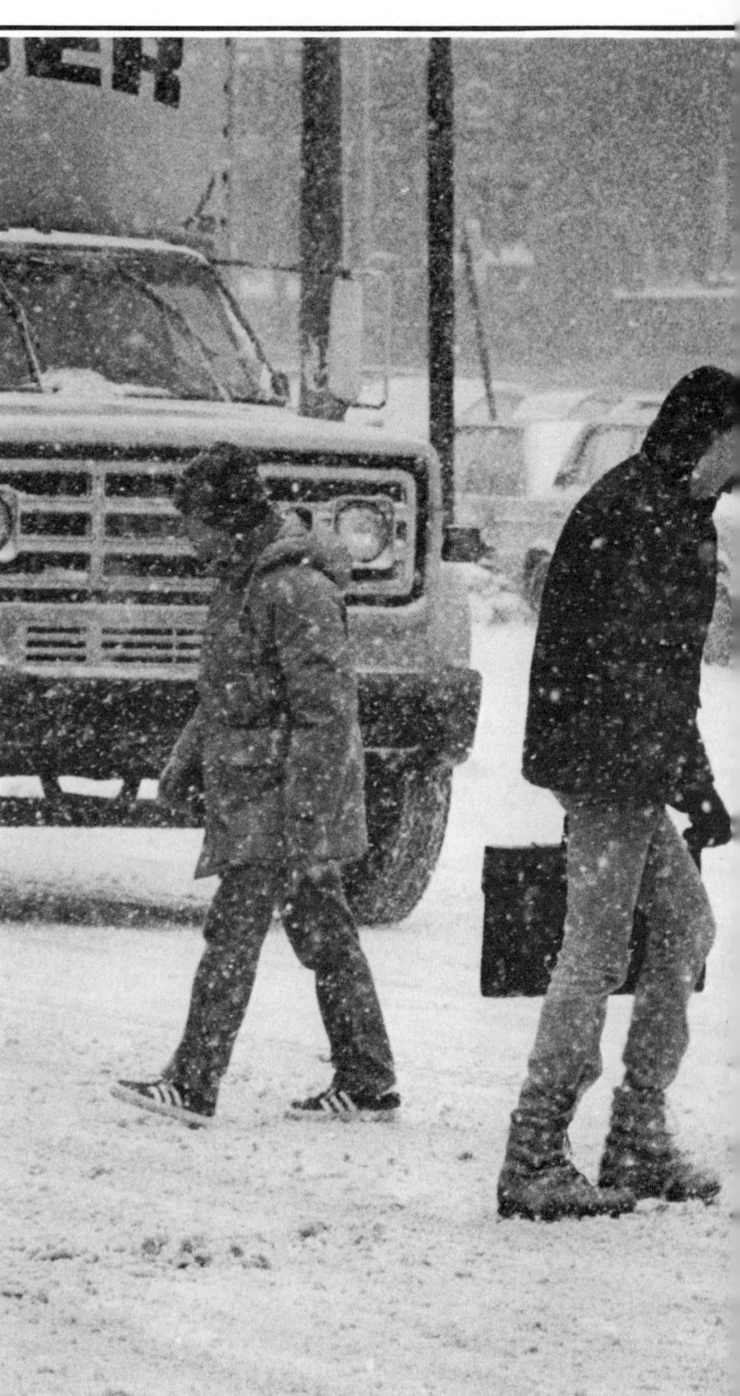

Today was suddenly cold, and it reminded me of last winter's snowstorm. Since I cannot use public transportation to travel, I have to use taxis. It is very difficult to get a cab when the weather is bad. It's very difficult to get a cab, period.

So I call the cab to pick me up. For that, you used to have to pay $3 over the meter rate; now it's $4. And that is the only way to get to school, to work, to wherever I have to go. I spend $40 or $50 a day . . . a day!!

When I was in school, when there was a snowstorm, I turned on the radio. If they said Barnard was open, I had to get to school. I could be the only one in the class—even the teacher wouldn't come in—but I had to get to school. I would ask myself, "Am I being superneurotic about this?" Or I would say, "The times are changing. Disabled people don't have to still prove they're superhuman, or do they?" I knew ninety-nine percent of the people would not be in class. How would they get home?

"When the school was empty because of a snowstorm, you could always count on somebody being there. Who? People with disabilities are always there. . . . In a way, those of us who have to be there laugh. We say, 'Look at this, the superhuman people; here we go again.'"

Well, that's my problem, too. How the hell would I get home, most of the time at night? That is, without saying to the cabbie, "I'll give you any amount of money you want if you'll just get me home." No one, I'm sure, except maybe someone who makes $50,000 a year or a single person with no dependents could afford this transportation system. I'm hardly poverty-stricken, but who can spend that kind of money every day? You figure one way to work, one way to school, one way back from school: five trips a day, minimum. That's twenty trips a week. With $4 over the

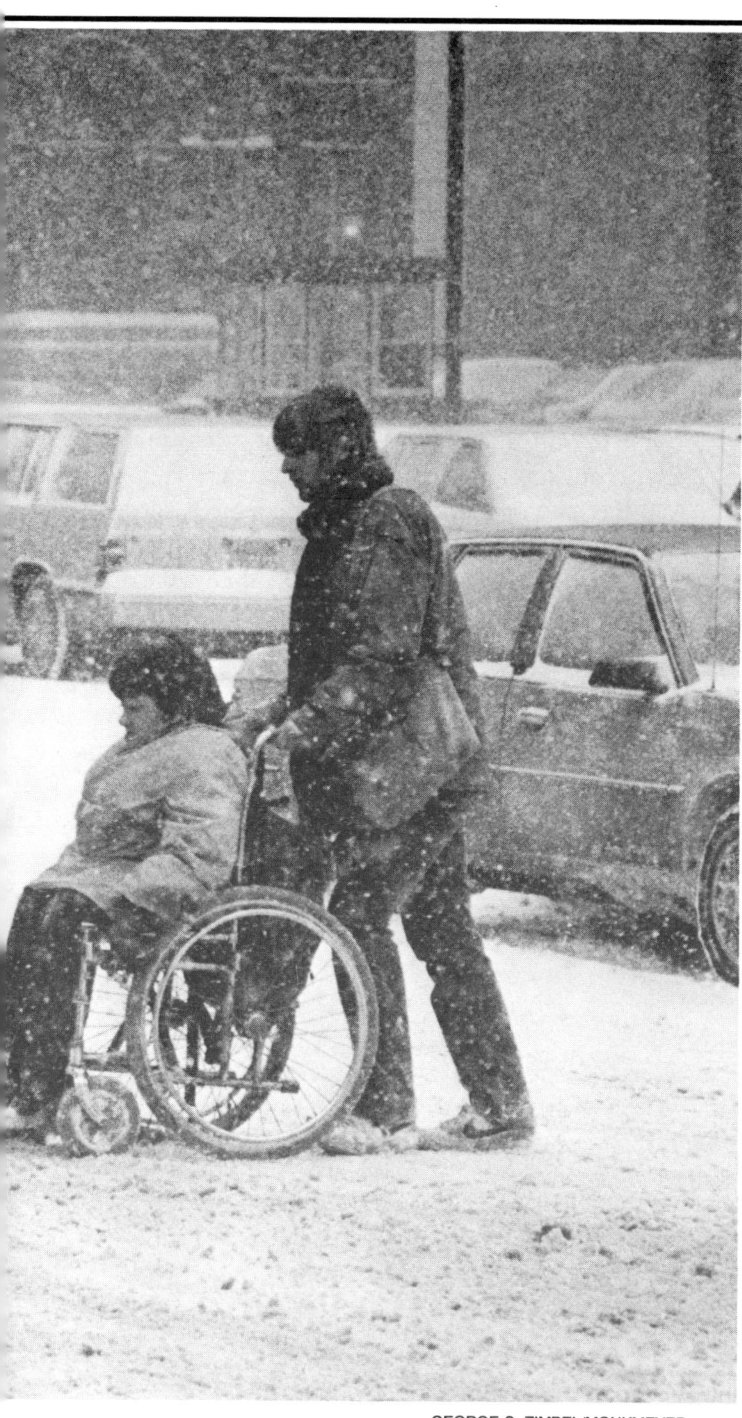
GEORGE S. ZIMBEL/MONKMEYER

meter every time. That's not considering how much the fare is.

On the average, I believe I spend $95 to $105 a week on transportation. That's when the weather is good and I don't have to call for a cab but can get one on the street. None of this, by the way, is tax deductible. For years, I spent all my money on transportation. I didn't buy any clothes; I would not spend on anything else. I have to work; I want to work; and the only way I can work is to spend this kind of money.

I earn more than $20,000 now. Years ago, of course, I earned far less. My mother doesn't think I'm a terrific saver, but I know I am if I can do all this and still pay for my needs. Recently, I had to take out loans for school, but almost everybody has to.

Figure that in addition to my having to be in school, I have to be at work. How many times am I at work when no one else is there? When it is snowing? When there is a strike of the transit workers? Anytime?

When the school was empty because of a snowstorm, you could always count on somebody being there. Who? People with disabilities are always there. We know we have to be there. In a way, those of us who have to be there laugh. We say, "Look at this, the superhuman people; here we go again."

We don't have to say anything, actually, because we know why we are there. We are constantly "proving." I think we have been brainwashed to the point that we do it as second nature. Not being there becomes very upsetting. It is like nothing can stop us; we just do it. *Realistically*, that is a problem to a certain degree because I don't think that there is a reason for me to have to do that. But *psychologically*, I think I have to do that. Of course, those people who are now in their 20s, they say, "Hey, I'm not going to do things that way. I don't have anything to prove."

They are totally different; they don't have to do anything. I'm not comparing them to the nondisabled; I'm comparing them to the older disabled person. In a way, I think they may be healthier. They may work out fine now, but because there are so many barriers, so many obstacles, for disabled people, if they don't try with that extra something, I don't know if they can "make it."

It is just so difficult. It seems if you take one step back, you are taking ten steps back. It is just not one step for us, it is much, much more. . . .

Jim Weisman

I once had a case where we represented nineteen blind transcribing typists—they listened to tapes on headphones and then typed what they heard. They were all employed by the same agency, worked in the five boroughs for the city of New York, and most of them were women. They had an average of fourteen years' experience.

The city was trying to reduce the number of its employees through attrition. It was cheaper to pension people off and not replace them, so attrition was up fifty-five percent in one year. The city was moving these people to one central location, taking them away from locations in which some of them had worked for twenty years. Now these are blind people who had fellow employees cashing their checks for them; local merchants knew them and delivered groceries to them; their trips to work had been established for many years. Moving to a new location was a tremendous hardship for them.

The city said the move was to make it easier for the administration. It seemed to us that it was intended to make things harder for the typists so that they would quit. Many of them thought that after working all these years in the same place, they would retire rather than move. It seemed unfair, and after exhaustive, unsuccessful efforts to resolve the issue, we decided to go to court. We tried to talk to the commissioner of this agency, but her attitude was "The hell with you." We ended up suing her.

"Banging his gavel, the judge said, 'Because they are blind, you do nothing because people are blind. What about because they are black, because they are women?' "

The name of the defendant was the commissioner of the Department of Social Services. When I called the case and as we were walking up to the counsel tables, the judge asked, "Is this a welfare case?" We said, "No, your honor. This is employment discrimination. The city is proposing to transfer fourteen transcribing typists from their present locations to one central location. Only the blind are being transferred."

The transfer notice was addressed to "Blind and Transcribing Typists," as if that is a job category.

I went on to say to the judge, "The city is proposing to transfer people just because they are blind." The judge said to the city's lawyer—at this point, still off the record—"Hey, you don't transfer people just because they are blind." And the lawyer said, "Well, your honor, because they are blind . . ." And that is as far as he got. Banging his gavel, the judge said, "Because they are blind, you do nothing because people are blind. What about because they are black, because they are women?; aren't these people in the union? Have you never heard of reverse order of seniority? Transfers are supposed to come in reverse order of seniority, not because they are blind! Now go ahead and present your case."

And so there was no case. The bottom line was that there was a messenger service that had existed for years, sending these tapes back and forth from the boroughs to the central office, and the city had wanted to fire the messengers!

Rehabilitation—A Do-It-Yourself Plan

Eugene Horcher

This is a do-it-yourself rehabilitation program. Why do it yourself? Why not rely on professionals? The professional often has many clients and little time and knows that failure with one will not hurt his career. The individual with a disability has only one client—a very important one—and more time to devote to his or her rehabilitation process. "Never rely solely on a professional" is a good rule of thumb. Consultation and advice are fine, but total reliance—on professionals, family, or friends—is not. Rehabilitating yourself means you are molding your life to an image of your own choosing.

" 'Never rely solely on a professional' is a good rule of thumb. . . . Rehabilitating yourself means you are molding your life to an image of your own choosing."

People who have disabilities face a bewildering world fraught with opportunities and barriers. Service delivery systems promise a lot but often provide delay, confusion, service delivery gaps, and disincentives. The individual seeking help may find that helpers (parents, friends, rehabilitation professionals, etc.) sometimes do more harm than good. The individual, whether disabled early in life or as an adult, usually faces this chaotic situation without a good understanding of his or her physical condition, intellectual and emotional capacities, and values.

The main objective and requirement in rehabilitating yourself is to gain control of your own life. Control over your own values, ideas, and behavior is a requirement of good mental health. This is true for nondisabled as well as disabled individuals.

Rehabilitation is a long-term process, one that requires determination and persistence. Patience, tolerance, and understanding are needed.

First, you must determine your own life-style goals. To rehabilitate yourself, you must know who you are, what you want out of life, and where you are going. You have to understand your physical condition, your intellectual ability, your specific aptitudes, your personality, and your values. Bookstores and libraries are full of information that will help you evaluate and understand yourself. Read, study, and then think about what you have learned. Find someone you trust and talk over your problems or difficulties. The person could be a friend or relative as long as he or she is frank and objective.

"The main objective and requirement in rehabilitating yourself is to gain control of your own life. Control over your own values, ideas, and behavior is a requirement of good mental health. This is true for nondisabled as well as disabled individuals."

Learn to listen to yourself and to others. Use a tape recorder or take notes so you can really understand what is said. Do not neglect history. Get copies of your school transcripts, list your hobbies and interests, write up a detailed work history as well as your own analysis of your physical capacities. Be specific and objective. Finally, after reviewing and analyzing this material, try to determine your values.

This process should yield a fairly accurate picture of you. Do not hesitate, however, to consult health care professionals if needed. If in doubt, consult. The time, effort, and money you spend on this study is an investment in your future. Write up a thorough summary of your findings. It will serve as an invaluable aid to you and to anyone who works with you.

Now you should understand yourself better, what you want out of life, and where you are going. You are, no doubt, aware that you will face various barriers and obstacles. The obvious ones for mobility impaired people are transportation and environmental barriers. You can't be a self-directing individual if you are unable to move about your house freely, can't move through your front door, across the street, and to accessible transportation with relative ease and independence. Ability to get to and use a work site, shopping, church, public facilities, restaurants, and friends also limits your way of life.

"Most of life consists of making judgments as to what you are willing to accept. The ideal is rarely, if ever, reached. Rather, a compromise solution is the standard way to resolve most problems. The goal to work toward is the best possible compromise under the circumstances."

Attitudinal barriers are usually more subtle but just as inhibiting. You must recognize these barriers, for instance, when someone else decides for you that you can't make it through college or vocational training or tells you who your friends should be or decides when you should go to bed or that you should not be hired because you will upset other workers. Once they are recognized, you have to figure out how to minimize or overcome these barriers. Then you must decide if the effort or "hassle" needed to overcome the barrier is worth the goal you are seeking. Most of life consists of making judgments as to what you are willing to accept. The ideal is rarely, if ever, reached. Rather, a compromise solution is the standard way to resolve most problems. The goal to work toward is the best possible compromise under the circumstances.

In order to overcome the barriers, you have to know how to use the information, resources, and services available to you as a person with a disability. These vary from community to community. An excellent source of information is the public library. Another is the daily newspaper. High schools and colleges have information in libraries and often have counseling centers. Social service organizations can also provide information, counseling, and medical and vocational services. Shelter workshops have many special information, referral, and independent living services.

Independent living centers are among the best sources of information and referral. Some states have special "hot lines" and information lines for people with disabilities. Private rehabilitation hospitals have information and referral services as well as medical and sometimes vocational services. Many hospitals have a rehabilitation unit, although these tend to have a medical orientation with limited information, referral, and vocational services.

All states have a department, bureau, or division of rehabilitation. This is the agency that most disabled adults are likely to contact once or more during their adult lives. Although touted as a source of comprehensive rehabilitation services, they frequently provide superficial services and limited information. Public aid and public employment offices are also sources of information and services.

In order to get good information, a thorough study should be made of these and all other available resources and services. The more you know, the better you will be able to plan your own rehabilitation.

Next, lay out a plan for action listing your goals, the barriers to those goals, and the services and actions needed to achieve those goals. Here you get down to specifics. If you need specialized housing, you have to locate (through newspapers, consumer publications and groups, information and referral sources) housing in your area that will meet your needs, as well as sources of funds (including your own savings and income) to pay the rent or mortgage.

The goal of employment involves the same process. You review your capacities and the job market. Then check with colleges, vocational schools, sheltered workshops, and employers to find out how you can get a job or training. You have to be especially realistic when employment is the goal. People will encourage you to get training and prepare for work but often those same people will feel no obligation to help you find a job once you are ready for work. For this reason, you should talk to employers and job placement counselors. Knowing you might return to them later for help or for a job, they will tend to be realistic. No one is guaranteed employment. Employment requires good planning, thorough training, persistence, and luck,

Attendant care might require contacting an independent living center, advertising in the newspaper, putting ads on school or hospital bulletin boards, and possibly interviewing and training an attendant on your own. Transportation could require a search for the right size and type of car, location of a driving instructor, finding vendors who sell and install hand controls, or arranging with local taxi or van services for appropriate transportation.

Your plan should cover all needed services, possible sources of funds, and a timetable for completing each part of the plan. Alternate solutions should be developed in case the first plan doesn't work out.

Once you have worked out a comprehensive plan, present it for evaluation to one or more people you trust. If you have disabled friends, talk it over with them. One good procedure is to find an individual with a similar disability who has reached a similar goal. This is one of the best ways of testing the viability of your plan. Sometimes you can locate a role model through consumer organizations or publications that are aimed at the disabled individual. Modify or alter your plan as needed after you get suggestions from friends, counselors, or role models.

You are now ready for the execution phase. This is a time-consuming process. You have to locate and arrange the services you need. The more agencies and services you have to coordinate, the more difficult it is to execute the plan. Public agencies, in particular, move slowly. Most public agency personnel are overworked, and they will probably be pleased that you have done all the preliminary work. Be ready to defend your plan. However, be prepared to fully consider the suggestions made by the agency representative and alter your plan if desirable and/or necessary.

If you have done your homework thoroughly, you will understand the services provided by the agency, the goals of the agency, its limitations, and the appeals process, if any. It is best to be candid and to cooperate as much as possible. Services take time, but the agency representatives should tell you how long it will take to determine eligibility and provide services. Contact them at frequent, regular intervals to make sure the program they lay out is progressing as promised. Also, volunteer to obtain documents and reports if you can get them.

State rehabilitation agencies need medical reports, hospital reports, school transcripts, GED diplomas and test scores, and proof of Social Security Disability and Supplementary Security Income status. You should know your income for the last year as well as current income and savings. It will save time to bring copies of all documents of this type to the initial interview.

Many agencies, including state rehabilitation agencies, will give you documents covering agency procedures, the appeals process, and a list of agency services, as well as your responsibilities as a client. Keep these records handy and read them over thoroughly. If you feel uncertain about the plan laid out by an agency, ask for a copy and get an appointment to come back after you have had time to review the program. Most agencies are flexible enough to allow you to modify a plan if circumstances change. Be flexible and tolerant. However, if you feel you have been treated unfairly by the counselor or other agency representative with whom you are dealing, use the appeals process. Avoid personal animosity if possible. The professional person may be "wrong" without being "bad." Keep notes on all contacts with the agency including dates, what was said, what happens next, etc.

The best plans can fail due to unforeseen circumstances. If your plan fails, review the situation as objectively as possible. Seek out a friend or counselor to get an independent opinion as to what went wrong. Learn from the failure. Disappointment is natural, but self-pity or blame is not. The solution is to evaluate the alternate plan you set up, revise it, if needed, and implement it, taking into account what you learned from the failure of your original plan.

Consumer groups and activities are a valuable aid in rehabilitating yourself. They are an excellent source of information about the latest laws, rules, developments, and services. They provide role models and mentors. Sometimes they function as therapy groups where individual and group problems can be worked out. They can act as your advocate in dealing with rehabilitation agencies or the community. They serve as pressure groups that can change laws and rules and influence rehabilitation agencies, community institutions, and the public in general. Utilizing the services offered by these groups can help you gain better control over your own life and environment.

Eugene Horcher, a rehabilitation counselor, is an advocate and ally. One year, he was given an award for being the most outstanding rehabilitation counselor in the state of Illinois. Equally important to him is his role as activist and the regard and respect of clients and disabled activists.

PEOPLE TAKING CHARGE

- *Speak to disabled individuals who are employed; ask them how they did it.*
- *Get as much training as possible in how to handle a job interview. Independent living centers, some rehabilitation institutes, Ys, and social service organizations prepare individuals.*
- *Appropriate clothing reflects professionalism. Enthusiasm can often win over a reluctant employer.*
- *Know about the company where you are being interviewed. Ask questions.*
- *Have confidence in your abilities and make clear to the employer any limitations you may have.*
- *Know the adaptations you need to perform your job.*
- *A survey of companies and job categories can be made by local organizations of disabled people.*
- *An on-site visit to potential employers can create better understanding of the capabilities of disabled people.*
- *Check the mayor's office for disabled individuals, Veterans Administration, state employment office, Goodwill Industries, independent living centers, and disabled consumer organizations for employment opportunities.*
- *If you receive financial assistance, know your Social Security representative, the telephone number, and the address of your local Social Security office.*
- *Before going to the Social Security office, telephone to check on its accessibility; ask what information you must bring with you.*
- *The wait at a Social Security office can be long. Bring medications, lunch, something to read, and, if possible, a friend.*
- *Know your rights about entitlements. Don't be intimidated by the attitudes of the "giving enemy." Ask the Social Security representative for literature.*
- *Should you feel that you have been wronged, request a fair hearing. Learn what it entails.*
- *Careful records about how you spend your money plus one year's bank statements and receipts should be available, if requested, for certification.*
- *Have an identification card, if requested—driver's license, credit cards, institution or employment I.D. are good.*
- *Learn banking procedures—how to write a check, how to make out a deposit or withdrawal slip, how to buy a money order.*
- *If you can't write your signature by hand, learn to write it, if possible, by mouth or any other way. Some banks offer signature stamps. Inquire at your bank.*

Handicapped
The U.S. Department of Health + Human Services
200 Independance Ave.
S.W Washington D.C.

To whom it may concern:

I am a twenty seven year old girl who has been diagnosed partially handicapped, but has been told she can still work. However, I have been applying all over the city of Toledo in cafeterias and restaurants. I stayed in Salina, Kansas for a year with my aunt and I had a job in a cafeteria out there for 6 months. When I came back home to live, I went down to the C.B.E.S., they helped me get a job at the counter in Arby's Roast Beef. I worked there for three weeks. The manager called me in her office + told me she had to let me go, because I was too slow.

I soon found out by the girls I worked with that the real reason was because I was handicapped and that their customers were complaining. Is there anyway I can find a decent + nice job? Without being criticized or having someone talking about your handicapped situation?

Please see if there is anyone or anything anyone can do to help me get a nice and decent job

Thank you for taking the time in reading my letter.

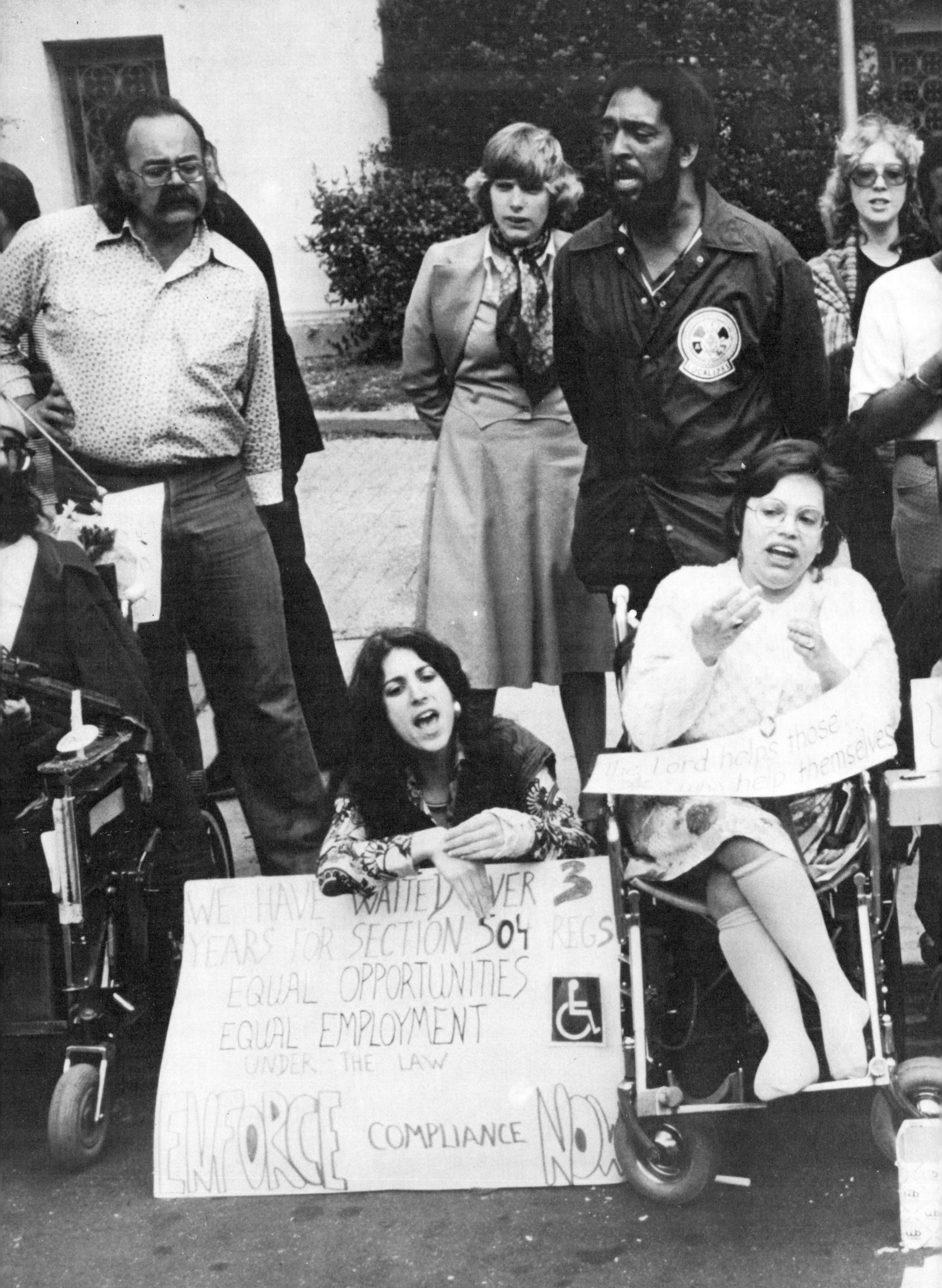
WE HAVE WAITED OVER 3
YEARS FOR SECTION 504 REGS
EQUAL OPPORTUNITIES
EQUAL EMPLOYMENT
UNDER THE LAW
ENFORCE COMPLIANCE NOW
The Lord helps those
help themselves

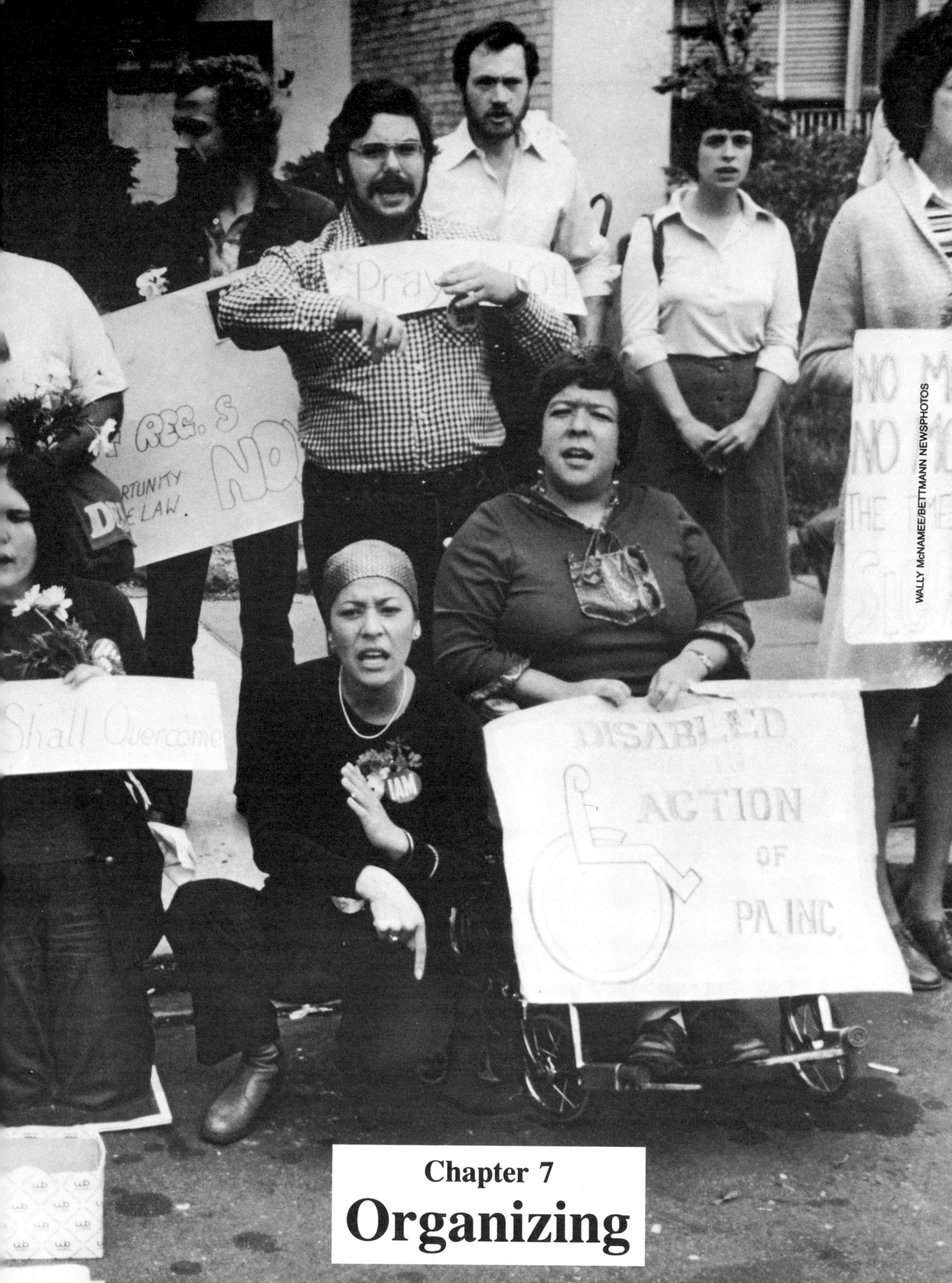

WALLY McNAMEE/BETTMANN NEWSPHOTOS

Chapter 7
Organizing

Organizations

Traditionally, the American approach to solving a problem is to create an organization. This attitude was the foundation of all the voluntary organizations that serve almost every disability category.

A good number of the organizations developed to serve various disability categories and have enlarged their services to include an active role in advocacy, ultimately benefiting all disabilities.

Local chapters might include rehabilitation facilities, diagnostic centers, employment training, and placement programs. They may make referrals or have on their staffs physicians, dentists, speech and hearing therapists, physical therapists, and sexuality counselors. An organization may have special transportation and maintain information on reliable sources for buying or renting equipment. They may organize social programs, parent support groups, and after-school activities, and some may have summer day and sleep-away camps.

The voluntary health organizations have in common an interesting history.

The National Association of the Deaf was founded in 1880 by a group of deaf men to protect the rights and privileges of the deaf. Until 1958, the association operated on a voluntary basis out of the homes of its officers.

Many people prominent in work for the blind in this country began to think and talk seriously about the need for a national organization in the early 1900s. Although the time did not seem ripe for formation of such an organization, the idea did not die. In 1921, H. Randolph Latimer, then president of the American Association of Workers for the Blind, agreed to lead a campaign to establish a national organization. The American Foundation for the Blind was incorporated "to aid the blind and partially blind of America and to cooperate with any organization, association, institution, or individual engaged in improving the condition of the blind and partially blind." The foundation was fortunate in having Helen Keller and Anne Sullivan Macy as enthusiastic supporters from the beginning.

The parents of children with cerebral palsy founded the United Cerebral Palsy Association, Inc., which officially came into being in 1949, to promote research, treatment, education, and rehabilitation and to subsidize professional training programs.

"A good number of the organizations developed to serve various disability categories have enlarged their services to include an active role in advocacy, ultimately benefiting all disabilities."

Very little was being done to encourage research in muscular dystrophy when small groups of parents in New York whose children had the disease organized the Muscular Dystrophy Association of America, Inc. in 1950. By 1959 a research center was built and supported by the association to do research in muscular dystrophy as well as related neuromuscular disorders.

The American Diabetes Association, which had been established as a professional society, decided to reorganize as a national voluntary health association in 1964 and involve everyone concerned with meeting the needs of individuals with diabetes.

About the same time, two national organizations, the

Epilepsy Association of America and the Epilepsy Foundation, merged to create a united national voluntary agency.

One voluntary health association changed its category. Franklin D. Roosevelt had established the National Foundation for Infantile Paralysis in 1938 at a time when it seemed impossible to prevent polio. The organization led the fight against polio, which resulted in the discovery of the Salk vaccine. This accomplished, the foundation decided to turn its efforts to arthritis and birth defects. By 1964, the Arthritis Foundation became a separate organization; and the National Foundation–March of Dimes now devotes itself exclusively to birth defects.

George Nelson Wright, in *Total Rehabilitation*, speaks about the voluntary health organizations:

> The traditional role of private agencies has been perpetuated by the limitations of public agencies. There are some things that government administration cannot do or does not do well. For example, private organizations are free to (1) give special considerations to selected groups of people, (2) provide services without delay pending investigation of legal eligibility, (3) accept high-risk cases, or (4) try unproved or unpopular methods.
>
> . . . The charity of humanity accounts for the voluntary movement. For the most part, the organizations were started by people who had a personal (or professional) interest from firsthand experience with the problem. And they prosper by providing concerned volunteers and contributors the opportunity to do something personally to help disabled people. Yet even a most generous and affluent society will not even begin to donate all of the money and help needed for complete human service programs. Government funds from general taxation are required. In fact, the state and federal rehabilitation budget far exceeds the combined financial resources raised by contributions to the voluntary organizations. This is not to suggest that the private sector can be charged with tokenism because relatively small budgets of voluntary health agencies do provide benefits unobtainable from public funds.

The Lion's share of the money raised by each voluntary organization must come from fund-raising efforts. Telethons and voluntary organizations go together in this society. (See page 169 for commentary on the mixed blessing of telethons.)

Voluntary Service Organizations and the Services They Provide

O.	NAME	ADVOCACY	ART THERAPY	ATTENDANT INFORMATION	CAMPS	CAREER TESTING	CLINICS	CONSUMER INFORMATION	EDUCATIONAL PROGRAMS	EMPLOYMENT REFERRAL	EQUIPMENT INFORMATION	FILMS	GENETIC COUNSELING	HOUSING INFORMATION	INDIVIDUAL COUNSELING	INSURANCE INFORMATION	JOB PLACEMENT	LOCAL CHAPTERS	OCCUPATIONAL THERAPY	PHYSICAL THERAPY	PUBLICATIONS	SCHOOL REFERRAL	SELF HELP PARENT GROUP	SEXUALITY COUNSELING	SPEECH & HEARING THERAPY	SPORTS ACTIVITIES	TRAVEL INFORMATION	VOCATIONAL TRAINING	VOLUNTEER
1	AIDS						●								●						●								
2	Al-Anon/Alateen Family Group														●						●								
3	Alcoholics Anonymous														●						●								
4	Alexander Graham Bell Association for the Deaf	●										●			●			●			●	●	●						
5	Alzheimer's Disease and Related Disorders							●							●						●								
6	American Cancer Society								●		●				●			●	●		●		●		●				●
7	American Cleft Palate Educ. Foundation																												
8	American Council of the Blind	●					●			●	●							●			●					●	●		
9	American Diabetes Association			●	●		●		●		●				●	●		●			●	●					●		●
0	American Foundation for the Blind	●			●			●	●		●	●						●			●						●		

NO.	NAME	ADVOCACY	ART THERAPY	ATTENDANT INFORMATION	CAMPS	CAREER TESTING	CLINICS	CONSUMER INFORMATION	EDUCATIONAL PROGRAMS	EMPLOYMENT REFERRAL	EQUIPMENT INFORMATION	FILMS	GENETIC COUNSELING	HOUSING INFORMATION	INDIVIDUAL COUNSELING	INSURANCE INFORMATION	JOB PLACEMENT	LOCAL CHAPTERS	OCCUPATIONAL THERAPY	PHYSICAL THERAPY	PUBLICATIONS	SCHOOL REFERRAL	SELF HELP PARENT GROUP	SEXUALITY COUNSELING	SPEECH & HEARING THERAPY	SPORTS ACTIVITIES	TRAVEL INFORMATION	VOCATIONAL TRAINING	VOLUNTEER
11	American Heart Association	●					●											●		●	●								
12	American Lung Association	●							●		●	●									●		●						
13	American Narcolepsy Association								●			●									●		●						
14	American Parkinson Disease Assoc.						●		●		●	●			●						●		●				●		
15	The Amyotrophic Lateral Sclerosis Association			●														●			●								
16	Arthritis Foundation	●			●		●	●	●		●	●						●	●	●	●		●						●
17	Assoc. for Children & Adults with Learning Disabilities	●		●	●	●			●	●								●			●	●	●						
18	Assoc. for Retarded Citizens											●			●	●		●			●								
19	Assoc. for the Severely Handicapped	●							●		●							●	●	●	●	●		●	●	●	●	●	
20	Asthma/Allergy Found. of American								●		●							●			●	●							●
21	Committee to Combat Huntington's Disease	●							●		●	●			●	●		●			●		●	●					
22	Cooley's Anemia Foundation	●										●				●		●			●		●						●
23	C. de Lange Syndrome Foundation	●																			●		●						
24	Cystic Fibrosis Foundation	●					●		●		●	●				●		●			●		●				●		●
25	Down's Syndrome Congress	●		●			●	●	●			●			●	●		●			●	●	●						●
26	Dysautonomia Foundation, Inc.						●											●											
27	Dystropic Epidermolysis Bullosa Research Association of America	●					●	●	●			●									●								
28	Epilepsy Foundation of American	●							●	●		●				●		●			●	●	●						
29	Foundation for Children with Learning Disabilities	●							●												●								
30	Friedreich's Ataxia Group								●												●		●						
31	Gaucher's Disease Registry								●												●								
32	Goodwill Industries of America	●						●		●					●	●		●										●	
33	Human Growth Foundation	●																●			●		●						
34	Ileitis and Colitis Foundation														●						●								
35	Intern'l Association Laryngectomees								●		●	●					●	●			●		●		●				●
36	Juvenile Diabetes Foundation International																	●			●								●
37	Leukemia Society of America									●					●			●			●		●			●			
38	Little People of America									●					●			●			●		●			●			●
39	Lupus Foundation of America	●		●											●		●	●			●		●						●
40	March of Dimes Birth Defects Found.	●							●	●		●						●			●		●						
41	Mental Health Association								●												●		●						

NO.	NAME	ADVOCACY	ART THERAPY	ATTENDANT INFORMATION	CAMPS	CAREER TESTING	CLINICS	CONSUMER INFORMATION	EDUCATIONAL PROGRAMS	EMPLOYMENT REFERRAL	EQUIPMENT INFORMATION	FILMS	GENETIC COUNSELING	HOUSING INFORMATION	INDIVIDUAL COUNSELING	INSURANCE INFORMATION	JOB PLACEMENT	LOCAL CHAPTERS	OCCUPATIONAL THERAPY	PHYSICAL THERAPY	PUBLICATIONS	SCHOOL REFERRAL	SELF HELP PARENT GROUP	SEXUALITY COUNSELING	SPEECH & HEARING THERAPY	SPORTS ACTIVITIES	TRAVEL INFORMATION	VOCATIONAL TRAINING	VOLUNTEER
42	Muscular Dystrophy Assoc.				●		●		●		●	●						●	●	●	●								
43	Myasthenia Gravis Foundation								●			●						●			●		●						
44	Narcotics Anonymous														●						●								
45	Nat'l. Alliance for the Mentally Ill						●				●				●			●					●						
46	Nat'l. Amputation Foundation									●							●				●								
47	Nat'l. Association for Hearing and Speech Action	●					●	●													●				●				
48	Nat'l Association for Sickle Cell Disease								●									●			●								
49	Nat'l. Assoc. for the Deaf-Blind	●						●													●		●						
50	Nat'l Assoc. for Visually Handicapped	●							●		●										●		●						
51	Nat'l. of Assoc. of Patients on Hemodialysis and Transplantation	●			●			●										●			●		●				●		
52	Nat'l. Assoc. of the Deaf	●			●												●				●							●	
53	Nat'l. Ataxia Foundation						●											●			●								
54	Nat'l. Council of Stutterers	●										●						●			●		●		●				
55	Nat'l. Council on Alcoholism	●							●									●			●								
56	Nat'l. Easter Seal Society	●									●										●								
57	Nat'l. Federation of the Blind	●							●						●			●			●		●						
58	Nat'l Foundation Jewish Genetic Diseases								●			●									●								
59	Nat'l. Head Injury Foundation	●													●			●			●								
60	Nat'l. Hemophilia Foundation											●				●		●			●						●		
61	Nat'l. Huntington's Disease Foundation	●					●	●	●			●			●			●			●		●						●
62	Nat'l. Kidney Foundation	●						●													●								
63	Nat'l. Multiple Sclerosis Society	●		●			●		●		●							●			●		●			●			
64	Nat'l. Neurofibromatosis Foundation							●	●				●																
65	Nat'l. Parkinson Foundation	●					●		●												●								
66	Nat'l. Retinitis Pigmentosa Foundation								●												●								
67	Nat'l. Reye's Syndrome											●									●								
68	Nat'l. Society for Children & Adults with Autism	●							●												●					●			
69	Nat'l. Spinal Cord Injury Assoc.	●						●	●	●	●			●			●	●			●								
70	Nat'l. Tay-Sachs & Allied Diseases Association						●						●								●								
71	Nat'l Tuberous Sclerosis Assoc.																				●		●						
72	Orton Dyslexia Society				●		●					●									●			●					●
73	Osteogenosis Imperfecta Foundation								●									●			●		●						●
74	Overeaters Anonymous														●						●								

NO.	NAME	ADVOCACY	ART THERAPY	ATTENDANT INFORMATION	CAMPS	CAREER TESTING	CLINICS	CONSUMER INFORMATION	EDUCATIONAL PROGRAMS	EMPLOYMENT REFERRAL	EQUIPMENT INFORMATION	FILMS	GENETIC COUNSELING	HOUSING INFORMATION	INDIVIDUAL COUNSELING	INSURANCE INFORMATION	JOB PLACEMENT	LOCAL CHAPTERS	OCCUPATIONAL THERAPY	PHYSICAL THERAPY	PUBLICATIONS	SCHOOL REFERRAL	SELF HELP PARENT GROUP	SEXUALITY COUNSELING	SPEECH & HEARING THERAPY	SPORTS ACTIVITIES	TRAVEL INFORMATION	VOCATIONAL TRAINING	VOLUNTEER
75	People First International																	●			●								
76	Polio Information Center	●						●													●		●						
77	Preder-Willi Syndrome Association																												
78	Society for Rehabilitation of the Facially Disfigured							●														●							
79	Spina Bifida Association of America						●														●								
80	Tourette Syndrome Assoc.	●								●			●					●											
81	United Cerebral Palsy Association	●					●		●			●						●			●								
82	United Ostomy Association	●						●										●			●								
83	United Way of America	●																●			●								
84	Vision Foundation	●																●			●								
85	Wilson's Disease Association	●																●											

VOLUNTARY HEALTH ORGANIZATIONS

1. **AIDS**
   Board of Health
   8 East 40th St.
   New York, NY 10010
   1-800-462-1884

2. **Al-Anon/Alateen Family Group Headquarters, Inc.**
   P.O. Box 182
   Madison Square Station
   New York, NY 10010
   or
   See local telephone book

3. **Alcoholics Anonymous World Services, Inc.**
   468 Park Avenue South
   New York, NY 10016
   or
   See local telephone book

4. **Alexander Graham Bell Association for the Deaf**
   3417 Volta Place, NW
   Washington, DC 20007

5. **Alzheimer's Disease and Related Disorders Association**
   70 East Lake Street
   Chicago, IL 60601

6. **American Cancer Society (ACS)**
   777 Third Avenue
   New York, NY 10017

7. **American Cleft Palate Educational Foundation**
   331 Salk Hall, University of Pittsburgh
   Pittsburgh, PA 15261

8. **American Council of the Blind (ACB)**
   Suite 304
   1211 Connecticut Avenue, NW
   Washington, DC 20036

9. **American Diabetes Association (ADA)**
   2 Park Avenue
   New York, NY 10016

10. **American Foundation for the Blind (AFB)**
    15 West 16th Street
    New York, NY 10011

11. **American Heart Association (AHA)**
    7320 Greenville Avenue
    Dallas, TX 75231

12. **American Lung Association (ALA)**
    740 Broadway
    New York, NY 10019

13. **American Narcolepsy Assocation (ANA)**
    Box 5846–0122
    Stanford, CA 94305

14. **American Parkinson Disease Association (APDA)**
    116 John Street
    New York, NY 10038

15. **The Amyotrophic Lateral Sclerosis Association**
    185 Madison Avenue
    New York, NY 10016

16. **Arthritis Foundation**
    3400 Peachtree Road, NE
    Suite 1101
    Atlanta, GA 30326

17. **Association for Children and Adults with Learning Disabilities (ACLD)**
    4156 Library Road
    Pittsburgh, PA 15234

18. **Association for Retarded Citizens (ARC)**
    National Headquarters
    2501 Avenue J
    Arlington, TX 76011

19. **Association for the Severely Handicapped (TASH)**
    7010 Roosevelt Way, NE
    Seattle, WA 98115

20. **Asthma and Allergy Foundation of America (AAFA)**
1707 N Street, NW
Suite 300
Washington, DC 20036

21. **Committee to Combat Huntington's Disease (CCHD)**
250 West 57th Street
Suite 2016
New York, NY 10147

22. **Cooley's Anemia Foundation**
105 East 22nd Street
Suite 911
New York, NY 10010

23. **Cornelia de Lange Syndrome Foundation**
60 Dyer Avenue
Collinsville, CT 06022

24. **Cystic Fibrosis Foundation (CFF)**
6000 Executive Boulevard
Suite 309
Rockville, MD 20852

25. **Down's Syndrome Congress (DSC)**
Central Office
1640 West Roosevelt Road
Chicago, IL 60608

26. **Dysautonomia Foundation**
570 Lexington Avenue
New York, NY 10017

27. **Dystrophic Epidermolysis Bullosa Research Assocation of America (D.E.B.R.A.)**
2936 Avenue W
Brooklyn, NY 11229

28. **Epilepsy Foundation of America**
4351 Garden City Drive
Suite 406
Landover, MD 20785

29. **Foundation for Children with Learning Disabilities (FCLD)**
99 Park Avenue
New York, NY 10016

30. **Friedreich's Ataxia Group in America (FAGA)**
P.O. Box 11116
Oakland, CA 94611

31. **Gaucher's Disease Registry (GDR)**
19856 Schoolcraft Street
Canoga Park, CA 91306

32. **Goodwill Industries of America (GIA)**
9200 Wisconsin Avenue
Bethesda, MD 20814

33. **Human Growth Foundation (HGF)**
4930 West 77th Street
Minneapolis, MN 55435

34. **Ileitis and Colitis Foundation, National Headquarters**
295 Madison Avenue
New York, NY 10017

35. **International Association of Laryngectomees (IAL)**
American Cancer Society
777 Third Avenue
New York, NY 10017

36. **Juvenile Diabetes Foundation International**
23 East 26th Street
New York, NY 10010

37. **Leukemia Society of America**
800 Second Avenue
New York, NY 10017

38. **Little People of America (LPA)**
Box 633
San Bruno, CA 94066

39. **Lupus Foundation of America**
4434 Covington Highway
Decatur, GA 30035

40. **March of Dimes Birth Defects Foundation**
1275 Mamaroneck Avenue
White Plains, NY 10605

41. **Mental Health Association (MHA)**
1800 North Kent Street
Arlington, VA 22209

42. **Muscular Dystrophy Assocation (MDA)**
810 Seventh Avenue
New York, NY 10019

43. **Myasthenia Gravis Foundation**
15 East 26th Street
New York, NY 10010

44. **Narcotics Anonymous**
25 St. Mark's Place
New York, NY 10010

45. **National Alliance for the Mentally Ill**
1234 Massachusetts Avenue
Suite 721
Washington, DC 20005

46. **National Amputation Foundation**
12–45 150th Street
Whitestone, NY 11357

47. **National Association for Hearing and Speech Action (NAHSA)**
10801 Rockville Pike
Rockville, MD 20852

48. **National Association for Sickle Cell Disease (NASCD)**
3460 Wilshire Boulevard
Suite 1012
Los Angeles, CA 90010

49. **National Association for the Deaf-Blind (NADB)**
2703 Forest Oak Circle
Norman, OK 73071

50. **National Association for Visually Handicapped (NAVH)**
305 East 24th Street
New York, NY 10010

51. **National Association of Patients on Hemodialysis and Transplantation (NAPHT)**
156 William Street
New York, NY 10038

52. **National Association of the Deaf (NAD)**
814 Thayer Avenue
Silver Spring, MD 20910

53. **National Ataxia Foundation**
6681 Country Club Drive
Minneapolis, MN 55247

54. **National Council of Stutterers (NCS)**
P.O. Box 8171
Grand Rapids, MI 49508

55. **National Council on Alcoholism (NCA)**
733 Third Avenue
New York, NY 10017

56. **National Easter Seal Society**
2023 West Ogden Avenue
Chicago, IL 60612

57. **National Federation of the Blind (NFB)**
1800 Johnson Street
Baltimore, MD 21230

58. **National Foundation for Jewish Genetic Diseases (NFJGD)**
609 Fifth Avenue
Suite 1200
New York, NY 10017

59. **National Head Injury Foundation**
280 Singletary Lane
Framingham, MA 01701

60. **National Hemophilia Foundation (NHF)**
19 West 34th Street
Room 1204
New York, NY 10001

61. **National Huntington's Disease Association (NHDA)**
128A East 74th Street
New York, NY 10021

62. **National Kidney Foundation (NKF)**
2 Park Avenue
New York, NY 10016

63. **National Multiple Sclerosis Society**
205 East 42nd Street
New York, NY 10017

64. **National Neurofibromatosis Foundation (NNFF)**
70 West 40th Street, 4th Floor
New York, NY 10018

65. **National Parkinson Foundation**
1501 NW Ninth Avenue
Miami, FL 33136

66. **National Retinitis Pigmentosa Foundation (RP Foundation)**
Rolling Park Building
8331 Mindale Circle
Baltimore, MD 21207

67. **National Reye's Syndrome (NRS)**
426 North Lewis
Bryan, OH 43506

68. **National Society for Children and Adults with Autism (NSAC)**
1234 Massachusetts Avenue, NW
Suite 1017
Washington, DC 20005–4599

69. **National Spinal Cord Injury Association**
369 Elliot Street
Newton Upper Falls, MA 02164

70. **National Tay-Sachs and Allied Diseases Assocation, Inc.**
92 Washington Avenue
Cedarhurst, NY 11516

71. **National Tuberous Sclerosis Association, Inc., (NTSA)**
P.O. Box 159
Laguna Beach, CA 92652

72. **Orton Dyslexia Society**
724 York Road
Baltimore, MD 21024

73. **Osteogenosis Imperfecta Foundation**
P.O. Box 428
Van Wert, OH 45891

74. **Overeaters Anonymous**
1940 Hempstead Turnpike
East Meadow, NY 11554

75. **People First International**
P.O. Box 12642
Salem, OR 97309

76. **Polio Information Center**
510 Main Street
Suite A446
Roosevelt Island, NY 10044

77. **Preder-Willi Syndrome Association**
5515 Malibu Drive
Edina, MN 55436

78. **Society for the Rehabilitation of the Facially Disfigured**
550 First Avenue
New York, NY 10016

79. **Spina Bifida Association of America (SBAA)**
343 South Dearborn Street
Suite 319
Chicago, IL 60604

80. **Tourette Syndrome Association (TSA)**
Bell Plaza Building
41–02 Bell Boulevard
Bayside, NY 11361

81. **United Cerebral Palsy Association (UCPA)**
66 East 34th Street
New York, NY 10016

82. **United Ostomy Association (UDA)**
2001 West Beverly Boulevard
Los Angeles, CA 90057

83. **United Way of America**
United Way Plaza
Alexandria, VA 22314

84. **Vision Foundation**
2 Mt. Auburn Street
Watertown, MA 02172

85. **Wilson's Disease Association**
P.O. Box 489
Dumfries, VA 22026

Telethons

"The telethon issue is ours alone," writes Anne Peters in her article "Telethon" (*Disability Rag*).

> It affects no other group of people. Telethons define us as special—unequal and inferior—and our problems as temporary; solvable with a cure. . . . Telethons are society's largest purveyor of what disabled people are like. The picture isn't very dignified. . . . It is difficult to view oneself with dignity when you are being patted on the head by a movie star several years your junior. . . . Telethons are what people give to help the less fortunate. They are the sanctioned way of dealing with the needs of this nation's disabled. Telethons raise money for equipment and other things we can't get any other way. . . . Talk of telethons brings controversy because people find good things happen as a result of telethons. . . .
>
> But the worst harm telethons do is create a mythology surrounding disability and disabled people. Beyond attributing false characteristics to the personalities of disabled people, telethons perpetuate the myth that our lives are controlled, overshadowed by our disability; . . . We still need the things telethons can give us, so we cannot afford to criticize them too much. If we do criticize, and because of our criticizing, the telethons stop, then where would we be? We realize the danger of this only too well, although we rarely articulate it. Disabled people know better. We don't bite the hand that feeds us. . . . But we criticize politicians who don't deliver their promises; we criticize government when it doesn't meet our needs. So why is it so hard to criticize a television presentation that provides us wheelchairs at a sacrifice of our dignity?

Protests of disability rights activists during a recent telethon were covered by several competing television stations. Those interviewed expressed concern regarding the paradox that exists in the disservice voluntary health organizations do to the image of disabled citizens at the same time they provide a wide range of needed services.

In an effort to answer these complaints, a few of the largest voluntary organizations have invited disabled citizens to serve as advisers in cities from which the telethons emanate.

Several changes have become apparent. Young children are no longer paraded across the stage to the accompaniment of "You'll Never Walk Alone." But the perspiring emcee, looking as much as possible like the image of a saint wearing a tuxedo, bereft of sleep, tie askew, smoking a never ending number of cigarettes, calling the children "his children," is still with us.

Telethons have been woven into the fabric of the American culture, an integral part of weekend holiday viewing, at a painful expense to most disabled citizens.

Organizations are sensitive to criticism. Changes can be brought about by contacting the public relations department of local chapters or national headquarters, giving specific details of the kinds of changes you would like to see. Both positive and negative comments could be effective.

Television stations are aware that criticism affects ratings and potential advertisers. Contact them, also, with specific suggestions of changes.

The money raised by every telethon is small in comparison to the state and federal rehabilitation budgets. However, state services vary, making geography an important factor in the service delivery system, so that voluntary health agencies provide services not available any place else.

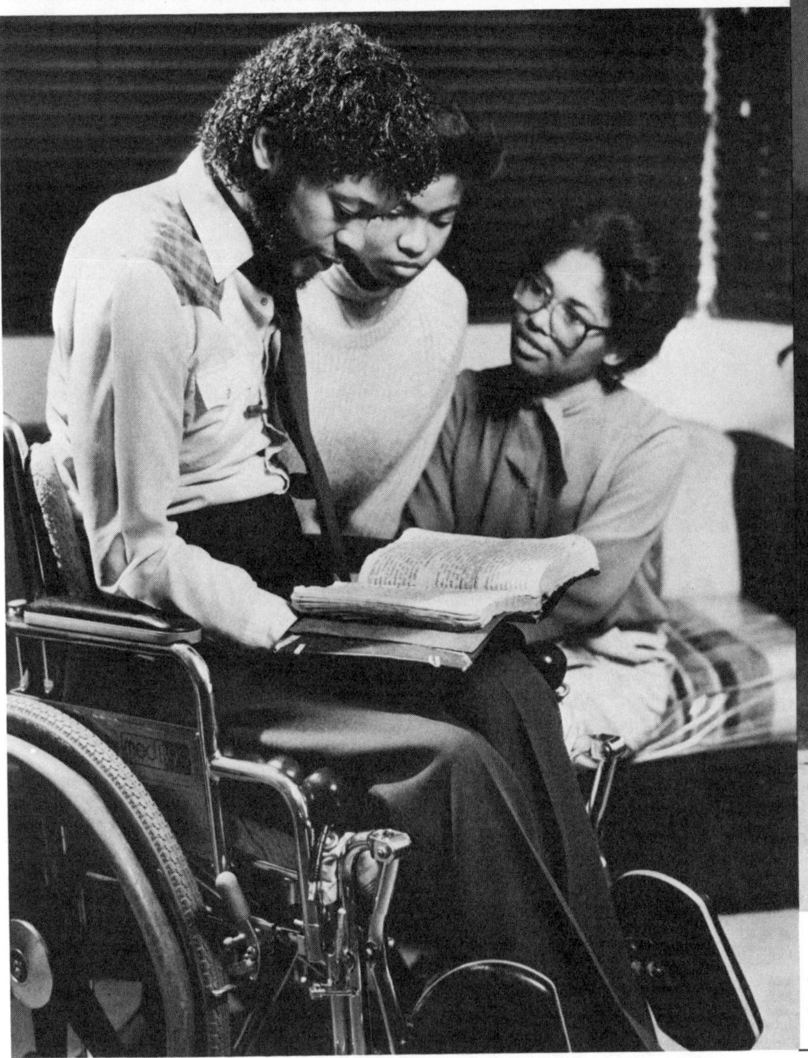

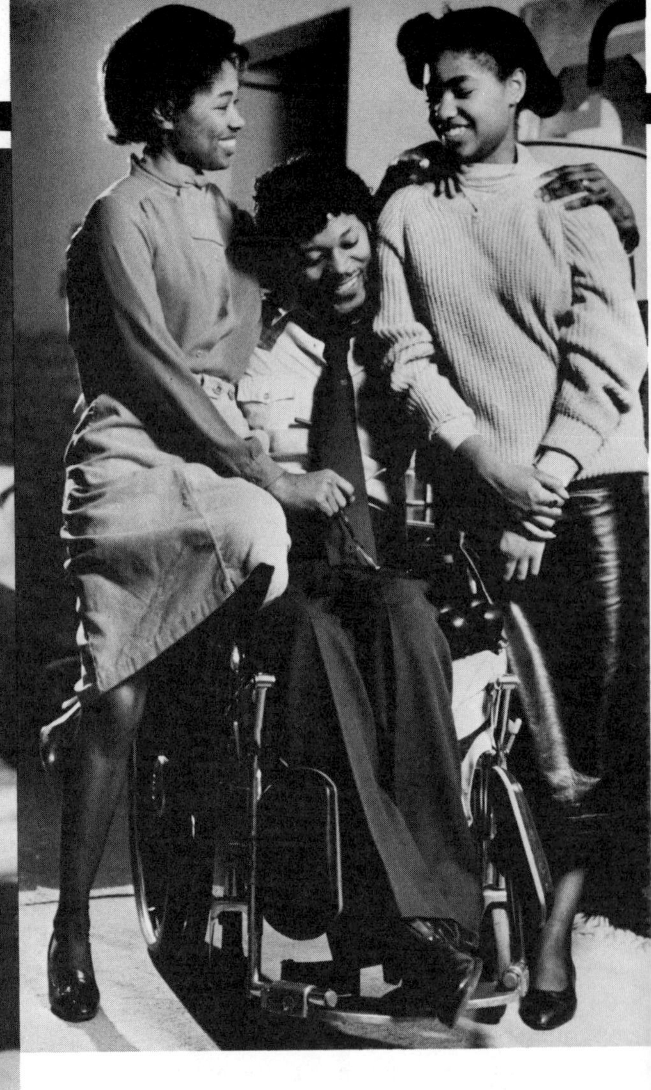

Fletcher Hickson and his wife Dolores and daughter Rene reading the Bible at their home on Roosevelt Island, New York. "The Bible comes first in our home," says Hickson.

ORGANIZATIONS/ DISABLED CITIZENS

Grass-roots organizing has been the trend since the 70s, so that now there are thousands of local and state organizations. Some of these groups are composed of parents of children with disabilities, veterans and their families, senior citizens with disabilities, independent living centers, and individuals with a similar disability.

Perhaps the best known national cross-disability organization is the American Coalition of Citizens with Disabilities, 1200 14th Street, N.W., Suite 201, Washington, D.C. 20005. The organization, with members from most disability organizations representing millions of individuals, seeks to obtain and protect the rights to education, housing, employment, transportation, and health care by securing comprehensive implementation of Section 504 of the Rehabilitation Act of 1973.

The Congress of Organizations of the Physically Handicapped, 16630 Beverly Avenue, Tinley Park, IL 60477, founded in 1958, is the oldest consumer organization with member clubs.

It has become clear to disability rights activists—those of us who have been a part of the movement for many years, and newcomers—that we need representation at local, city, state, and federal levels.

Our voices must be heard beyond disability interest organizations: from local school boards to the transit authorities, from city planners to the unions, from political organizations, right to the voting booth.

Relationships with the Public

William T. Snyder

The information function of an organization is an activity that must be recognized and integrated in the total operation. It is important that the person responsible for disseminating information is highly respected within the organization and is one of the key decision-making and policy-making persons.

A long-standing definition of public relations, first used by the editors of *Public Relations News*, is:

> Public relations is the management function that evaluates public attitudes, identifies the policies and procedures of an individual or an organization with the public interest, and plans and executes a program of action to earn public understanding and acceptance.

In addition to information, advocacy has been added to the responsibilities of your organization's communications specialist. Information pertains to the collection and dissemination of knowledge on specific facts or circumstances. Advocacy involves the acts of pleading for, supporting, and recommending—in other words, justification of the effort that is being undertaken.

Some of the characteristics that apply to all good information communicators include:

Curiosity

Ability to interpret technical data in lay language

Understanding of both the written and spoken language, including basic knowledge of grammar

An evident interest in, and obvious enthusiasm for, the job

No matter what other qualifications a candidate may have, if he or she falls short in any of these abilities, the person will not be totally suited to serve as an organization's communicator.

An essential tool to every organization is the basic newsletter. One or more newsletters may be published, and they may be in any format from a single page, informal memorandum to a slick, illustrated magazine.

This workhorse information piece is the regularly scheduled, timely, informative organization-to-audience communication.

The content of the newsletter may be determined by the audience to be reached. Careful thought should be given to evaluating the newsletter content. Will others be interested? Can it help broaden interest in the organization? Will it gain new adherents to your cause?

The value of a regularly scheduled newsletter is that its content can be varied. As long as regularity has been established so that recipients can anticipate receiving information regularly, the newsletter may be devoted to one specific, timely topic or relate to a vast variety of subjects. It can fully detail a single issue or serve as a source guide for further information on many subjects. It can announce specific meetings, publicize fund-raisers, urge action on legislation, announce a scientific breakthrough, and solicit tax-deductible gifts. In addition, it can urge and advocate positive actions or identify known positions of opposition.

Whatever it does, a newsletter should always be credible, accurate, informative, and as dependably on schedule

"An essential tool to every organization is the basic newsletter."

as your morning newspaper or your favorite weekly magazine.

Every issue of your newsletter should contain an invitation to "write in for further information" or other incentives to have readers contact the editor. Response from readers to newsletter articles can serve as a guide to policy and action. Reader response is a reaction to something already determined and published. But reader reaction can serve as an indication of interest in special phases of your organization's activities.

The communication specialist who edits the newsletter is responsible for finding the material for use in the newsletter. The communicator must have contact with every phase of the organization's programs and the ability to evaluate the various activities and projects undertaken.

Through two-way communication, newsletter readers can help form policy for an organization. The newsletter can become a working communication medium between the organization and interested readers in different parts of the United States.

Other responsibilities of the organization's information officer are meetings, displays, and exhibitions. These are techniques through which direct response to the message

"The most important and time-consuming part of your information communicator's job is establishing and maintaining good relationships with the mass media. Members of the mass media include radio, television, and printed matter."

conveyed can be measured. All three are carefully planned to concentrate attention on an activity or phase of a program. For clear identification, we'll consider that meetings are either of a general membership and policy nature or are planned to bring authorities on subjects of special interest to the attention of specific audiences.

These activities can be used effectively to get new members—invite people to join the organization, offer to volunteer for specific duties, request additional information, make contributions in support, help organize a local chapter, or any of the dozens of other ways in which an organization hopes to win friends and adherents.

The most important and time-consuming part of your information communicator's job is establishing and maintaining good relationships with the mass media. Member of the mass media include radio, television, and printe matter. Materials in print include national publications, re gional and local weeklies, daily newspapers, specialize journals, billboards, posters, and other forms of printe material that are available to the total population—whethe these readers have an interest in your activities or not. Be cause the mass media are nonselective in the audience the reach, your use of them should be carefully planned to mee your information and advocacy needs.

As each medium is unique in its appeal to the public specialized attention should be given to preparation of ma terials.

When a newspaper is fortunate enough to carry a larg amount of advertising, it also has a proportionate amoun of space to fill with news, information, and feature articles

The information officer has two basic methods c working with daily newspaper staffs. First, general infor mation is best handled through a press release. This is prepared news story provided to the proper department c a newspaper. It is advisable to prepare a factual summary which can be discussed with an appropriate editor of th paper. This editor may wish to assign a staff person or tea to develop the story. Clear professional photographs shoul be offered to daily newspapers, but these papers should als be offered the opportunity to take their own photographs.

Any information provided to a daily newspaper ma be suited to some needs of community weeklies. But pe sonality stories, local fund-raising and promotional activi ties, and related topics may be better suited for use i community weeklies than in daily newspapers.

Newspapers are the medium for content and detai Full background statements can be developed. Controversie can be covered with balanced statements from all points c view.

The *Washington Post* in recent years issued a sma brochure for use by amateur and professional publicist The publication is called "What's Your Story?" and contair a few precautions that are worth consideration by all info mation communicators. They include:

- DO begin each release with the most newsworthy item items.
- DON'T submit the same story to several different edito without informing each of them that you are doing it.
- DO keep your release factual and concise.
- DON'T use jargon familiar only to people in your orga ization.

- DO identify all company, department, or operation abbreviations when they are first mentioned.
- DON'T call the newspaper to add to your release, only to correct or cancel it. A reporter will call you if more information is needed.
- DO be prepared to provide additional facts and data if and when a reporter calls.
- DON'T break a paragraph or a sentence at the bottom of a page. (Each page may go to a different typesetter.)
- DO type each release individually or duplicate mechanically.
- DON'T send carbon copies as they smudge and are hard to read.

Target areas can usually be selected for news stories. As a general rule, both community weeklies and daily newspapers cover areas larger than the city in which the newspaper is published. News wire services bring world and national news to subscribing media in your community. Similarly, wire services are dependent on news releases furnished to them, material secured by their own staff members, or information published in local newspapers. The information communicator's best means of gaining national attention for a really important news or feature story is through the news services. Even in the local area, for spot news breaks, the wire services should be kept informed. In addition to servicing newspapers, wire services provide the digests of news used by radio and television.

National publications, specialized journals, and other publications that may be interested in the work of an agency usually prefer receiving a succinct news release or an inquiry about the specific topic to be covered. In most cases, these publications want to assign a qualified writer to handle specialized stories; however, there are occasions when a well-prepared news release is acceptable to them.

In general, when appealing to the mass media for coverage of stories about an organization, it should be remembered that radio is the medium for sound and concise messages; television is the medium for visual presentation of action-oriented projects; and newspapers are the medium for detailed stories, full information, and good still photographs. A good information specialist works with all media.

Radio is by far the most popular medium of communications. All licenses to operate radio stations are granted by the Federal Communications Commission to serve the public interest, convenience, and necessity of the listening audience. One measure of how stations meet this requirement is the station's record of public service. This includes carrying messages of an informational nature about activities and services available to the community. Most stations are pleased to carry public service announcements about timely activities and programs; and they will also feature recorded informational programs or interviews of a timely nature. Professionally prepared broadcast material always is chosen over "time filling" material. Almost every radio broadcast outlet has a person on the staff who is responsible for "public service" and will assist an organization with information about acceptable broadcast material. Concise information announcements, known as "spots," are preferred by most broadcasters and offer the most effective service to charitable organizations.

"In general, when appealing to the mass media for coverage of stories about an organization, it should be remembered that radio is the medium for sound and concise messages; television is the medium for visual presentation of action-oriented projects; and newspapers are the medium for detailed stories, full information, and good still photographs. A good information specialist works with all media."

Some "all news" radio stations and a few other broadcast stations maintain news departments with reporters who work in the field. These people should be contacted when special events are planned. Before contacting a radio station with specific material, much time and effort can be saved if you will familiarize yourself with the station's programming and personalities. Then speak to the public service director with specific ideas about the message you want to convey. Because most radio stations are extremely local in their appeal, they are usually cooperative in supporting local agencies and activities.

Television is an entirely different medium from radio. Because it involves both sight and sound, it attracts more concentrated attention than radio. Yet despite the fact that television stations are also licensed to serve the public interest, convenience, and necessity of the audience, programming formats restrict the amount of time available for information about community services and programs.

Despite these limitations, the staffs of commercial television stations want to serve their communities with coverage. They are always looking for news stories and features, and they are aware of their obligation to serve the public interest. It should always be remembered that television is a visual medium. It requires pictures—and pictures are most effective when they show action.

Every commercial television station has individuals in two key posts that relate to the community. Information communicators should be familiar with the individuals who act as community relations director and news assignment director at each television station serving your community. The community relations director is usually the station's information communicator. He is responsible for the public relations of the station. If it can be made visual, the same type of information used for radio spots should be made available to the station's community service director. He will know if this can be adapted to TV use. Perhaps a single slide, with a voice announcement, can convey your message. Better still, if 10-second or 20-second picture stories can be developed, he is the person who can assist you in preparing these film spots or refer you to people who can produce them for you.

It is also good to know the schedule of camera crews and times when these crews may have open schedules. For example, television is essentially a five-day week business. Television stations usually have a rigid Monday through Friday program schedule. This means that Saturday and Sunday events are much less likely to get live camera coverage than similar activities on weekdays. Also, if your station carries local news at 6:00 and 11:00 P.M., it is entirely likely that camera crews and news personalities will be restricted in their ability to cover any activity in your community between the hours of 4:30 and 7:00 P.M. or after 9:30 P.M. This means that functions and activities scheduled for late afternoon, dinner time, and late in the evening have a poor chance at local television coverage.

Part of planning any activity or function should relate to this timing schedule. Another part of planning should involve a contact with the news assignment director of your TV station a week in advance of the activity with a brief news release or a summary of the event with time, date, and place as the most important part of the information. A check back 24 hours before the event should be made.

Part of the job is to create something involving action that is photogenic. Be sure that every individual who may be in an action picture is fully informed about the subject or event. There is no time or place on news film for pauses or equivocations. Statements must be pertinent, direct, and accurate. Full responses to inquires must be made clearly and factually. On television, "No comment" or the commentator's statement that "Officials were unavailable for comment," invariably comes through to the viewer as "They must have done something wrong."

Network television offers opportunities for a good information communicator to have feature stories and personalities viewed. A variety of talk shows featuring celebrity hosts is produced by syndicating organizations and networks. Initial contacts for appearances on these shows are usually made by letter, in which the subject or person to be featured is concisely described. Unique and unusual ideas are welcomed by producers of talk shows. Morning network news and feature shows operate in a similar way. Shows that are produced by network news departments are usually planned over long periods of time. Content is predetermined by the network news department. However, it is possible to submit ideas for investigation and televising.

Cable television brings clear television directly into homes in many communities that are distant from television broadcasting stations. Many of these systems provide an information channel that carries a limited amount of local news coverage. Charity functions are frequently important activities in smaller communities, and camera coverage for use of cable systems should be part of planning in such areas. When a message can be condensed to a single slide, it is often possible to have this slide part of the news and weather visual presentation on cable TV systems.

The work of getting your message across is a never ending, often unrewarding, task. It is, however, one of the most effective ways of being listened to. From your effort may come a sense that the goal you hope to achieve is closer to becoming a reality.

William T. Snyder, a disability rights activist, a public relations practitioner who had his own company in Baltimore, Maryland, and an active delegate of the American Foundation for the Blind and the American Coalition of Citizens with Disabilities, wrote this article so that organizations could better understand how to work with the media. Bill died before he could see this article in print, but he leaves us his words.

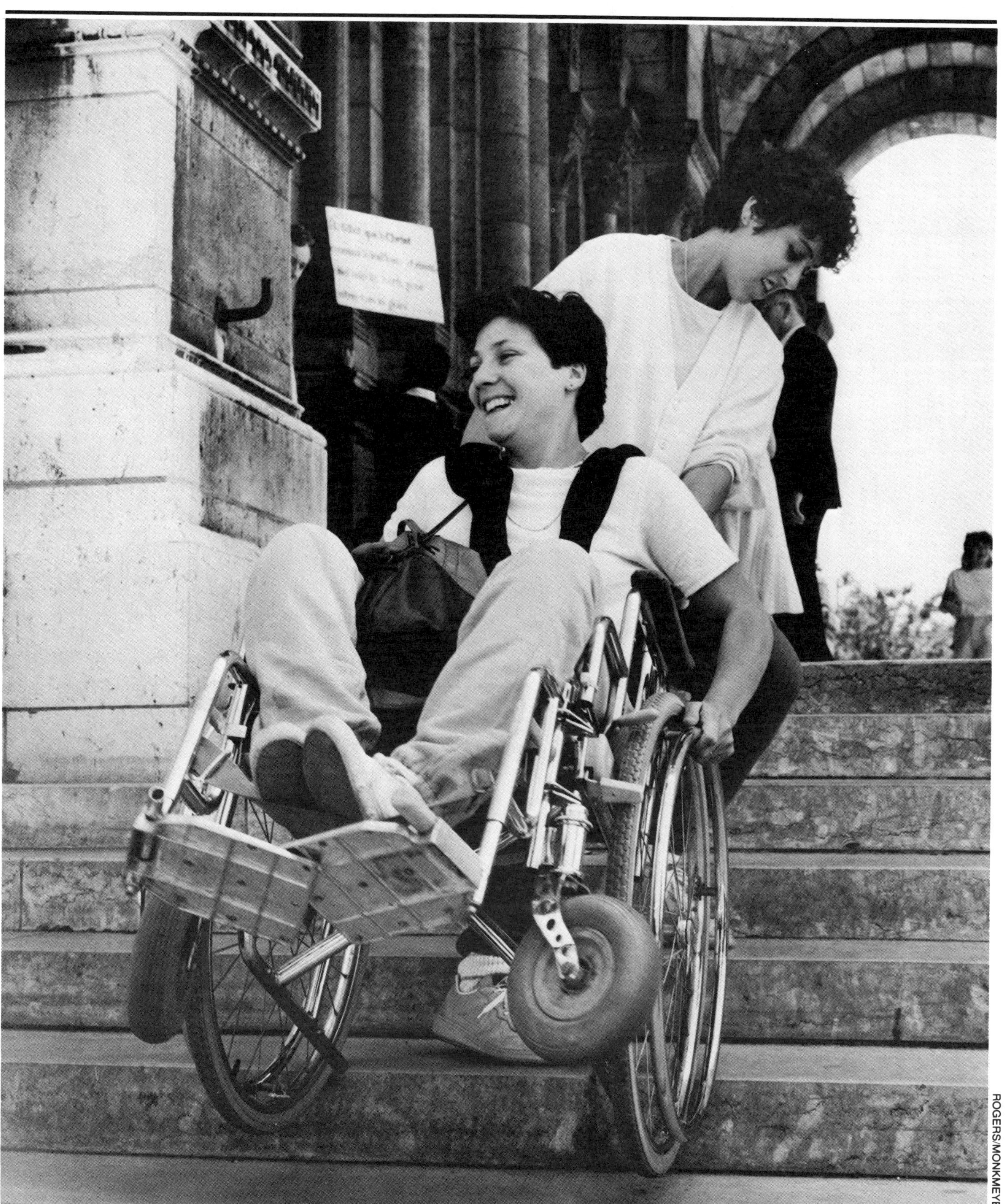

ROGERS/MONKMEYER

Bibliography

"Advice and Affirmation For and About Children Who Are Disabled or Ill." *Ms.* 13 (October 1984): 131–32.

Airport Operators Council International. *Access Travel: Airports: A Guide to Accessiblity of Terminals.* 2d ed. Washington, DC: Federal Aviation Administration, 1977.

Anderson, H. "Don't Stare—I'll Tell You Later." *The Exceptional Parent* (December 1980): 45–48.

"Are You The One With A Handicap? [Views of G. Jewell]." *McCalls* III (May 1984): 72+.

Baker, B.L.; Brightman, A.J.; and Hinshaw, S.P. *Toward Independent Living.* Champaign, IL: Research Press, 1980.

Barish, F. *Frommer's: A Guide for the Disabled Traveler.* New York: Frommer/Pasmantier Publishers, 1984.

Berger, L. "How to Behave with Handicapped People." *Seventeen* 39 (October 1980): 78.

Brown, C. *Down All the Days.* New York: Stein and Day, 1970.

Bruck, L. *Access: The Guide to a Better Life for Disabled Americans.* New York: Random House, 1978.

Burgdorf, R.L., ed. *The Legal Rights of Handicapped Persons: Cases, Materials and Text.* Baltimore: Paul H. Brooks, 1980.

Cary, J.R. *How to Create Interiors for the Disabled: A Guide for Family and Friends.* New York: Pantheon Books, 1978.

Chipouras, S.; Cornelius, D.; Daniels, S.M.; and Makas, E. *Who Cares? A Handbook on Sex Education and Counseling Services for Disabled People.* Washington DC: George Washington University, 1979.

Cornelius, D.A., ed. *Barrier Awareness: Attitudes Toward People with Disabilities.* Washington, DC: George Washington University, 1981.

Dailey, A.T. "Physically Handicapped Women." *Counseling Psychologist* 8i (1979): 41–42.

Debro, D. *Learning to Live With Disability: A Guidebook for Families.* Virginia: Institute for Information Studies, 1980.

DeJong, G. *Movement for Independent Living: Ideology, and Implications for Disability Research.* Occasional Paper no. 2. Tufts University Medical Rehabilitation Research and Training Center and Michigan State University Centers for International Rehabilitation, 1979.

DeLoach, C., and Greer, G. *Adjustment to Severe Disabilities.* New York: McGraw-Hill Co., 1981.

Eisenberg, J.G.; Griggens, C.; and Duval, R.J., eds. *Springer Series on Rehabilitation.* Vol. 2: *Disabled People as Second Class Citizens.* New York: Springer, 1982.

Enley, G. *Let There Be Love: Sex and the Handicapped.* New York: Taplinger Publishing Co., Inc., 1975.

Fay, F.A., and Minch, J. *Access to Recreation: A Report on the National Hearing on Recreation for Handicapped Persons for Architectural and Transportation Barriers Compliance Board.* Massachusetts: Tufts University Medical Rehabilitation Research and Training Center, n.d.

Frieden, L. "IL" Movement and Programs." *American Rehabilitation* 3 (1978): 6–9.

Gliedman, J., and Roth, W. "Unexpected Minority." *New Republic* 182 (February 2, 1980): 26–30.

Goffman, E. *Behavior in Public Places.* New York: The Free Press, MacMillan Publishing Co., Inc., 1963.

Goffman, E. *Stigma: Notes on the Management of Spoiled Identity.* Englewood Cliffs, NJ: Prentice-Hall, 1963.

Gollay, E., and Bennett, A. *The College Guide for Students with Disabilities: A Detailed Directory of Higher Education Services, Programs, and Facilities Accessible to Handicapped Students in the United States.* Lanham, MD: University Press of America, Inc., 1976.

Hale, G., ed. *The Source Book for the Disabled.* New York: Paddington Press Ltd., 1979.

"Handicapped Passengers Aids Studied [American Airlines]." *Aviation World* 114 (February 16, 1981): 33.

"Help For Disabled Drivers [Illustrated]." *Changing Times* 39 (August 1985): 55+.

Kellogg, M.A., and McGee, H. "Next Minority." *Newsweek* 88 (December 20, 1976): 74–75.

Kessler, H.H. *The Crippled and the Disabled: Rehabilitation of the Physically Handicapped in the United States*. New York: Columbia University Press, 1935.

Kilmartin, M. "Disabled Doesn't Mean No Sex." *Ms*. 12 (May 1984): 114+.

"Knowledge in Motion—Workshop—American Coalition of Citizens with Disabilities, Inc." *Public Transportation for Disabled People*. New York, January 1982.

Koestler, F.A. *The Unseen Minority: A Social History of Blindness in America*. New York: David McKay, 1976.

Krents, H. *The Human Dimension to Affirmative Action for the Handicapped*. U.S. Department of Labor Employment Standards Administration. Office of Federal Contract Compliance, April 1980.

Larson, M.R., and Snobl, D.E. *Attendant Care Manual*. Marshall, MN: Southwest State University, n.d.

Laurie, G. *Housing and Home Services for the Disabled: Guidelines and Experiences in Independent Living*. New York: Harper and Row, 1977.

Lifchez, R., and Winslow, B. *Design for Independent Living: The Environment and Physically Disabled People*. New York: Whitney Library of Design, Watson-Guptill Publications, 1979.

Lunt, S. *A Handbook for the Disabled*. New York: Charles Scribners, 1982.

Macaluso, V. "Will Disabled People Miss the Boat on Affirmative Action?" *The Coalition*, vol. 4, no. 1 (Spring 1982): 1, 4.

Mehan, H.; Hertweck, A.L.; and Meihls, J.L. *Handicapping the Handicapped: Decision Making in Students' Educational Careers*. Stanford, CA: Stanford University Press, 1986.

Meyer, D.J.; Vadasy, P.F.; and Fewell, R.R. *Living with a Brother or Sister with Special Needs: A Book for Sibs*. Seattle, WA: University of Washington Press, 1985.

Mims, F.M. "Personal Computers For The Disabled [Illustrated]." *Creative Computing* 11 (August 1985): 78–81.

Mistler, S.; Cornelius, D.; and Daniels, S. *The Invisible Battle: Attitudes Towards Disability*. Washington, D.C.: George Washington University, 1978.

Norman, M. "Let Your Fingers Do The Talking [Speech Synthesizers]." *Psychology Today* 18 (September 1984): 66.

Office for Handicapped Individuals, Clearinghouse for the Handicapped. *Directory of National Information Sources on Handicapping Conditions and Related Services*. 2d ed. Washington, DC: Office for Handicapped Individuals, Clearinghouse for the Handicapped. Government Printing Office, 1980.

Olson, K. "Nervous Acknowledgment Is Better Than None." *Psychology Today* 14 (June 1980): 108.

Park, E. "Around the Mall and Beyond." *Smithsonian* 12 (June 1981): 22.

Power, P.W., and Dell Orto, A.E., eds. *Role of the Family in the Rehabilitation of the Physically Disabled*. Baltimore: University Park Press, 1980.

President's Committee on Employment of the Handicapped. *Getting Through College with a Disability: A Summary of Services Available on 500 Campuses for Students with Handicapping Conditions*. Washington, DC: President's Committee on Employment of the Handicapped, 1977.

Redden, M.; Fortunato R.; Schwandt, W.; and Brown, J.W. *Barrier Free Meetings: A Guide for Professional Associations*. Washington, DC: American Association for the Advancement of Science, n.d.

Rehabilitation World. *International Directory of Access Guides*. Rehabilitation World, 1978.

Reich, A.A. "Conquering a New American Frontier: Changing Attitudes Toward the Disabled." *USA Today* 113 (May 1985): 60–64.

Royse, R.E. *CIL (Center for Independent Learning): Design for Success*. Kansas: University of Kansas, Kansas Center for Mental Retardation and Human Development, 1980.

Rusk, H.A., and Taylor, E.J. *New Hope for the Handicapped: The Rehabilitation of the Disabled from Bed to Job*. New York: Harper and Row, 1949.

Turnbull, A., and Turnbull, R. *Parents Speak Out: Then and Now*. Westerville, OH: Charles E. Merrill Publishing Co., 1984.

Velleman, R.A. *Serving Physically Disabled People: An Information Handbook for All Libraries*. New York: R.R. Bowker, 1979.

Weiner, F. *Help for the Handicapped Child*. New York: McGraw Hill, 1973.

Westerwelk, V.D., and McKinney, J.D. "Effects of a Film on Nonhandicapped Children's Attitudes Toward Handicapped Children." *Exceptional Children* 46 (1980): 294–296.

White House Conference on Handicapped Individuals. *White House Conference on Handicapped Individuals: Del-*

egate Workbook: Workshop V: Social Concerns 3: Architectural, Transportation, Communication: Washington, DC, May 23–27, 1977. Washington, D.C.: White House Conference on Handicapped Individuals, 1977.

Wolfensberger, W. *Citizen Advocacy for the Handicapped, Impaired and Disadvantaged: An Overview.* Washington, D.C.: U.S. Department of Health, Education and Welfare, 1972.

Wright, B.A. *Physical Disability—A Psychological Approach*. New York: Harper and Row, 1960.

Wright, G. *Total Rehabilitation*. Boston: Little Brown and Company, 1980.

Yuker, H.E. "Attitudes of the General Public Toward Handicapped Individuals." *White House Conference on Handicapped Individuals: Vol. 1: Awareness Papers*. N.p., 1977.

Yuker, H.E. "Public Attitudes Towards Americans with Disabilities: What Should be Done?" *IYDP Report* (August/September 1980): 7.

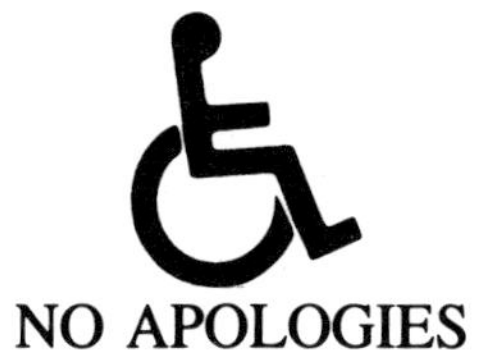

NO APOLOGIES

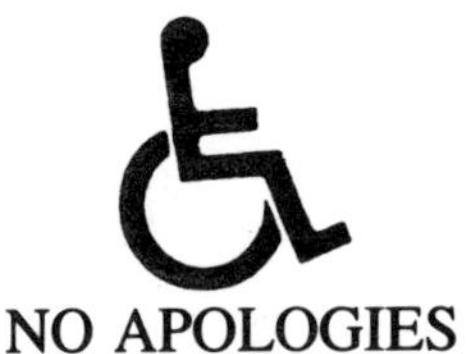

Index

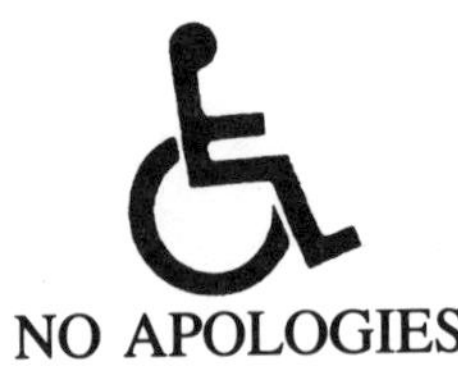

NO APOLOGIES

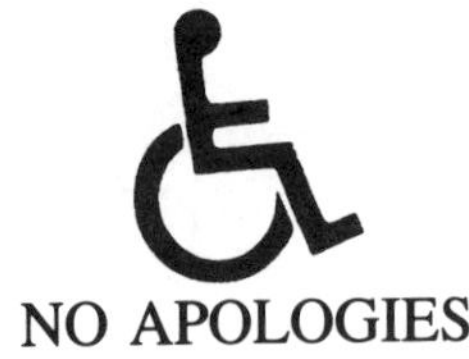
NO APOLOGIES

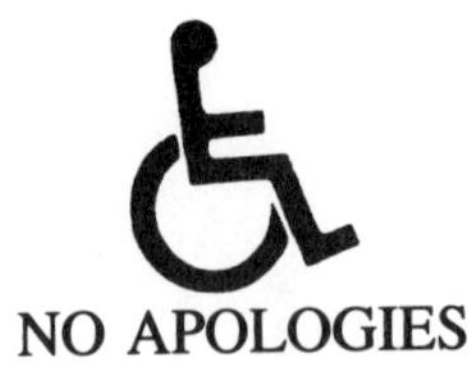
NO APOLOGIES

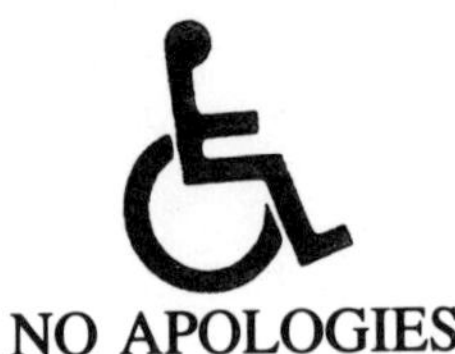
NO APOLOGIES